LAW & ETHICS for Medical Careers

FIFTH EDITION

Law & Ethics
for Medical Careers

Karen Judson, B.S.

Carlene Harrison, Ed.D., C.M.A.

Mc
Graw
Hill **Higher Education**

Boston   Burr Ridge, IL   Dubuque, IA   New York   San Francisco   St. Louis
Bangkok   Bogotá   Caracas   Kuala Lumpur   Lisbon   London   Madrid   Mexico City
Milan   Montreal   New Delhi   Santiago   Seoul   Singapore   Sydney   Taipei   Toronto

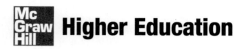
Higher Education

LAW & ETHICS FOR MEDICAL CAREERS

Published by McGraw-Hill, a business unit of The McGraw-Hill Companies, Inc., 1221 Avenue of the Americas, New York, NY, 10020. Copyright ©2010 by The McGraw-Hill Companies, Inc. All rights reserved. Previous editions © 1994, 1999, 2003, and 2006. No part of this publication may be reproduced or distributed in any form or by any means, or stored in a database or retrieval system, without the prior written consent of The McGraw-Hill Companies, Inc., including, but not limited to, in any network or other electronic storage or transmission, or broadcast for distance learning.

Some ancillaries, including electronic and print components, may not be available to customers outside the United States.

This book is printed on acid-free paper.

1 2 3 4 5 6 7 8 9 0 DOW/DOW 0 9

ISBN 978-0-07-340206-2
MHID 0-07-340206-0

Vice president/Editor in chief: *Elizabeth Haefele*
Vice president/Director of marketing: *John E. Biernat*
Senior sponsoring editor: *Debbie Fitzgerald*
Developmental editor: *Connie Kuhl*
Executive marketing manager: *Roxan Kinsey*
Lead media producer: *Damian Moshak*
Media producer: *Marc Mattson*
Director, Editing/Design/Production: *Jess Ann Kosic*
Lead project manager: *Susan Trentacosti*
Senior production supervisor: *Janean A. Utley*
Senior designer: *Srdjan Savanovic*

Lead photo research coordinator: *Carrie K. Burger*
Media project manager: *Mark A. S. Dierker*
Cover design: *George Kokkonas*
Interior design: *Jeanne Calabrese*
Typeface: *10/12 Garamond Book*
Compositor: *Laserwords Private Limited*
Printer: *R. R. Donnelley*
Cover credit: *Scales: © Don Farrall,Gettyimages; Stethoscope: ©Shirley Hu/Dreamstime.com*
Credits: The credits section for this book begins on page 357 and is considered an extension of the copyright page.

Library of Congress Cataloging-in-Publication Data

Judson, Karen, 1941-
 Law & ethics for medical careers/Karen Judson, Carlene Harrison. — 5th ed.
  p. ; cm.
 Rev. ed. of: Law and ethics for medical careers/Karen Judson, Carlene Harrison, Sharon Hicks. 4th ed. c2006.

 Includes index.

 ISBN-13: 978-0-07-340206-2 (alk. paper)
 ISBN-10: 0-07-340206-0 (alk. paper)

 1. Medical ethics. 2. Medical jurisprudence. 3. Medical assistants—Professional ethics.
4. Medical assistants—Legal status, laws, etc. I. Harrison, Carlene. II. Judson, Karen, 1941-
Law and ethics for medical careers. III. Title. IV. Title: Law and ethics for medical careers.
 [DNLM: 1. Legislation, Medical–United States. 2. Ethics, Medical—United States.
3. Health Personnel—United States. W 32.5 AA1 J93L 2010]

R725.5.J83   2010
174.2—dc22   2008048702

Law & Ethics for Medical Careers, Fifth Edition, is an educational tool, not a law practice book. Since the law is in constant change, no rule or statement of law in this text should be relied upon for any service to any client. The reader should always consult standard legal sources for the current rule or law. If legal counseling or other expert advice is needed, the services of appropriate professionals should be sought. Between the time that Web site information is gathered and published, it is not unusual for some sites to have closed. Also, the transcription of the URLs can result in typographical errors. Text changes will be made in reprints when possible.

The Internet addresses listed in the text were accurate at the time of publication. The inclusion of a Web site does not indicate an endorsement by the authors or McGraw-Hill, and McGraw-Hill does not guarantee the accuracy of the information presented at these sites.

www.mhhe.com

BRIEF TABLE OF CONTENTS

TABLE OF CONTENTS

ABOUT THE AUTHORS

Karen Judson, B.S. Karen Judson taught biology laboratories at Black Hills University in Spearfish, South Dakota, high school sciences in Idaho, and grades one and three in Washington state. She is also a former laboratory and X-ray technician and completed two years of nurses' training while completing a degree in Biology.

Karen has worked as a science writer since 1983. She has written relationship, family, and psychology articles for a variety of magazines, including a series of high school classroom magazines, making a total of 500 articles published. Karen writes science and relationship books for teenagers (Enslow and Marshall Cavendish publishers). Her book for teens, *Sports & Money: It's a Sell Out* made the New York City Public Library's list of best books for teens in 1995. Her book for teens, *Genetic Engineering,* was chosen by the National Science Teachers' Association as one of the best science books for children in 2001 and was featured on the NSTA Web site.

Carlene Harrison, Ed.D., C.M.A. Carlene Harrison is the Dean of the School of Allied Health at Hodges University and is also currently serving as Acting Chair of the Health Administration Program. She has been a member of the faculty at Hodges University since 1992, but came on board full time in 2000, serving first as chair of the Medical Assisting Program. As Dean of the School of Allied Health, she has overall responsibility for four degree programs: Health Administration, Health Studies, Medical Assisting, and Health Information Technology. Her doctorate is from Argosy University. Her dissertation research looked at improvement in critical thinking in adult learners.

Before becoming a full-time educator, she worked for over 20 years in the health care field as an administrator. Employed mostly in the outpatient setting, she has worked for for-profit, not-for-profit, and public health organizations.

TO THE STUDENT

As you study to become a health care practitioner, you have undoubtedly realized that patients are more than the sum of their medical problems. In fact, they are people with loved ones, professions, worries, hobbies, and daily routines that are probably much like your own. However, because patients' lives and well-being are at stake as they seek and receive health care, in addition to seeing each patient as an individual you must carefully consider the complex legal, moral, and ethical issues that will arise as you practice your profession, and you must learn to resolve such issues in an acceptable manner.

Law & Ethics for Medical Careers, Fifth Edition, provides an overview of the laws and ethics you should know to help you give competent, compassionate care to patients that is also within acceptable legal and ethical boundaries. The text can also serve as a guide to help you resolve the many legal and ethical questions you may reasonably expect to face as a student and, later, as a health care practitioner.

To derive maximum benefit from *Law & Ethics for Medical Careers,* Fifth Edition:

- Review the Learning Outcomes and Key Terms at the beginning of each chapter for an overview of the material included in the chapter.
- Complete all Check Your Progress questions as they appear in the chapter and correct any incorrect answers.
- Review the legal cases to see how they apply to topics in the text, and try to determine why the court ruled as it did.
- Study the Ethics Issues at the end of each chapter, and answer the discussion questions.
- Complete the Review questions at the end of the chapter, correct incorrect answers and review the material again.
- Review the Case Studies and use your critical-thinking skills to answer the questions.
- Complete the Internet Activities at the end of the chapter to become familiar with online resources and to see what additional information you can find about selected topics.
- Study each chapter until you can answer questions posed by the Learning Outcomes, Check Your Progress, and Chapter Review questions correctly.

CHAPTER STRUCTURE

Each chapter begins with a page that previews topics you will study.

Learning Outcomes The learning outcomes describe the basic knowledge you can acquire by studying the chapter. Their importance to you is to indicate what general categories of knowledge you should derive from the chapter.

Key Terms This alphabetic list is of important vocabulary terms found in the chapter. This is a list of key words that you should be familiar with after reading each chapter. The terms are printed in boldface type when they first appear in the chapter text and are listed in the margin of the page on which the term is introduced to provide you with a quick definition of each term.

Ethics Issues This feature at the end of each chapter is based on interviews conducted with ethics counselors within the professional organizations for health care practitioners, and interviews with bioethics experts. The discussion questions are derived from real-life experiences and ethical dilemmas from a variety of health care practitioners. Read the Ethics Issues and decide how they are relevant to the health care profession you will practice. Answer the discussion questions to help clarify your personal ethical viewpoint concerning each situation.

Chapter Review Each chapter review includes Applying Knowledge questions that review facts presented and points made in the text. Use these questions to test your comprehension of the material then review appropriate sections of the text as necessary to reinforce the learning outcomes.

Case Study Each case study is followed by exercises that allow you to practice your critical-thinking skills and use knowledge gained from reading the text in order to decide how to resolve the real-life situations or theoretical scenarios presented.

Internet Activities Each activity includes exercises that are designed to increase your knowledge of topics related to the chapter material and to gain expertise in using the Internet as a research tool. Keep a resource notebook to record useful Web sites as they are found. To locate new Web sites, conduct a subject search as needed to help you answer the questions that follow each activity.

TEXT FEATURES

The following special features are found in the student text/workbook for *Law & Ethics for Medical Careers,* Fifth Edition. These features are designed to stimulate classroom discussion, provide supplementary facts and examples to the text material, introduce you to Internet research, and provide a review of the text material covered.

Voice of Experience This feature illustrates real-life experiences that are related to the text. Each quotes health care practitioners in various locations throughout the United States as they encounter problems or situations relevant to the material discussed in the text.

Check Your Progress This feature is a short quiz that allows you to test your comprehension of the material just read. Answer the questions, correct incorrect answers, and then review appropriate sections to be sure you understand the material.

Court Case Each case summarizes a lawsuit that illustrates points made in the text. In each case, consider the relevance of the case to your health care specialty area and note the outcome. Determine why the court made its particular ruling. The legal citations at the end of each court case indicate where to find the complete text of a case. "Classic" cases are those that established ongoing precedent.

WHAT'S NEW

1. The Ethics Guide at the end of each chapter is revised and retitled Ethics Issues. This feature contains ethical dilemmas and discussion questions taken from interviews with a variety of medical ethics experts and health care practitioners.

2. Chapter 12, "Health Care Trends and Forecasts," is new content and is substituted for the old Chapter 12, "Ethics for Health Care Practitioners." This new chapter discusses issues that are critical to the health care environment and to health care practitioners as we move into the twenty-first century—such as health care costs, access, and quality—and what lies ahead in medical technology and in health information technology.

3. All statistics are updated, as well as content relevant to laws passed since the fourth edition, court cases, and lists in the appendixes.

4. New case studies are added. We made an effort to include a variety of allied health professions in case studies and other examples throughout the text, even more so than in previous editions of the book.

5. A new four-color design makes the text more appealing, and interesting photos are added to enhance the student's learning experience.

TEACHING AND LEARNING SUPPLEMENTS

Online Learning Center www.mhhe.com/judson5e The Online Learning Center offers an extensive array of learning and teaching tools. The student's side includes quizzes, case studies, and PowerPoint presentations for each chapter, links to professional associations and Web sites, and flashcards for vocabulary reinforcement.

A new feature—30-second video vignettes—showcases a problem or situation common to health care and asks students to respond. This interactive element will provide the students with immediate feedback to the situation seen in each video and will be available to both students and instructors.

The instructor's resources on this site include Test Bank and PowerPoint presentations for each chapter, links to professional associations and Web sites, and the Instructor's Manual. The **Instructor's Manual** provides instructors with guidance in how to interpret court case citations, helpful Web site links, correlation charts, course syllabi, teaching strategies, answers to "Check Your Progress," answers to Ethics Issue discussion questions, and answers to Applying Your Knowledge, Case Study, and Internet Activities questions.

ACKNOWLEDGMENTS

Author Acknowledgments

Karen Judson Thank you to Connie Kuhl, McGraw-Hill developmental editor, the entire production staff at McGraw-Hill, and all the reviewers and sources who contributed their time and expertise to making the fifth edition of *Law & Ethics for Medical Careers* the best ever. Thank you, too, Carlene, for joining the team and working hard to achieve our shared goal of excellence.

Carlene Harrison A big thank you to Karen Judson for getting me started on this marvelous adventure called writing. To our reviewers, your contributions really make a difference. To Connie Kuhl and the entire production staff at McGraw Hill thank you for patience when I kept asking dumb questions. And last, to my husband Bill, your support and love keeps me going.

Reviewer Acknowledgments

Thomas Ankeney, BA, RCP, RRT, CPFT, AE-C, NCPT
Maric College

Shkelzen Badivuku
Gibbs College

Julette Barta, CphT, BSIT
SJVC

Rebecca Britt
Northwestern State University

Lou Brown
Wayne Community College

Rita Bulington, RN, AS
Ivy Tech Community College

Christine M. Cole, CCA
Williston State College

Barbara Desch
San Joaquin Valley College, Inc.

Terri Fleming
Ivy Tech Community College

Tammy B. Foles
Antonelli College

William D. Goren, J.D., L.L.M.
Northwestern Business College

Beulah A. Hofmann, RN, MSN
Ivy Tech Community College

Carol Lee Jarrell
Brown Mackie College

Karmon Kingsley, CMA, CHI
Cleveland State Community College

Christine Malone, MHA
Everett Community College

Lynne M. Muñoz, M.Ed.
Everett Community College

Matthew R. Panzio, MD
Gibbs

Cindy Pavel
Ivy Tech Community College

Pamela B. Primrose, MLFSC, ABD, MT, ASCP
Ivy Tech Community College

Pat Stettler, CMT, FAAMT
Everett Community College

Carol Adams-Turner
Lamar State College-Orange

Constance Winter
Bossier Parish Community College

Previous Reviewers

Cindy A. Abel, BS, CMA, PBT (ASCP)
Ivy Tech State College

Barbara C. Berger BSN, RN, CMA, MS
Northwestern Connecticut Community College

Amelia Broussard, PhD, RN, MPH,
Associate Professor
Clayton College & State University

Christine M. Cole
Williston State College

Dawn Felice Dannenbrink, MHA
High-Tech Institute

Dena A. Evans, BSN, MPH, RN, CMA
Richmond Community College

Kim Ford, CMA
Catawba Valley Community College

Gardiner M. Haight, B.S. Comm., J.D.
Bryant and Stratton College

Janet K. Henderson, CMA, AAT
North Georgia Technical College

Beulah A. Hofmann
Ivy Tech State College

Joyce S. Johnson, Department Head,
Office Systems Technology
Alamance Community College

Lynda M. Konecny
New York City College of Technology

Norma Mercado, MAHS, RHIA
Austin Community College

Helen L. Myers
Hagerstown Community College

Michael W. Posey, Ph.D
Franklin University

Joan Renner, B.S.N, R.N.B.C. Adjunct Faculty
Cecil Community College

Sharon M. Roberts MBA, MS, PTA
Newbury College

Diane P. Roche, CMA, BSHCA, MSA
South Piedmont Community College

James Steen, MBA, SS, RHIA
San Jacinto College North

Rita Stoffel, BS, MT, MBA
Red Rocks Community College

Nina Thierer, CMA, BS, CPC
Ivy Tech State College-Fort Wayne

Geraldine M. Todaro, MSTE, CMA, CLPlb
Stark State College of Technology

Tova R. Wiegand-Green
Ivy Tech State College

VISUAL GUIDE TO *LAW & ETHICS FOR MEDICAL CAREERS*, 5/E

Learning Outcomes and **Key Terms** at the beginning of each chapter introduce you to the chapter and help prepare you for the information that will be presented.

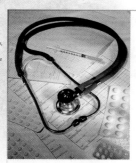

CHAPTER 1

Introduction to Law and Ethics

Learning Outcomes

After studying this chapter, you should be able to:

1. Explain why knowledge of law and ethics is important to health care practitioners.

2. Recognize the importance of professional codes of ethics.

3. Distinguish among law, ethics, bioethics, etiquette, and protocol.

4. Define *moral values* and explain how they relate to law, ethics, and etiquette.

5. Describe at least three bioethical issues of concern for your chosen profession.

Key Terms

American Medical Association Principles	defendant	liable
bioethicists	ethics	litigious
bioethics	ethics committees	medical ethicists
code of ethics	ethics guidelines	moral values
common sense	etiquette	plaintiff
compassion	fraud	precedent
courtesy	health care practitioners	protocol
critical thinking	Hippocratic oath	summary judgment
	law	

2

Voice of Experience features real-life situations that you can relate to in various occupations.

NEW!! Four-color design

Voice of Experience
Nurse Tends Dying Patients

Angela has been a registered nurse for 14 years. Just as some hospital nurses are drawn to surgery, the emergency room, or the intensive care unit, Angela prefers hospice and palliative care. "Broadly speaking," Angela explains, "medicine is about repairing, extending, and medicating, while end-of-life care is more about the patient as an individual, about basic human needs. In addition, it isn't just the patient you are caring for; you are caring for the entire family group—everybody needs you.

"We live in a time when death has been removed from family and home for the most part," Angela continues, "and people generally have less understanding of the process than a hundred years ago. . . . The family most often feels helpless and confused. The hospice nurse is able to help not just the patient, but the family, too, through a sad and often frightening time."

Sometimes family members are hesitant about approaching a dying loved one. For example, Angela remembers a situation where the mother of two siblings in their 30s was dying. "When I arrived they were practically plastered against the walls of the room, clearly unsure of what they should be doing." Angela encouraged the two family members to come to their mother's bedside and comfort her. "The son pulled a chair to the side of the bed and held his mother's hand. The daughter climbed onto the bed and cradled her mother . . . . I like to think that because I urged them to take a more active part in her passing that they found comfort after their mother was gone."

Angela also recalls a patient in his 80s whose 32 family members joined him in his hospice room. "It was almost a living wake. They talked for hours about his life and the experiences they had each shared with him. They laughed and they cried and it was wonderful. This sharing in their loved one's death was a beautiful experience for those left behind, and I hope it helped him in some way as well."

Court Cases are actual lawsuits that illustrate points made in the text. These cases help you consider the relevance of each case for your chosen profession.

"The real-life court cases are great because these bring the laws to an understandable level for someone new to health care."
— Christine Malone, MHA, Everett Community College

Court Case
Patient Can Contribute to Negligence

A man who was a detainee at a county jail was taken to a county hospital emergency room when he complained of pain in his lower abdomen, nausea, and vomiting of blood for two weeks. An RN took the man's vital signs, finding his blood pressure to be 159/106 and his pulse to be fast. The nurse also drew blood and ordered initial lab work. A physician saw the patient and ordered that a nasogastric tube be inserted to check for blood in the stomach. The nurse tried to insert the tube, but the patient complained that it was extremely painful and said he did not want the tube inserted. The nurse explained why the tube was necessary, but the patient declined, insisting that his problems were due to his appendix. He signed a form indicating that he was refusing medical treatment against medical advice. The man was returned to the jail, where he died one week later of gastrointestinal hemorrhaging.

Blood test results that came back after the patient left the hospital were abnormal, indicating a life-threatening condition. Since the patient had signed himself out of the hospital, and the hospital claimed it no longer had a duty to him, his test results were not forwarded to the physician who examined the patient or to the patient.

The administrator of the patient's estate filed a malpractice suit against the nurse and the hospital. A trial jury found for the defendants, under the defense of contributory negligence. The administrator appealed, but the appellate court affirmed the lower court's judgment.

Lyons v. Walker Regional Medical Center, Inc., and Hunter, Supreme Court of Alabama, 2003 Ala. LEXIS 104.

📖 **executive order** A rule or regulation issued by the President of the United States that becomes law without the prior approval of Congress.

📖 **checks and balances** The system established by the U.S. Constitution that keeps any one branch of government from assuming too much power over the other branches.

The President of the United States is the chief executive of the *executive branch* of government, which is responsible for administering the law. Through his or her ability to issue **executive orders**, the president has limited legislative powers. Executive orders become law without the prior approval of Congress. They are usually issued for one of three purposes: to create administrative agencies or change the practices of an existing agency, to enforce laws passed by Congress, or to make treaties with foreign powers.

The United States Supreme Court heads the *judicial branch* of government, which also includes federal judges and courts in every state. The judicial branch interprets the law and oversees the enforcement of laws.

The division of powers and responsibilities among three branches of government ensures that a system of **checks and balances** will keep any one branch from assuming too much power. See Figure 3-1.

State Governments

State governments also have three branches: *legislative, executive,* and *judicial.* The number of state legislators a state may elect is based upon the number of political districts in each state, since citizens elect legislators from the various districts. Therefore, the numbers of members of state legislatures are not the same as the number of members in the United States Congress.

State legislative branches also consist of two chambers: the Senate and the House of Representatives. In some states, the House of Representatives is called the Assembly or General Assembly. Terms served may be the same

Marginal Key Terms provide a quick definition of the important words that you should be familiar with at the end of each chapter.

"The definitions in the margins and the use of the terms in the text were placed in such a way that they were more understandable within the text."
— Carol Lee Jarrell: Brown Mackie College.

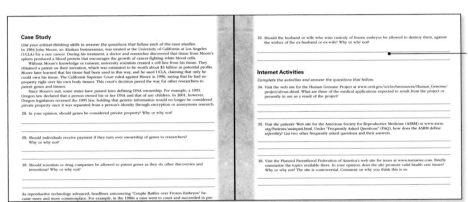

TABLE 3-1 Exclusive Powers of the National Government and State Governments

National Government	State Governments
Print money	Issue licenses
Regulate interstate (between states) and international trade	Regulate intrastate (within the state) businesses
Make treaties and conduct foreign policy	Conduct elections
Declare war	Establish local governments
Provide an army and navy	Ratify amendments to the Constitution
Establish post offices	Take measures for public health and safety
Make laws necessary and proper to carry out the above powers	May exert powers the Constitution does not delegate to the national government or prohibit the states from using

Tables within each chapter summarize important information for you.

CHECK YOUR PROGRESS

1. Define *medical record*.

2. List five purposes served by a patient's medical record.

3. As the person responsible for charting in a medical office, would you record a patient's statement that she often feels "woozy" and thinks she has "dropsy"? Why or why not?

4. If a reconstructive surgeon wants to publish "before" and "after" photographs of patients in a brochure left in the waiting room for distribution to prospective patients, what must she do?

5. If a patient makes critical remarks to you, a medical assistant, about your physician/employer, would you record the remarks in the patient's medical record? Why or why not?

Check Your Progress are short quizzes located at intervals throughout the chapter to allow you to review important material that you just learned.

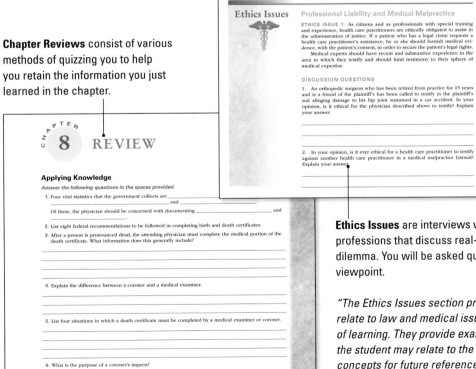

Case Study

Use your critical-thinking skills to answer the questions that follow each of the case studies.
In 1984 John Moore, an Alaskan businessman, was treated at the University of California at Los Angeles (UCLA) for a rare cancer. During his treatment, a doctor and researcher discovered that tissue from Moore's spleen produced a blood protein that encourages the growth of cancer-fighting white blood cells.
Without Moore's knowledge or consent, university scientists created a cell line from his tissue. They obtained a patent on their invention, which was estimated to be worth about $3 billion in potential profits. Moore later learned that his tissue had been used in this way, and he sued UCLA, claiming that only he could own his tissue. The California Supreme Court ruled against Moore in 1990, saying that he had no property right over his own body tissues. This court's decision paved the way for other researchers to patent genes and tissues.
Since Moore's suit, some states have passed laws defining DNA ownership. For example, a 1995 Oregon law declared that a person owned his or her DNA and that of any children. In 2001, however, Oregon legislators reversed the 1995 law, holding that genetic information would no longer be considered private property once it was separated from a person's identity through encryption or anonymous research.

28. In your opinion, should genes be considered private property? Why or why not?

29. Should individuals receive payment if they turn over ownership of genes to researchers? Why or why not?

30. Should scientists or drug companies be allowed to patent genes as they do other discoveries and inventions? Why or why not?

As reproductive technology advanced, headlines announcing "Couple Battles over Frozen Embryos" became more and more commonplace. For example, in the 1980s a man went to court and succeeded in pre-

33. Should the husband or wife who wins custody of frozen embryos be allowed to destroy them, against the wishes of the ex-husband or ex-wife? Why or why not?

Internet Activities

Complete the activities and answer the questions that follow.

34. Visit the web site for the Human Genome Project at www.ornl.gov/sci/techresources/Human_Genome/project/about.shtml. What are three of the medical applications expected to result from the project or presently in use as a result of the project?

35. Visit the patients' Web site for the American Society for Reproductive Medicine (ASRM) at www.asrm.org/Patients/mainpati.html. Under "Frequently Asked Questions" (FAQ), how does the ASRM define *infertility*? List two other frequently asked questions and their answers.

36. Visit the Planned Parenthood Federation of America's web site for teens at www.teenwire.com. Briefly summarize the topics available there. In your opinion, does the site promote valid health care issues? Why or why not? The site is controversial. Comment on why you think this is so.

At the end of each chapter you have **Case Study** that will help you practice your critical thinking skills, **and Internet Activities** that will increase your knowledge of topics related to the allied health field.

Chapter Reviews consist of various methods of quizzing you to help you retain the information you just learned in the chapter.

CHAPTER 8 REVIEW

Applying Knowledge

Answer the following questions in the spaces provided.

1. Four vital statistics that the government collects are _____, _____, and _____.
   Of these, the physician should be concerned with documenting _____ and _____

2. List eight federal recommendations to be followed in completing birth and death certificates.

3. After a person is pronounced dead, the attending physician must complete the medical portion of the death certificate. What information does this generally include?

4. Explain the difference between a coroner and a medical examiner.

5. List four situations in which a death certificate must be completed by a medical examiner or coroner.

6. What is the purpose of a coroner's inquest?

Ethics Issues | Professional Liability and Medical Malpractice

ETHICS ISSUE 1: As citizens and as professionals with special training and experience, health care practitioners are ethically obligated to assist in the administration of justice. If a patient who has a legal claim requests a health care practitioner's assistance, he or she should furnish medical evidence, with the patient's consent, in order to secure the patient's legal rights.
Medical experts should have recent and substantive experience in the area in which they testify and should limit testimony to their sphere of medical expertise.

DISCUSSION QUESTIONS

1. An orthopedic surgeon who has been retired from practice for 15 years and is a friend of the plaintiff's has been called to testify in the plaintiff's suit alleging damage to his hip joint sustained in a car accident. In your opinion, is it ethical for the physician described above to testify? Explain your answer.

2. In your opinion, is it ever ethical for a health care practitioner to testify against another health care practitioner in a medical malpractice lawsuit? Explain your answer.

Ethics Issues are interviews with individuals in various professions that discuss real-life experience and an ethical dilemma. You will be asked questions to help clarify your ethical viewpoint.

"The Ethics Issues section provides a look at how ethical issues relate to law and medical issues the student is in the process of learning. They provide examples of concepts and thus the student may relate to the ethical issues to remember the concepts for future reference."
— Constance Winter,
Bossier Parish Community College

LAW & ETHICS for Medical Careers

PART

1

The Foundations of Law and Ethics

CHAPTER 1

Introduction to Law and Ethics

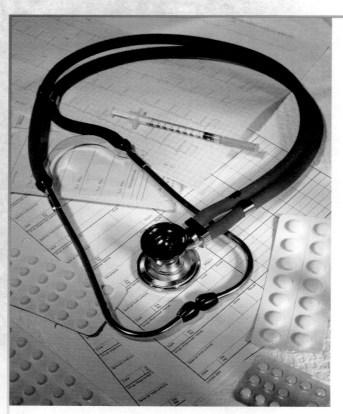

Learning Outcomes

After studying this chapter, you should be able to:

1. Explain why knowledge of law and ethics is important to health care practitioners.

2. Recognize the importance of professional codes of ethics.

3. Distinguish among law, ethics, bioethics, etiquette, and protocol.

4. Define *moral values* and explain how they relate to law, ethics, and etiquette.

5. Describe at least three bioethical issues of concern for your chosen profession.

Key Terms

American Medical Association Principles

bioethicists

bioethics

code of ethics

common sense

compassion

courtesy

critical thinking

defendant

ethics

ethics committees

ethics guidelines

etiquette

fraud

health care practitioners

Hippocratic oath

law

liable

litigious

medical ethicists

moral values

plaintiff

precedent

protocol

summary judgment

Barbara, an experienced certified medical assistant (CMA) in a medical office with a walk-in clinic, advises new employees in the reception area of the office to follow the medical office procedures whenever possible and prudent, but, above all, to use common sense in dealing with patients.

Barbara had told a new receptionist in the medical office to politely ask walk-in patients why they needed to see a doctor. An elderly man who was hard of hearing was obviously too embarrassed to reply, but the receptionist persisted. When he finally shouted, "I can't pee," all heads in the busy waiting room turned toward the receptionist and the patient. The red-faced receptionist turned to arrange for the man to see a physician, but he quickly left the building. Barbara criticized the receptionist's patient-handling technique, but the crux of the matter was that the patient left without seeing a doctor for his medical problem.

"Patients' needs always trump office routine," Barbara emphasizes. "If we somehow hurt or hinder a patient while doggedly sticking to a set routine, we may have risked legal liability, but more important, we haven't done our job."

WHY STUDY LAW AND ETHICS?

There are two important reasons for you to study law and ethics:

- To help you function at the highest possible professional level, providing competent, compassionate health care to patients.
- To help you avoid legal entanglements that can threaten your ability to earn a living as a successful **health care practitioner.**

health care practitioners Those who are trained to administer medical or health care to patients.

litigious Prone to engage in lawsuits.

We live in a **litigious** society, where patients, relatives, and others are inclined to sue health care practitioners, health care facilities, manufacturers of medical equipment and products, and others when medical outcomes are not acceptable. This means that every person responsible for health care delivery is at risk of being involved in a health care–related lawsuit. It is important, therefore, for you to know the basics of law and ethics as they apply to health care, so you can recognize and avoid those situations that might not serve your patients well, or that might put you at risk of legal liability.

In addition to keeping you at your professional best and helping you to avoid litigation, knowledge of law and ethics can also help you gain perspective in the following three areas:

1. *The rights, responsibilities, and concerns of health care consumers.* Health care practitioners not only need to be concerned about how law and ethics impact their respective professions, but they must also understand how legal and ethical issues affect the patients they treat. With the increased complexity of medicine has come the desire of consumers to know more about their options and rights and more about the responsibilities of health care providers. Today's health care consumers are likely to consider themselves partners with health care practitioners in the healing process and to question fees and treatment modes. They may ask such questions as, Do I need to see a specialist? If so, which specialist can best treat my condition? Will I be given complete information about my condition? How much will medical treatment cost? Will a physician treat me if I have no health insurance?

In addition, as medical technology has advanced, patients have come to expect favorable outcomes from medical treatment, and when expectations are not met, lawsuits may result.

2. *The legal and ethical issues facing society, patients, and health care practitioners as the world changes.* Nearly every day the media report news events concerning individuals who face legal and ethical dilemmas over biological/medical issues. For example, a grief-stricken husband must give consent for an abortion in order to save the life of his critically ill and unconscious wife. Parents must argue in court their decision to terminate life-support measures for a daughter whose injured brain no longer functions. Patients with HIV/AIDS fight to retain their right to confidentiality.

   While the situations that make news headlines often involve larger social issues, legal and ethical questions are resolved daily, on a smaller scale, each time a patient visits his or her physician, dentist, physical therapist, or other health care practitioner. Questions that must often be resolved include these: Who can legally give consent if the patient cannot? Can patients be assured of confidentiality, especially since telecommunication has become a way of life? Can a physician or other health care practitioner refuse to treat a patient? Who may legally examine a patient's medical records?

   Rapid advances in medical technology have also influenced laws and ethics for health care practitioners. For example, recent court cases have debated these issues: Does the husband or the wife have ownership rights to a divorced couple's frozen embryos? Will a surrogate mother have legal visitation rights to the child she carried to term? Should modern technology be used to keep those patients alive who are diagnosed as brain-dead and have no hope of recovery? How should parenthood disputes be resolved for children resulting from reproductive technology?

3. *The impact of rising costs on the laws and ethics of health care delivery.* Rising costs, both of health care insurance and of medical treatment in general, lead to questions concerning access to health care services and allocation of medical treatment. For instance, should the uninsured or underinsured receive government help to pay for health insurance? And should everyone, regardless of age or lifestyle, have the same access to scarce medical commodities, such as organs for transplantation or highly expensive drugs?

Court Cases Illustrate Risk of Litigation

As you will see in the court cases used throughout this text, sometimes when a lawsuit is brought, the trial court or a higher court must first decide if the **plaintiff** has a legal reason to sue, or if the **defendant** is **liable.** When a court has ruled that there is a standing (reason) to sue and that a defendant can be held liable, the case may proceed to resolution. Often, once liability and a standing to sue have been established, the two sides agree on an out-of-court settlement. Depending on state law, an out-of-court settlement may not be published. For this reason, the final disposition of a case is not always available from published sources. The cases that have decided liability, however, are still case law, and such cases have been used in this text to illustrate specific points.

In addition, sometimes it takes time after the initial trial for a case to be settled. For example, perhaps a patient dies after surgery in 1998, and the family files a wrongful death suit soon after. The case may go through several appeals and finally be settled in 2001.

plaintiff The person bringing charges in a lawsuit.

defendant The person or party against whom criminal or civil charges are brought in a lawsuit.

liable Accountable under the law.

precedent Decisions made by judges in the various courts that become rule of law and apply to future cases, even though they were not enacted by a legislature; also known as case law.

summary judgment A decision made by a court in a lawsuit in response to a motion that pleads there is no basis for a trial.

fraud Dishonest or deceitful practices in depriving, or attempting to deprive, another of his or her rights.

It is also important to remember that while the final result of a case is important to the parties involved, from a legal standpoint the most important aspect of a court case is not the result, but whether or not the case represents good law and will be persuasive as other cases are decided.

While the most recent cases published have been sought for illustration in this text, sometimes a dated case (1995, 1985, 1970, etc.) is used because it established important **precedent.**

Court cases appear throughout each chapter of the text, to illustrate how the legal system has decided complaints brought by or against health care service providers and product manufacturers. Some of these cases involve **summary judgment.** Summary judgment is the legal term for a decision made by a court in a lawsuit in response to a motion that pleads there is no basis for a trial because there is no genuine issue of material fact. In other words, a motion for summary judgment states that one party is entitled to win as a matter of law. Summary judgment is available only in a civil action. (Chapter 3 distinguishes between criminal and civil actions.)

The following court cases illustrate that a wide variety of legal questions can arise for those engaged directly in providing health care services, whether in a hospital, in a medical office setting, or in an emergency situation. Health care equipment and product dealers and manufacturers can be held indirectly responsible for defective medical devices and products through charges of the following types:

- Breach of warranty.
- Statements made by the manufacturer about the device or product that are found to be untrue.
- Strict liability, for cases in which defective products threaten the personal safety of consumers.
- **Fraud** or intentional deceit. (Fraud is discussed in further detail in Chapter 3.)

The extent of liability for manufacturers of medical devices and products may be changing, however, since a 2008 U.S. Supreme Court decision held that makers of medical devices such as implantable defibrillators or breast implants are immune from liability for personal injuries as long as the Food and Drug Administration (FDA) approved the device before it was marketed and it meets the FDA's specifications. (See the *Medtronic Inc.* case below.)

Drugs and medical devices are regulated under separate federal laws; as of February 2008, the same immunity from liability had not yet been extended to drug manufacturers. However, the United States Supreme Court was scheduled to hear another FDA preemption case during its second session of 2008: *Warner-Lambert Co. v. Kent* a case involving certain Michigan residents who claimed injury by the diabetes drug Rezulin. In this case, the question before the Court was this: Does a federal law prohibiting fraudulent communications to government agencies preempt a state law permitting plaintiffs to sue for faulty products that would not have reached the market absent the fraud?

Examples of how drug manufacturers could be held legally responsible before any Supreme Court decision protecting them from liability were the many lawsuits recently filed against Merck & Company, a pharmaceutical firm that manufactured the drug Vioxx, once widely recommended for pain relief for arthritis sufferers. The drug was suspected of causing heart attacks and strokes in some patients, and from 1999, the year Vioxx went on the market, to 2007, Merck faced lawsuits from 47,000 plaintiffs, including patients, health providers, unions, and insurers. Many of the lawsuits

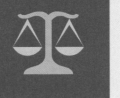
Patient Sues Hospital

In August 1997, a patient admitted to a Louisiana medical center for the treatment of bronchitis and back pain called the nurses' station to ask for someone to fix the television set and the window blinds. In response, two maintenance workers came to the patient's room and removed the television set. The workers examined the blinds, but informed the patient they could not fix them. The workers then left, promising to replace the television set, but not commenting on the window blinds.

The patient continued to ask for someone to adjust the window blinds to keep out the sun. She said that when she was in pain, light was unpleasant to her. No one came to fix the blinds.

The patient eventually tried to close the blinds herself. Dressed in street clothes and sandals, she climbed on a recliner chair with lockable wheels located in her room, and reached high above her head in an attempt to turn the slats of the blinds. The patient fell off the chair and sustained an injury to her left shoulder, upper back, and cervical spine.

The patient then sued the medical center for the injuries she had suffered. An appeals court overturned a circuit court's decision to dismiss and sent the case back for further proceedings. The appeals court determined: "It is not unforeseeable that a patient experiencing discomfort due to bright light entering the room, and who has obtained no relief through repeated requests for aid, might decide to take matters into her own hands and attempt to close the broken blinds. Furthermore, because the top of the blinds is located above the easy reach of the average person, it is not unforeseeable that the patient would attempt to use a chair to reach the top of the blinds."

Lichti v. Schumpert Medical Center, 2000 LA.App.LEXIS 61 (Court of Appeal of Louisiana, Second Circuit, Jan. 26, 2000).

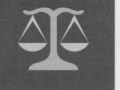
County Liable in Ambulance Delay

In 1991 an Indiana man suffered a heart attack while mowing the lawn. He took two nitroglycerin tablets while his wife called an ambulance. The emergency operator took the wife's call at 2:10 PM and said an ambulance would be dispatched. Seven minutes later the ambulance had not arrived, so the wife called a nearby fire station, where the local branch of the emergency medical squad was holding a meeting. An ambulance was sent immediately when this call was received, and it arrived at the patient's house in one minute.

The patient later learned that the emergency operator who had first been called had never dispatched an ambulance to his home. The chief deputy sheriff of the county explained that the officer taking emergency calls was inexperienced as a dispatcher. The officer had been the only one assigned to monitor the emergency line on that day because the sheriff's department was having its annual picnic.

The patient sued the county for negligence in operating the 911 emergency service. He claimed he had suffered permanent heart damage because of the operator's failure to promptly dispatch an ambulance.

The county moved for summary judgment based on the fact that it had no relationship with the man that created a duty of care to him. The trial court granted the motion, but an appellate court reversed the judgment. It held that the call to the emergency operator, in which the man's wife spoke of her husband's heart attack and the immediate need for an ambulance, was sufficient to establish knowledge that inaction could be harmful.

When the operator said an ambulance would be dispatched, he established that the county explicitly agreed to assist the patient. Accordingly, the court held, the county had assumed a private duty to the man and could be held liable for failure to dispatch an ambulance.

Kober v. Dial, 653 N.E.2d 524 (Ind. Ct. of App., July 26, 1995).

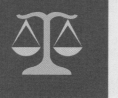
Supreme Court Shields Medical Devices from Lawsuits

An angioplasty was performed on a patient, Charles Riegel, in New York. During the procedure, the catheter used to dilate the patient's coronary artery failed, causing serious complications. The patient sued the catheter's manufacturer, Medtronic Inc., under New York state law, charging negligence in design, manufacture, and labeling of the device, which had received FDA approval in 1994. Medtronic argued that Riegel could not bring state law negligence claims, because the company was preempted from liability under Section 360k(a) of the Medical Device Amendments (MDA) of the U.S. Food, Drug, and Cosmetic Act.

The case reached the United States Supreme Court, where the question to be decided was this: Does Section 360k(a) of the Medical Device Amendments to the Food, Drug, and Cosmetic Act preempt state law claims seeking damages for injuries caused by medical devices that received premarket approval from the Food and Drug Administration?

In February 2008, the U.S. Supreme Court held that makers of medical devices are immune from liability for personal injuries as long as the Food and Drug Administration (FDA) approved the device before it was marketed and it meets the FDA's specifications.

Riegel v. Medtronic, Inc., 552 U.S. February 20, 2008.

alleged that Merck knew of the drug's potentially harmful side effects when the company placed the drug on the market.

In November 2007, Merck agreed to settle most of the lawsuits relating to Vioxx for a total of $4.85 billion. The settlement was open to plaintiffs who filed cases before November 8, 2007, who could provide medical proof of their heart attack or stroke, and who could prove they had used at least 30 Vioxx pills within 14 days prior to their illness.

Merck anticipated that some plaintiffs would opt out of the settlement, continuing to fight the company on a case-by-case basis. The company projected that remaining claims could cost the firm between $2 billion and $3 billion.

COMPARING ASPECTS OF LAW AND ETHICS

In order to understand the complexities of law and ethics, it is helpful to define and compare a few basic terms. Table 1-1 summarizes the terms described in the following sections.

law Rule of conduct or action prescribed or formally recognized as binding or enforced by a controlling authority.

Law

A **law** is defined as a rule of conduct or action prescribed or formally recognized as binding or enforced by a controlling authority. Governments enact laws to keep society running smoothly and to control behavior that could threaten public safety. Laws are considered the minimum standard necessary to keep society functioning.

Enforcement of laws is made possible by penalties for disobedience, which are decided by a court of law or are mandatory as written into the law. Penalties vary with the severity of the crime. Lawbreakers may be fined, imprisoned, or both. Sometimes lawbreakers are sentenced to probation.

TABLE 1-1   Comparing Aspects of Law and Ethics

	Law	Ethics	Moral Values
Definition	Set of governing rules	Principles, standards, guide to conduct	Beliefs formed through the influence of family, culture, and society
Main Purpose	To protect the public	To elevate the standard of competence	To serve as a guide for personal ethical conduct
Standards	Minimal—promotes smooth functioning of society	Builds values and ideals	Serves as a basis for forming a personal code of ethics
Penalties of Violation	Civil or criminal liability. Upon conviction: fine, imprisonment, revocation of license, or other penalty as determined by courts	Suspension or eviction from medical society membership, as decided by peers	Difficulty in getting along with others

	Bioethics	Etiquette	Protocol
Definition	Discipline relating to ethics concerning biological research, especially as applied to medicine	Courtesy and manners	Rules of etiquette applicable to one's place of employment
Main Purpose	To allow scientific progress in a manner that benefits society in all possible ways	To enable one to get along with others	To enable one to get along with others engaged in the same profession
Standards	Leads to highest standards possible in applying research to medical care	Leads to pleasant interaction	Promotes smooth functioning of workplace routines
Penalties for Violation	Can include all those listed under "Law," "Ethics," and "Etiquette"; as current standards are applied and as new laws and ethical standards evolve to govern medical research and development, penalties may change	Ostracism from chosen groups	Disapproval of one's professional colleagues; possible loss of business

Other penalties appropriate to the crime may be handed down by the sentencing authority, as when offenders must perform a specified number of hours of volunteer community service or are ordered to repair public facilities they have damaged.

Many laws affect health care practitioners, including criminal and civil statutes as well as state medical practice acts. Medical practice acts apply specifically to the practice of medicine in a certain state. Licensed health care professionals convicted of violating criminal, civil, or medical practice laws may lose their licenses to practice. (Medical practice acts are discussed further in Chapter 2. Laws and the court system are discussed in more detail in Chapter 3.)

Ethics

ethics Standards of behavior, developed as a result of one's concept of right and wrong.

moral values One's personal concept of right and wrong, formed through the influence of the family, culture, and society.

An illegal act by a health care practitioner is always unethical, but an unethical act is not necessarily illegal. **Ethics** are concerned with standards of behavior and the concept of right and wrong, over and above that which is legal in a given situation. **Moral values**—formed through the influence of the family, culture, and society—serve as the basis for ethical conduct.

The United States is a culturally diverse country, with many residents who have grown up within vastly different ethnic environments. For example, a Chinese student in the United States brings to his or her studies a unique set of religious and social experiences and moral concepts that will differ from that of a German, Japanese, Korean, French, Italian, or even Canadian classmate. Therefore, moral values and ethical standards can differ for health care practitioners, as well as patients, in the same setting.

In the American cultural environment, however, acting morally toward another usually requires that you put yourself in that individual's place. For example, when you are a patient in a physician's office, how do you like to be treated? As a health care provider, can you give care to a person whose conduct or professed beliefs differ radically from your own? In an emergency, can you provide for the patient's welfare without reservation?

Codes of Ethics and Ethics Guidelines

code of ethics A list of principles intended to govern behavior—here, the behavior of those entrusted with providing care to the sick.

While most individuals can rely upon a well-developed personal value system, organizations for the health occupations also have formalized **codes of ethics** to govern behavior of members and to increase the level of competence and standards of care within the group. Included among these are the American Nurses' Association Code for Nurses, American Medical

CHECK YOUR PROGRESS

1. Name two important reasons for studying law and ethics.

_____

_____

2. Which state laws apply specifically to the practice of medicine?

_____

_____

3. What purpose do laws serve?

_____

_____

4. How is the enforcement of laws made possible?

_____

_____

5. What factors influence the formation of one's personal set of ethics and values?

_____

_____

Association's Code of Medical Ethics, American Health Information Management Association's Code of Ethics, American Society of Radiologic Technologists Code of Ethics, and the Code of Ethics of the American Association of Medical Assistants. Codes of ethics generally consist of a list of general principles, and are often available to laypersons as well as members of health care practitioner organizations.

Many professional organizations for health care practitioners also publish more detailed **ethics guidelines,** usually in book form, for members. Generally, ethics guideline publications detail a wide variety of ethical situations that health care practitioners might face in their work and offer principles for dealing with the situations in an ethical manner. They are routinely available to members of health care organizations, and are typically available to others for a fee.

One of the earliest medical codes of ethics, the code of Hammurabi, was written by the Babylonians around 2250 B.C.E. This document discussed the conduct expected of physicians at that time, including fees that could be charged.

Sometime around 400 B.C.E., Hippocrates, the Greek physician known as the Father of Medicine, created the **Hippocratic oath,** a pledge for physicians that remains influential today (see Figure 1-1).

Percival's Medical Ethics, written by the English physician and philosopher Thomas Percival in 1803, superseded earlier codes to become the definitive guide for a physician's professional conduct. Earlier codes did not

ethics guidelines Publications that detail a wide variety of ethical situations that professionals (in this case, health care practitioners) might face in their work and offer principles for dealing with the situations in an ethical manner.

Hippocratic oath A pledge for physicians, developed by the Greek physician Hippocrates circa 400 B.C.E.

I swear by Apollo, the physician, and Aesculapius, and Health, and Allheal, and all the gods and goddesses, that, according to my ability and judgment, I will keep this oath and stipulation, to reckon him who taught me this art equally dear to me as my parents, to share my substance with him and relieve his necessities if required; to regard his offspring as on the same footing with my own brothers, and to teach them this art if they should wish to learn it, without fee or stipulation, and that by precept, lecture, and every other mode of instruction, I will impart a knowledge of the art to my own sons and to those of my teachers, and to disciples bound by a stipulation and oath, according to the law of medicine, but to none other.

I will follow that method of treatment which, according to my ability and judgment, I consider for the benefit of my patients, and abstain from whatever is deleterious and mischievous. I will give no deadly medicine to anyone if asked, nor suggest any such counsel; furthermore, I will not give to a woman an instrument to produce abortion.

With purity and holiness I will pass my life and practice my art. I will not cut a person who is suffering with a stone, but will leave this to be done by practitioners of the work. Into whatever houses I enter I will go into them for the benefit of the sick and will abstain from every voluntary act of mischief and corruption; and further from the seduction of females or males, bond or free.

Whatever, in connection with my professional practice, or not inconnection with it, I may see or hear in the lives of men which ought not to be spoken abroad, I will not divulge, as reckoning that all such should be kept secret.

While I continue to keep this oath unviolated, may it be granted to me to enjoy life and the practice of the art, respected by all men at all times, but should I trespass and violate this oath, may the reverse be my lot.

FIGURE 1-1 Hippocratic Oath

American Medical Association Principles A code of ethics for members of the American Medical Association, written in 1847. (American Medical Association, Council on Ethical and Judicial Affairs, *Codes of Medical Ethics,* 2002–2003 Edition, p. xiv.)

address concerns about experimental medicine, but according to Percival's code, physicians could try experimental treatments when all else failed, if such treatments served the public good.

When the American Medical Association met for the first time in Philadelphia in 1847, the group devised a code of ethics for members based upon Percival's code. The resulting **American Medical Association Principles,** currently called the *American Medical Association Principles of Medical Ethics,* have been revised and updated periodically to keep pace with changing times (see Figure 1-2). The *American Medical Association Principles of Medical Ethics* briefly summarizes the position of the American Medical Association (AMA) on ethical treatment of patients, while the more extensive *Code of Medical Ethics: Current Opinions with Annotations* provides more detailed coverage.

Preamble

The medical profession has long subscribed to a body of ethical statements developed primarily for the benefit of the patient. As a member of this profession, a physician must recognize responsibility to patients first and foremost, as well as to society, to other health professionals, and to self. The following Principles adopted by the American Medical Association are not laws, but standards of conduct which define the essentials of honorable behavior for the physician.

I. A physician shall be dedicated to providing competent medical care, with compassion and respect for human dignity and right.

II. A physician shall uphold the standards of professionalism, be honest in all professional interactions, and strive to report physicians deficient in character or competence, or who engage in fraud or deception, to appropriate entities.

III. A physician shall respect the law and also recognize a responsibility to seek changes in those requirements which are contrary to the best interests of the patient.

IV. A physician shall respect the rights of patients, colleagues, and other health professionals and shall safeguard patient confidences and privacy within the constraints of the law.

V. A physician shall continue to study, apply, and advance scientific knowledge, maintain commitment to medical education, make relevant information available to patients, colleagues, and the public, obtain consultation, and use the talents of other health professionals when indicated.

VI. A physician shall, in the provision of appropriate patient care, except in emergencies, be free to choose whom to serve, with whom to associate, and the environment in which to provide care.

VII. A physician shall recognize a responsibility to participate in activities contributing to the improvement of the community and the betterment of public health.

VIII. A physician shall, while caring for a patient, regard responsibility to the patient as paramount.

IX. A physician shall support access to medical care for all people.

FIGURE 1-2 American Medical Association *Principles of Medical Ethics*
Source: American Medical Association, *Code of Medical Ethics, Current Opinions with Annotations,* current issue.

The Code of Ethics of AAMA shall set forth principles of ethical and moral conduct as they relate to the medical profession and the particular practice of medical assisting.

Members of AAMA dedicated to the conscientious pursuit of their profession and thus desiring to merit the high regard of the entire medical profession and the respect of the general public which they serve, do pledge themselves to strive always to:

A. render service with full respect for the dignity of humanity;
B. respect confidential information obtained through employment unless legally authorized or required by responsible performance of duty to divulge such information;
C. uphold the honor and high principles of the profession and accept its disciplines;
D. seek to continually improve the knowledge and skills of medical assistants for the benefit of patients and professional colleagues;
E. participate in additional service activities aimed toward improving the health and well-being of the community.

Creed

- I believe in the principles and purposes of the profession of medical assisting.
- I endeavor to be more effective.
- I aspire to render greater service.
- I protect the confidence entrusted to me.
- I am dedicated to the care and well-being of all people.
- I am loyal to my employer.
- I am true to the ethics of my profession.
- I am strengthened by compassion, courage, and faith.

FIGURE 1-3 Code of Ethics of the American Association of Medical Assistants (AAMA)

When members of professional associations such as the AMA and the AAMA are accused of unethical conduct, they are subject to peer council review and may be censured by the organization (see Figure 1-3). Although a professional group cannot revoke a member's license to practice, unethical members may be expelled from the group, suspended for a period of time, or ostracized by other members. Unethical behavior by a medical practitioner can result in loss of income and eventually the loss of a practice if, as a result of that behavior, patients choose another practitioner.

bioethics A discipline dealing with the ethical implications of biological research methods and results, especially in medicine.

Bioethics

Bioethics is a discipline dealing with the ethical implications of biological research methods and results, especially in medicine. As biological research has led to unprecedented progress in medicine, medical practitioners have had to grapple with issues such as these:

▮ What ethics should guide biomedical research? Do individuals own all rights to their body cells, or should scientists own cells they have altered?

Is human experimentation essential, or even permissible, to advance biomedical research?

- What ethics should guide organ transplants? Although organs suitable for transplant are in short supply, is the search for organs dehumanizing? Should certain categories of people have lower priority than others for organ transplants?
- What ethics should guide fetal tissue research? Some say such research, especially stem cell research, is moral because it offers hope to disease victims, while others argue that it is immoral.
- Do reproductive technologies offer hope to the childless, or are they unethical? Are the multiple births that sometimes result from taking fertility drugs an acceptable aspect of reproductive technology, or are those multiple births too risky for women and their fetuses and even immoral in an allegedly overpopulated world?
- Should animals ever be used in research?
- How ethical is genetic research? Should the government regulate it? Will genetic testing benefit those at risk for genetic disease, or will it lead to discrimination? Should the cloning of human organs for transplantation be permitted? Should cloning of human beings ever be permitted?

Society is attempting to address these questions, but because the issues are complicated, many questions may never be completely resolved.

The Role of Ethics Committees

Health care practitioners may be able to resolve the majority of the ethical issues they face in the workplace from their own intuitive sense of moral values and ethics. Some ethical dilemmas, however, are not so much a question of right or wrong but more a question like "which of these alternatives will do the most good and the least harm?" In these more ambiguous situations, health care practitioners may want to ask the advice of a medical ethicist or members of an institutional ethics committee.

medical ethicist or bioethicist Specialists who consult with physicians, researchers, and others to help them make difficult ethical decisions regarding patient care.

Ethics committee Committee made up of individuals who are involved in a patient's care, including health care practitioners, family members, clergy, and others, with the purpose of reviewing ethical issues in difficult cases.

Medical ethicists or **bioethicists** are specialists who consult with physicians, researchers, and others to help them make difficult decisions, such as whether to resuscitate brain-damaged premature infants or what ethics should govern privacy in genetic testing. Hospital or medical center **ethics committees** usually consist of physicians, nurses, social workers, clergy, a patient's family, members of the community, and other individuals involved with the patient's medical care. A medical ethicist may also sit on the ethics committee if such a specialist is available. When difficult decisions must be made, any one of the individuals involved in a patient's medical care can ask for a consultation with the ethics committee. Larger hospitals have standing ethics committees, while smaller facilities may form ethics committees as needed.

When a case is referred to the ethics committee, the members meet and review the case. The committee does not make binding decisions, but helps the physician, nurse, patient, patient's family, and others clarify the issue and understand the medical facts of the case and the alternatives available to resolve the situation. Ethics committees may also help with conflict resolution among parties involved with a case. They do not, however, function as institutional review boards or morals police looking for health care workers who have committed unethical acts.

Etiquette

While professional codes of ethics focus upon the protection of the patient and his or her right to appropriate, competent, and humane treatment,

etiquette Standards of behavior considered to be good manners among members of a profession as they function as individuals in society.

etiquette refers to standards of behavior that are considered good manners. Every culture has its own ideas of common courtesy. Behavior considered good manners in one culture may be bad manners in another. For example, in some Middle Eastern countries it is extremely discourteous for one male acquaintance to ask another, "How is your wife?" In Western culture, such a question is well received. Similarly, within nearly every profession, there are recognized practices considered to be good manners for members.

Most health care facilities have their own policies concerning professional etiquette that staff members are expected to follow. Policy manuals written especially for the facility can serve as permanent records and as guidelines for employees in these matters.

By the same token, health care practitioners are expected to know **protocol,** standard rules of etiquette applicable specifically to their place of employment. For example, when another physician telephones, does the receptionist put the call through without delay? Is a physician who is also a patient billed at the same rate as other patients who are not physicians?

protocol A code prescribing correct behavior in a specific situation, such as a situation arising in a medical office.

Within the health care environment, all health care practitioners are, of course, expected to treat patients with the same respect and courtesy afforded others in the course of day-to-day living. Politeness and appropriate dress are mandatory.

QUALITIES OF SUCCESSFUL HEALTH CARE PRACTITIONERS

Successful health care practitioners have a knowledge of techniques and principles that includes an understanding of legal and ethical issues. They must also acquire a working knowledge of and tolerance for human nature and individual characteristics, since daily contact with a wide variety of individuals with a host of problems and concerns is a significant part of the work. Courtesy, compassion, and common sense are often cited as the "three Cs" most vital to the professional success of health care practitioners.

Courtesy

courtesy The practice of good manners.

The simplest definition of **courtesy** is the practice of good manners. Most of us know how to practice good manners, but sometimes circumstances make us forget. Maybe we're having a rotten day—we overslept and dressed in a hurry but were still late to work; the car didn't start so we had to walk, making us even more late; we were rebuked at work for coming in late . . . and on and on. Perhaps we're burned out, stressed out, or simply too busy to think. Regardless of a health care practitioner's personal situation, however, patients have the right to expect courtesy and respect, including self introduction. ("Hi, I'm Maggie and I'll be taking care of you," is one nursing assistant's way of introducing herself to new patients in the nursing home where she works.)

Think back to experiences you have had with health care practitioners. Did the receptionist in a medical office greet you pleasantly, or did he or she make you feel as though you were an unwelcome intruder? Did the laboratory technician or phlebotomist who drew your blood for testing put you at ease or make you more anxious than you already were? If you were hospitalized, did health care practitioners carefully explain procedures and treatments before performing them, or were you left wondering what was

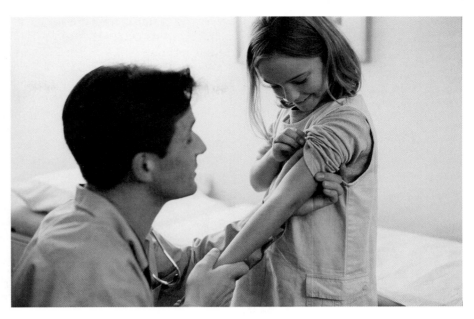

FIGURE 1-4 Empathy is a stronger emotion than sympathy.

happening to you? Chances are that you know from your own experiences how important common courtesy can be to a patient.

Compassion

compassion The identification with and understanding of another's situation, feelings, and motives.

Compassion is empathy—the identification with and understanding of another's situation, feelings, and motives (Figure 1-4). In other words, compassion is temporarily putting oneself in another's shoes. It should not be confused with sympathy, which is feeling sorry for another person's plight—typically a less deeply felt emotion than compassion. While "I know how you feel" is not usually the best phrase to utter to a patient (it too often earns the retort, "No, you don't"), compassion means that you are sincerely attempting to know how the patient feels.

Common Sense

common sense Sound practical judgment.

Common sense is simply sound practical judgment. It is somewhat difficult to define, because it can have different meanings for different people, but it generally means that you can see which solution or action makes good sense in a given situation. For example, if you were a nursing assistant and a gasping, panicked patient told you he was having trouble breathing, common sense would tell you to immediately seek help. You wouldn't simply enter the patient's complaint in his medical chart and wait for a physician or a nurse to see the notation. Likewise, if a patient spilled something on the floor, common sense would tell you to wipe it up (even if you were not a member of the housekeeping staff) before someone stepped in it and possibly slipped and fell. While it's not always immediately obvious that someone has common sense, it usually doesn't take long to recognize its absence in an individual.

Additional capabilities that are helpful to those who choose to work in the health care field include those that are listed below under the headings, "People Skills" and "Technical Skills."

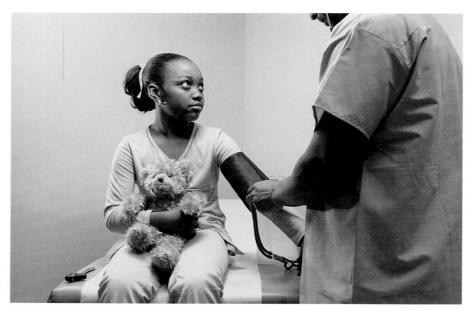

FIGURE 1-5   The health care practitioner taking the girl's vital signs has put her at ease.

People Skills

People skills are those traits and capabilities that allow you to get along well with others and to relate well to patients or clients in a health care setting. They include such attributes as the following:

- A relaxed attitude when meeting new people.
- An understanding of and empathy for others.
- Good communication skills, including writing, speaking, and listening.
- Patience in dealing with others and the ability to work as a member of a health care team (see Figure 1-5).
- Tact.
- The ability to impart information clearly and accurately.
- The ability to keep information confidential.
- The ability to leave private concerns at home.
- Trustworthiness and a sense of responsibility.

Technical Skills

Technical skills include those abilities you have acquired in your course of study, including but not limited to the following:

- Computer literacy.
- Proficiency in English, science, and mathematics.
- A willingness to learn new skills and techniques.
- An aptitude for working with the hands.
- Ability to document well.
- Ability to think critically.

Critical Thinking Skills

When faced with a problem, most of us worry a lot before we finally begin working through the problem effectively, which means using fewer emotions

critical thinking The ability to think analytically, using fewer emotions and more rationality.

and more rational thinking skills. As a health care practitioner, you will be expected to approach a problem at work in a manner that lets you act as ethically, legally, and helpfully as possible. Sometimes solutions to problems must also be found as quickly as possible, but solutions must always be within the scope of your training, licensure, and capabilities. This problem-solving process is called **critical thinking.** Here is a five-step aid for approaching a problem using critical thinking:

1. **Identify and clarify the problem.** It's impossible to solve a problem unless you know the exact nature of the problem. For example, imagine that patients in a medical office have frequently complained that the wait to see physicians is too long, and several have protested loudly and angrily that their time "is valuable too." Rhea is the waiting room receptionist and the person who faces angry patients first, so she would like to solve this problem as quickly as possible. Rhea has recognized that a problem exists, of course, but her apologies to patients have been temporary fixes, and the situation continues.

2. **Gather information.** In the above situation, Rhea begins to gather information. She first checks to see exactly why patients have been kept waiting, and considers the following questions: Are all the physicians simply oversleeping and beginning the day behind schedule? (Not likely, but an easy solution if this were the case would be to buy the physicians new alarm clocks.) Are the physicians often delayed in surgery or because of hospital rounds? Is the clinic understaffed? How long, on average, has each patient who has complained been left waiting beyond his or her appointment time?

3. **Evaluate the evidence.** Rhea evaluates the answers she has gathered to the above questions and determines that too many patients are, indeed, waiting too long beyond appointment times to see their physicians. The next step in the critical thinking process is to consider all possible ways to solve the problem.

4. **Consider alternatives and implications.** Rhea has determined that the evidence supports the fact that a problem exists and begins to formulate alternatives by asking herself these questions: Could the waiting room be better supplied with current reading material or perhaps television sets and a children's corner, so that patients both with and without children are less likely to complain about waiting? Is the waiting room cheery and comfortable, so waiting does not seem interminable? What solution would best serve the goals of physicians, other medical office personnel, and patients? Rhea must consider costs of, objections to, and all others' opinions of each alternative she considers.

5. **Choose and implement the best alternative.** Rhea selects an alternative and implements it. As a medical office receptionist, she cannot act alone, but she has brought the problem to the attention of those who can help, and her suggestions have been heard. As a result of Rhea's research, acceptable solutions to patients' complaints that they are forced to wait too long to see physicians might include the following:

   ▮ Patients are asked to remind receptionists when they have been waiting over 15 minutes so receptionists can check to see what is causing the delay.
   ▮ Additional personnel are hired to see patients.
   ▮ The waiting room is stocked with current news publications, television sets, and/or a child play center for patient comfort while waiting.

Critical thinking is not easy, but, like any skill, it improves with practice.

The health care practitioner who demonstrates the above qualities, coupled with a working knowledge of law and ethics, is most likely to find success and job satisfaction in his or her chosen profession.

CHECK YOUR PROGRESS

6. Tell how each of the following characteristics relates to law and ethics in the health care professions:

The ability to be a good communicator and listener.

_____

_____

The ability to keep information confidential.

_____

_____

The ability to impart information clearly and accurately.

_____

_____

The ability to think critically.

_____

_____

Ethics Issues

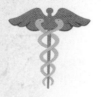

Introduction to End-of-Chapter Ethics Discussions

Learning Outcomes for the Ethics Issues Feature at the End of Each Chapter

After studying the material in each chapter's Ethics Issues feature you should be able to:

1. Discuss current ethical issues of concern to health care practitioners.
2. Compare ethical guidelines to the law as discussed in each chapter of the text.
3. Practice critical thinking skills as you consider medical, legal, and ethical issues for each situation presented.
4. Relate the ethical issues presented in the text to the health care profession you intend to practice.

Health care practitioners are bound by state and federal laws, but they are also bound by certain ethical standards—both personal standards and those set forth by professional codes of ethics and ethical guidelines, and by bioethicists. Many professional organizations for health care practitioners employ an ethics consultant who is available to speak with organization members who need help with an ethical dilemma. "We serve as a third party who can stand outside a situation and facilitate communication," says Dr. Carmen Paradis, an ethics consultant with the Cleveland Clinic's Department of Bioethics. At the Cleveland Clinic, ethics consultations are available to health care practitioners, patients, family members, and others involved with patient decisions.

Medical facility ethics committees can also serve as consultants. In larger health care facilities such committees usually deal with institutional matters, but in smaller communities where ethics consultants may not be available, members of an ethics committee may also function as ethics consultants.

Keep in mind as you read the Ethical Issues feature for each chapter that ethical guidelines are not law, but deal solely with ethical conduct for health care practitioners. Most guidelines published for professional health care practitioner organizations emphasize this difference. For example, as stated in *Guidelines for Ethical Conduct for the Physician Assistant Profession,* "Generally, the law delineates the minimum standard of acceptable behavior in our society. Acceptable ethical behavior is usually less clearly defined than law and often places greater demands on an individual. . . .

"Ethical guidelines for health care practitioners are not meant to be used in courts of law as legal standards to which practitioners will be held. Ethical guidelines are, rather, meant to guide health care practitioners and to encourage them to think about their individual actions in certain situations."

The ethical guidelines for various health care professions have several points in common, but first and foremost is that health care practitioners are obligated to provide the best care possible for every patient, and to protect the safety and welfare of every patient.

State and federal law may differ somewhat from an ethical principle. For example, a state's law may not require physicians to routinely inquire about physical, sexual, and psychological abuse as part of a patient's medical history, but the physician may feel an ethical duty to his or her patients to do so.

Furthermore, the fact that a health care practitioner who has been charged with illegal conduct is acquitted or exonerated does not necessarily mean that the health care practitioner acted ethically.

The term *ethical* as used here refers to matters involving the following:

1. Moral principles or practices.
2. Matters of social policy involving issues of morality in the practice of medicine.

The term *unethical* refers to professional conduct that fails to conform to these moral standards or policies.

The ethical issues raised are from the real-life experiences of a variety of health care practitioners and are recounted throughout the text to raise awareness of the ethical dilemmas many practitioners face daily, and to stimulate discussion.

Ethics Issues

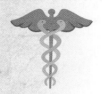

Introduction to Law and Ethics

ETHICS ISSUE 1: A physician assistant in a medical practice with several physicians contacts his professional association, the American Academy of Physician Assistants (AAPA), to report that he is being pressured to sign a document stating that he agrees with the use of expired medications in the ACLS (crash cart) drug box. He knows the practice is an attempt to save money, but he feels uncomfortable signing such a document and, in fact, calls the issue a "job breaker." The PA's state laws do not specifically prohibit this practice, but he strongly suspects it is unethical.

DISCUSSION QUESTIONS

1. Might a legal issue arise if a code went badly and there were a question about the use of outdated medications? Explain your answer.

_____

_____

2. In your opinion, is it ethical for the medical practice to use outdated medications? Is it ethical to require the PA to sign a document affirming his agreement with the practice? Explain your answers.

_____

_____

ETHICS ISSUE 2: A registered nurse calls her professional organization's ethics consultant to ask for resources she can present to her employing medical clinic to support her intention to quit working with a physician she feels is providing sloppy and possibly dangerous care.

DISCUSSION QUESTIONS

1. What is the most important principle for the nurse to consider here?

_____

_____

2. In your opinion, are there legal issues inherent in this situation, as well as ethical issues? Explain your answer.

_____

_____

ETHICS ISSUE 3: A physician assistant is planning a trip abroad with a medical relief agency. The physician who was to be his supervisor cancels at the last minute. Should he go alone, the PA asks, when he will have no physician supervisor? (The destination country has no physician assistants and, therefore, no laws regarding their practice.)

DISCUSSION QUESTION

1. While it will not be illegal, in the destination country, for the PA to complete the medical relief mission on his own, will it be ethical? Explain your answer.

_____

_____

ETHICS ISSUE 4: Family members of a certified medical assistant (CMA) employed by a medical clinic in a small community often ask the CMA for medical advice. Two of her family members have asked her to bring antibiotic samples home for them.

DISCUSSION QUESTION

1. In your opinion, would it be ethical for the CMA to give medical advice to her own family members? To bring drug samples home for them? Explain your answers.

_____

_____

ETHICS ISSUE 5: A radiology technician practicing in a small community is interested in dating a person he has seen as a patient.

_____

_____

DISCUSSION QUESTION

1. In your opinion, would it be ethical for the patient to date one of his patients? Would it be ethical for him to date a coworker? Explain your answers.

_____

_____

 Go to www.mhhe.com/judson5e to practice your case review skills. Then read on for more information.

1 REVIEW

Applying Knowledge

Answer the following questions in the spaces provided.

1. List three areas where health care practitioners can gain insight through studying law and ethics.

_____

_____

_____

2. Define *summary judgment.*

_____

_____

3. Define *bioethics.*

_____

_____

4. Define *law.*

_____

_____

5. Define *ethics.*

_____

_____

6. How is unethical behavior punished?

_____

_____

7. Define *etiquette.*

_____

_____

8. How are violations of etiquette handled?

_____

_____

9. What is the purpose of a professional code of ethics?

_____

_____

10. Name five bioethical issues of concern in today's society.

_____

_____

11. What duties might a medical ethicist perform?

_____

_____

12. Decisions made by judges in the various courts and used as a guide for future decisions are called

_____

_____

Circle the correct answer for each of the following multiple-choice questions.

13. Written codes of ethics for health care practitioners:
    a. Evolved primarily to serve as moral guidelines for those who provided care to the sick
    b. Are legally binding
    c. Did not exist in ancient times
    d. None of the above

14. A Greek physician who is known as the Father of Medicine:
    a. Hippocrates
    b. Percival
    c. Hammurabi
    d. Socrates

15. A pledge for physicians that remains influential today:
    a. Code of Hammurabi
    b. Babylonian Ethics Code
    c. Hippocratic oath
    d. None of the above

16. This ethics code superseded earlier codes to become the definitive guide for a physician's professional conduct:
    a. Code of Hammurabi
    b. Percival's Medical Ethics
    c. Hippocratic oath
    d. Babylonian Ethics Code

17. Unethical behavior is always:
    a. Illegal
    b. Punishable by legal means
    c. Unacceptable
    d. None of the above

18. Unlawful acts are always:
    a. Unacceptable
    b. Unethical
    c. Punishable by legal means
    d. All of the above

19. Violation of a professional organization's formalized code of ethics:
    a. Always leads to prosecution in a court of law
    b. Is ignored if one's membership dues in the organization are paid
    c. Can lead to expulsion from the organization
    d. None of the above

20. Law is:
    a. The minimum standard necessary to keep society functioning smoothly
    b. Ignored if transgressions are ethical, rather than legal
    c. Seldom enforced by controlling authorities
    d. None of the above

21. Conviction of a crime:
    a. Cannot result in loss of license unless ethical violations also exist
    b. Is always punishable by imprisonment
    c. Always results in expulsion from a professional organization
    d. Can result in loss of license

22. The basis for ethical conduct includes:
    a. One's morals
    b. One's culture
    c. One's family
    d. All of the above

23. Sellers and manufacturers can be held legally responsible for defective medical devices and products through charges of:
    a. Fraud
    b. Breach of warranty
    c. Misrepresentation of the product through untrue statements made by the manufacturer or seller
    d. All of the above

24. Bioethics is concerned with:
    a. Health care law
    b. Etiquette in medical facilities
    c. The ethical implications of biological research methods and results
    d. None of the above

25. Critical thinking skills include:
    a. Assessing the ethics of a situation
    b. First clearly defining a problem
    c. Determining the legal implications of a situation
    d. None of the above

Case Study

Use your critical thinking skills to answer the questions that follow each of the case studies. Indicate whether each situation is a question of law, ethics, protocol, or etiquette.
You are employed as an assistant in an ophthalmologist's office. Your neighbor asks you to find out for him how much another patient was charged for an eye examination at the eye clinic that employs you. Your neighbor also asks you how much the patient was charged for his prescription eyeglasses (the eye clinic also sells lenses and frames).

26. Can you answer either of your neighbor's questions? Explain your answer.

_____

_____

A physician employs you as a medical assistant. Another physician comes into the medical office where you work and asks to speak with your physician/employer.

27. Should you seat the physician in the waiting room, or show her to your employer's private office? Why?

_____

_____

You are employed as a licensed practical nurse (LPN) in a small town. (In California and Texas, the term for this profession is "licensed vocational nurse"—abbreviated as LVN.) A woman visits the clinic where you work, complaining of a rash on her body. She says she recently came in contact with a child who had the same symptoms, and she asks, "What did this child see the doctor for, and what was the diagnosis?" She explains that she needs to know, so that she can be immunized if necessary. You explain that you cannot give out this information, but another LPN overhears, pulls the child's chart, and gives the woman the information she requested.

28. Did both LPNs in this scenario act ethically and responsibly? Explain your answer.

_____

_____

A physician admitted an elderly patient to the hospital, where she was treated for an irregular heartbeat and chest pain. The patient was competent to make her own decisions about a course of treatment, but her opinionated and outspoken daughter repeatedly second-guessed the physician's recommendations with medical information she had obtained from the Internet.

29. In your opinion, what responsibilities, if any, does a physician or other health care practitioner have toward difficult family members or other third parties who interfere with a patient's medical care?

_____

_____

30. What might the physician in the above situation have said to her patient's daughter to help resolve the situation?

_____

_____

Internet Activities

Complete the activities and answer the questions that follow.

31. Use a search engine to conduct a search for Web sites on the Internet concerned with bioethics. Name two of those sites you think are reliable sources of information. Explain your choices. How does each site define the term *bioethics?*

_____

_____

32. Locate the Web site for the organization that represents the health care profession you intend to practice. Does the site provide guidance on ethics? If so, how? Does the site link to other sites concerning ethics? If so, list three ethics links; then explore these links.

_____

_____

33. Visit the Web site sponsored by the National Institutes of Health called "Bioethics Resources" (http://bioethics.od.nih.gov/casestudies.html). Scroll down to case studies. Pick a case study and review it. Do you agree or disagree with the conclusions reached about the issue? Explain your answer.

_____

_____

2

Working in Health Care

Learning Outcomes

After studying this chapter, you should be able to:

1. Define licensure, certification, registration, and accreditation.

2. Demonstrate an understanding of how physicians are licensed, how physicians are regulated, and the purpose of a medical board.

3. Define four types of medical practice management systems.

4. Discuss two federal acts that prohibit fraud and abuse in health care billing.

5. Define three types of managed care health plans.

6. Define *telemedicine, cybermedicine,* and *e-health,* and discuss their roles in today's health care environment.

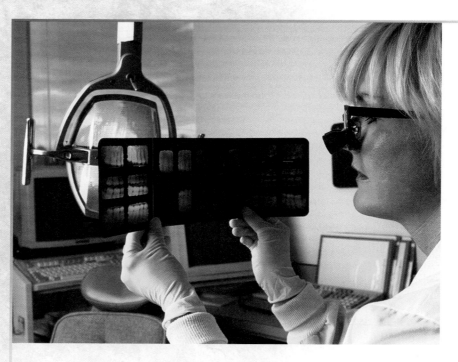

Key Terms

accrediation

allopathic

ambulatory care setting

associate practice

certification

corporation

cybermedicine

e-health

endorsement

Federal False Claims Act

gatekeeper physician

group practice

Health Care Quality Improvement Act of 1986 (HCQIA)

Healthcare Integrity and Protection Data Bank (HIPDB)

Health Insurance Portability and Accountability Act of 1996 (HIPAA)

health maintenance organization (HMO)

indemnity

individual (or independent) practice association (IPA)

licensure

managed care

medical boards

medical practice acts

National Practitioner Data Bank (NPDB)

open access

partnership

physician-hospital organization (PHO)

point-of-service (POS) plan

preferred provider association (PPA)

preferred provider organization (PPO)

primary care physician (PCP)

reciprocity

registration

respondeat superior

sole proprietorship

telemedicine

tertiary care settings

Voice of Experience
Audiologist Hears Patients' Concerns

Louise had worked with the hearing impaired in public schools for 10 years when she decided to become an audiologist. Upon receiving her master's degree in audiology and obtaining national certification and a state audiology license, Louise worked first as a school audiologist and then as an audiologist in a Midwestern ear, nose and throat clinic, where she presently practices. Louise performs clinical audiological evaluations for the physicians in the clinic, and she also dispenses hearing aids.

"Be prepared for years of study," Louise advises anyone considering a career as an audiologist, "the doctorate in audiology, AuD, will soon be mandatory.

"And remember that, regardless of which aspect of audiology you choose, you will be working with people. You need to have patience and understanding with all age groups, and you need to remember that you will never know it all. . . . Audiology is not an exact science, no matter how sophisticated our testing instruments have become.

When we are working with hearing loss we cannot 'fix' the system; we can only work with what is left. We need to be realistic in what we can do."

Patients who research hearing loss on the Web can be trying, Louise admits. "They sometimes come armed with a complete diagnosis and plan based on what they read on the Internet." Some patients or their families may have unrealistic expectations, Louise adds, and at times her job involves "knowing that you really can't help someone."

But when help is possible, the job can be exhilarating. For example, when Louise was a public school audiologist, she tested a five-year-old and realized that the child had a severe sensorineural hearing loss. She dreaded telling the child's mother, but was relieved when the woman said, "Thank you. You are the first person to confirm what I have been telling doctors for several years." The lesson she learned from this experience, Louise says, is that "it is important for professionals to trust a mother's instincts; they are usually correct."

LICENSURE, CERTIFICATION, REGISTRATION, AND ACCREDITATION

With increased medical specialization have come more exacting professional requirements for health care practitioners. Members of the health care team today are usually licensed, registered, or certified to perform specific duties, depending on job classification and state requirements. Furthermore, programs for educating health care practitioners are often accredited. Accreditation is a process education programs may complete that ensures certain standards have been met. Managed care plans may also earn accreditation or certification for excellence.

Licensure is a mandatory credentialing process established by law, usually at the state level. Licenses to practice are required in every state for all physicians and nurses and for many other health care practitioners as well. Individuals who do not have the required license are prohibited by law from practicing certain health care professions.

Certification is a voluntary credentialing process, usually national in scope, and is most often sponsored by a nongovernmental, private-sector group. Certification by a professional organization, usually through an examination, signifies that an applicant has attained a certain level of knowledge and skill. Since the process is voluntary, lack of certification does not prevent an employee from practicing the profession for which he or she is otherwise qualified.

Registration is an entry in an official registry or record, listing the names of persons in a certain occupation who have satisfied specific requirements. The list is usually made available to health care providers. One way to become registered is simply to add one's name to the list in the registry. Under this method of registration, unregistered persons are not prevented from working in a field for which they are otherwise qualified.

licensure A mandatory credentialing process established by law, usually at the state level, that grants the right to practice certain skills and endeavors.

certification A voluntary credentialing process whereby applicants who meet specific requirements may receive a certificate.

registration A credentialing procedure whereby one's name is listed on a register as having paid a fee and/or met certain criteria within a profession.

A second way to become registered in a health occupation is to attain a certain level of education and/or pay a registration fee. Under this second method, when there are specific requirements for registration, unregistered individuals may be prevented from working in a field for which they are otherwise qualified.

Under no circumstances may persons claim to be licensed, certified, or registered if they are not.

Accreditation is the process by which health care practitioner education programs, health care facilities, and managed care plans are officially authorized. Two examples of accrediting agencies for health care practitioner education programs are the Commission on Accreditation of Allied Health Education Programs (CAAHEP), discussed in more detail on page 32, and the Accrediting Bureau of Health Education Schools (ABHES). Accreditation is usually voluntary, but accredited programs for various disciplines must maintain certain standards to earn and keep accreditation. Most accredited programs for health care education also include an internship or externship (practical work experience) that lasts for a specified period of time.

The Joint Commission on Accreditation of Healthcare Organizations (JCAHO) accredits health care organizations that meet certain standards. As of 2004, the Joint Commission evaluated and accredited over 16,000 health care organizations and programs in the United States, including the following:

- General, psychiatric, children's, and rehabilitation hospitals.
- Critical access hospitals.
- Health care networks, including health maintenance organizations (HMOs), preferred provider organizations (PPOs), integrated delivery networks, and managed behavioral health care organizations.
- Home care organizations, including those that provide home health services, personal care and support services, home infusion and other pharmacy services, durable medical equipment services, and hospice services.
- Nursing homes and other long-term care facilities, including subacute care programs, dementia special care programs, and long-term care pharmacies.
- Assisted living facilities.
- Behavioral health care organizations.
- Ambulatory care providers, such as outpatient surgery facilities, rehabilitation centers, infusion centers, and group practices, as well as office-based surgery.
- Clinical laboratories, including independent or freestanding laboratories, blood transfusion and donor centers, and public health laboratories.

To earn and maintain JCAHO accreditation, an organization must undergo an on-site survey by a JCAHO survey team at least every three years. Laboratories must be surveyed every two years.

A recognized accrediting agency for managed care plans is the National Commission for Quality Assurance (NCQA), an independent, nonprofit organization that evaluates and reports on the quality of the nation's managed care organizations. NCQA evaluates managed care programs in three ways:

1. Through on-site reviews of key clinical and administrative processes.
2. Through the Health Plan Employer Data and Information Set (HEDIS)—data used to measure performance in areas such as immunization and mammography screening rates.
3. Through use of member satisfaction surveys.

Participation in NCQA accreditation and certification programs is voluntary. The organization reported in 2004 that about half of the nation's HMOs were NCQA-accredited. NCQA began including preferred provider organizations (PPOs) in its accreditation programs in 2000, and in 2004 just "a handful" had undergone NCQA evaluation to become accredited.

RECIPROCITY

reciprocity The process by which a professional license obtained in one state may be accepted as valid in other states by prior agreement without reexamination.

For those professions that require a state license, such as physician, registered nurse, or licensed practical/vocational nurse, **reciprocity** may be granted. This means that a state licensing authority will accept a person's valid license from another state as proof of competency without requiring reexamination.

If a state license is required and reciprocity is not granted when moving to another state, then the health care practitioner must apply to the state licensing authority to take required examinations in order to obtain a valid license to practice in the new state.

MEDICAL PRACTICE ACTS AND MEDICAL BOARDS

medical practice acts State laws written for the express purpose of governing the practice of medicine.

In all 50 states, **medical practice acts** have been established by statute to govern the practice of medicine. Primary mandates of medical practice acts are to

1. Define what is meant by "practice of medicine" in each state.
2. Explain requirements and methods for licensure.
3. Provide for the establishment of medical licensing boards.
4. Establish grounds for suspension or revocation of license.
5. Give conditions for license renewal.

Medical practice acts were first passed in colonial times, but were repealed in the 1800s, when citizens decided that the United States Constitution gave anyone the right to practice medicine. Quackery became rampant, and for the protection of the public, medical practice acts were reenacted.

Although laws are in place to protect consumers against medical quackery, even today unscrupulous people attempt to circumvent the law by hawking devices, potions, and treatments they say are "guaranteed" to cure any ailment or infirmity. Each state periodically revises its medical practice acts to keep them current with the times. Medical practice acts can be found in the code of each state, which consists of laws for that state. A copy of the state code is available in most public libraries, in some university libraries, and, in some cases, on the Internet.

medical boards Bodies established by the authority of each state's medical practice acts for the purpose of protecting the health, safety, and welfare of health care consumers through proper licensing and regulation of physicians and other health care practitioners.

Each state's medical practice acts also mandate the establishment of **medical boards**, whose purpose is to protect the health, safety, and welfare of health care consumers through proper licensing and regulation of physicians and, in some jurisdictions, other health care practitioners. Board membership is composed of physicians and others who are, in most cases, appointed by the state's governor. Some boards act independently, exercising all licensing and disciplinary powers, while others are part of larger agencies such as departments of health. Funding for state medical boards comes from licensing and registration fees. Most boards include an executive officer, attorneys, and investigators. Some legal services may be provided by the state's office of the attorney general.

1. Define *registration*.

_____

_____

2. Define *licensure*.

_____

_____

3. Define *certification*.

_____

_____

4. Define *accreditation*.

_____

_____

5. Define *reciprocity*.

_____

_____

Through licensing, each state medical board ensures that all health care practitioners who work in areas for which licensing is required have adequate and appropriate education and training and that they follow high standards of professional conduct while caring for patients. Applicants for license must generally

▮ Provide proof of education and training.
▮ Provide details about work history.
▮ Pass an examination designed to assess their knowledge and their ability to apply that knowledge and other concepts and principles important to ensure safe and effective patient care.
▮ Reveal information about past medical history (including alcohol and drug abuse), arrests, and convictions.

Each state's medical practice acts also define unprofessional conduct for medical professionals. Laws vary from state to state, but examples of unprofessional conduct include

▮ Physical abuse of a patient.
▮ Inadequate record keeping.
▮ Failure to recognize or act on common symptoms.
▮ The prescription of drugs in excessive amounts or without legitimate reason.
▮ Impaired ability to practice due to addiction or physical or mental illness.
▮ Failure to meet continuing education requirements.
▮ The performance of duties beyond the scope of a license.
▮ Dishonesty.

- Conviction of a felony.
- The delegation of the practice of medicine to an unlicensed individual.

Minor disagreements and poor customer service do not fall under the heading of misconduct.

See Appendix 1 for a list of medical board addresses and telephone numbers in all 50 states. Facsimile (fax) numbers and Web site or e-mail addresses are included where available.

CHECK YOUR PROGRESS

6. Define *medical practice acts*.

_____

_____

7. Where can you find the medical practice acts for your state?

_____

_____

8. What is the primary responsibility of state medical boards?

_____

_____

Court Case

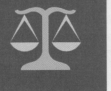

Physician Disciplined by Board of Medical Examiners

A licensed pharmacist and a state pharmacy board investigator called a state's Board of Medical Examiners to express concern about a physician's prescription practices. The board investigated and found the physician had deviated from accepted standard of care by

- Inadequately evaluating patients before prescribing antidepressants and failing to document reasons for prescriptions or following up on patient's use of the prescribed medications.
- Prescribing antibiotics for prolonged periods as treatment for urinary tract infections without determining that the infections had recurred or documenting the recurrence of the infections. The physician had also prescribed several antibiotics to a patient at once, allowing the patient to choose which antibiotic was the most effective.
- Prescribing narcotic and anxiolytic medications (drugs that relieve anxiety) to patients with nonterminal chronic pain without adequately pursuing and documenting use of available alternatives to narcotics and controlled medications.

Based on the above findings, the Board of Medical Examiners placed the physician on probation for two years and ordered him to secure 60 hours of continuing education in the treatment of urinary tract infections, medical treatment of the elderly, management of chronic pain patients, and record keeping. He was also ordered to make prescription records available at all times for board inspection and was directed to stop making telephone refills for prescriptions of controlled medications.

Miller v. Board of Medical Examiners, 609 N.W.2d 478, 2000 Iowa Sup. LEXIS 68.

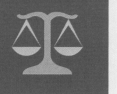
Board Upheld in Permanently Revoking Physician's License

In 1995 an Ohio appellate court ruled that the state medical board had the authority to revoke a physician's license permanently.

The physician was convicted on two felony counts of theft. Afterward, the state medical board held a hearing and revoked the physician's license. The physician appealed, and a court affirmed.

On further appeal, the case was remanded to the board for further consideration. The board again voted to revoke the physician's license and this time specifically noted that the revocation was permanent. The physician again appealed. The trial court reversed, ruling that the board did not have the statutory authority to revoke the physician's license permanently.

The appellate court overturned the trial court's decision. It held that the board's authority to revoke a license to practice medicine included the authority to revoke such a license *permanently*.

Roy v. Medical Board of Ohio, 655 N.E.2d 771 (Ohio Ct. of App., Feb. 23, 1995).

The previous court case established legal precedent for a state medical board's authority to *permanently* revoke a physician's license to practice medicine. It continues to be cited as precedent in cases where a state medical board *permanently* revokes a physician's license and the physician appeals the board's decision.

HEALTH CARE PROFESSIONS

Today a growing number of specialized medical practitioners work with physicians as part of the health care team. Nonphysician members of the health care team, called allied health care practitioners, have certain professional characteristics in common. They

- Share responsibility for delivery of health services.
- Generally have received a certificate, associate's degree, bachelor's degree, master's degree, doctoral degree, or postbaccalaureate training in a science related to health care and have met all state requirements concerning licensure, certification, and registration.

Listed below are a few of the licensed, certified, and registered health care practitioners who work with physicians, dentists, and/or other professionals in providing services to patients in medical offices, dental offices, hospitals, clinics, hospices, extended-care facilities, community programs, schools, and other health care settings. A brief description of each profession is given. When both technicians and technologists are included in the description of a profession, technologists perform duties at a higher level of expertise than technicians. They have either taken a more extensive course of study than technicians or acquired qualifying experience. Since educational and credentialing requirements are subject to change, this information should be obtained from the national organization representing a profession and/or from state credentialing authorities.

The Commission on Accreditation of Allied Health Education Programs (CAAHEP) was established in 1994. CAAHEP accredits more than 2,000 programs in 19 allied health professions throughout the United States and Canada. CAAHEP provides information concerning duties, education requirements, and sources for further information about allied health professions and the location of schools offering the accredited programs. Professions marked with an asterisk below are currently included in the list of CAAHEP-accredited programs.

*Anesthesiologist Assistant.** The anesthesiologist assistant assists the anesthesiologist in developing and implementing an anesthesia care plan. Duties can include preoperative and postoperative tasks, as well as operating room assistance.

Athletic Trainer. The athletic trainer works with attending and/or consulting physicians as an integral part of the health care team associated with physical training and sports.

Audiologist. Audiologists are educated in the science of hearing and are qualified to test patients' hearing and to prescribe some types of therapy for hearing problems. Positions require a minimum of a master's degree, plus national certification and state licensing. In 2007, education requirements were moving toward a minimum of a doctorate in audiology (AuD).

*Cardiovascular Technologist.** The cardiovascular technologist works under the supervision of physicians to perform diagnostic and therapeutic examinations in the cardiology (heart) and vascular (circulation) areas.

*Cytotechnologist.** Cytology is the study of the structure and function of cells. Cytotechnologists work with pathologists to microscopically examine body cells in order to detect changes that may help to diagnose cancer and other diseases.

Dental Hygienist. Dental hygienists perform clinical and educational duties related to hygiene of the mouth and teeth, usually for dentists within a dental office. They may work for one dentist or dental clinic or for several dentists at varying locations.

*Diagnostic Medical Sonographer.** The diagnostic medical sonographer administers ultrasound examinations under the supervision of a physician responsible for the use and interpretation of ultrasound procedures.

Dietician and Nutritionist. These specialists work closely with physicians and other medical practitioners to educate and assist patients with special dietary and nutritional needs.

ECG Technician. Electric activity of the heart is measured and recorded by electrocardiographic equipment operated by ECG (electrocardiogram) technicians under the supervision of physicians.

EEG Technician and Technologist. Electroencephalography is the recording and study of the electrical activity of the brain. EEG (electroencephalogram) technicians and technologists work under the supervision of physicians to operate EEG equipment used to perform patient diagnostic tests.

*Electroneurodiagnostic Technologist.** Electroneurodiagnostic technology involves the study and recording of the electrical activity of the brain and nervous system. Electroneurodiagnostic technologists work in collaboration with EEG technicians and technologists.

*Emergency Medical Technician (Paramedic). Emergency medical technicians (EMTs), or paramedics, most often work from an ambulance or in a hospital emergency room, providing life-support care to critically ill and injured patients.

*Exercise Physiologist. The exercise physiologist is a professional competent in graded exercise testing, exercise prescription, exercise leadership, emergency procedures, and health education for patients with cardiovascular, pulmonary, and metabolic diseases, as well as other diseases and disabilities. These positions require a minimum of a master's degree.

*Exercise Scientist. Exercise scientists work in positions where exercise is used either as a modality in rehabilitation or as a preventive measure in any number of programs intended for the development and or maintenance of physical fitness. In preparation, they have studied the basic human sciences and have had intensive clinical experiences. Positions require a degree in exercise science.

Health and Fitness Specialist. Health and fitness specialists are professionals qualified to assess, design, and implement individual and group exercise and fitness programs for healthy people and people with controlled diseases. The profession requires a minimum of an associate's degree.

Health Information Administrator. Entry-level jobs depend upon education, work experience, and place of employment. (Most health information administrators have worked as health information technicians.) Duties are related to the management of health information and systems used to collect, store, process, retrieve, analyze, disseminate, and communicate health information. A health information administrator position requires a four-year bachelor's degree. The professional certification requires successful completion of a national exam administered by the American Health Information Management Association (AHIMA).

Health Information Technician. Health information technicians must have a two-year associate's degree. Common job titles for health information technicians include coder, medical record technician, abstractor, and supervisor. The professional certification requires successful completion of a national exam administered by the American Health Information Management Association (AHIMA).

*Kinesiotherapist. Kinesiology is the study of muscles and muscle movement. Kinesiotherapists work under a physician's supervision, using therapeutic exercise and education to treat the effects of disease, injury, and congenital disorders on body movement.

Licensed Practical Nurse (LPN)/Licensed Vocational Nurse (LVN). LPNs, called LVNs in California and Texas, perform many of the same duties as registered nurses, with some exceptions, depending upon state law. LPNs and LVNs work under the supervision of physicians and registered nurses.

*Medical Assistant. Medical assistants perform administrative and clinical duties for physician/employers, usually within an **ambulatory care setting,** such as a medical office, clinic, or outpatient surgical center. The certified medical assistant (CMA) credential is earned through the certifying board of the American Association of Medical Assistants. The registered medical assistant (RMA) credential is obtained through

ambulatory care setting
Facility, such as a medical office, clinic, or outpatient surgical center, that provides medical care for patients who can walk and are not bedridden.

the American Medical Technologists (AMT) organization. Both credentials involve specific educational requirements and require applicants to pass an examination assessing knowledge and skills. The CMA credential also requires continuing education in order to maintain the certification.

*Medical Illustrator. Medical illustrators create illustrations for science and medical texts and other publications, and they also function in administrative, consultative, and advisory capacities. They must be knowledgeable in the biological sciences, anatomy, physiology, pathology, general medical knowledge, and the visual arts.

Medical Laboratory Technician and Medical Technologist. Duties of medical technicians include performing simple tests in hematology, serology, blood banking, urinalysis, microbiology, and clinical chemistry. Medical technologists have completed a longer training course than laboratory technicians. They supervise technicians and assistants and perform more complicated analytical laboratory tests. Several organizations provide certification, which is often a condition of employment. In addition, many states require licensing of medical technicians and technologists.

A new title has recently been adopted for professionals who traditionally have been called "medical technicians" or "medical technologists." This new title is "clinical laboratory scientist." (See the U.S. Department of Labor's Bureau of Labor Statistics Web site at this address: www.bls.gov/oco/ocos096.htm.)

Medical Massage Therapist. Massage therapists learn techniques to relieve pain from injuries, illnesses, or chronic conditions; to increase range of motion in joints; and to otherwise help patients with recovery and rehabilitation through body massage. National Certification in Therapeutic Massage and Bodywork requires at least 500 hours of formal training at an established school of massage therapy and passing the national examination offered by the National Certification Board for Therapeutic Massage and Bodywork. Medical massage therapists are supervised by physicians and employed by medical offices, hospitals, clinics, rehabilitation facilities, and other health care businesses. Licensed massage therapists may also establish their own businesses.

Medical Transcriptionist. Medical transcriptionists key material dictated by physicians to be placed with patients' medical records. They must have preparation in English grammar, anatomy and physiology, and pharmacology. They work in medical records departments in hospitals, managed care plan facilities, nursing homes, and ambulatory care facilities such as clinics, medical offices, and outpatient surgical centers. Transcriptionists with advanced skills may be self-employed.

Nurse Practitioner. Those individuals who have earned a registered nurse (RN) license may complete masters or doctoral degree university programs to become nurse practitioners. Nurse practitioners are skilled in physical diagnosis, psychosocial assessment, and primary health care management. They may work independently, in collaboration with a physician, or under the supervision of a physician.

Nursing Assistant. Nursing assistants provide basic patient care under the supervision of registered nurses. Routine duties include changing bed linens; taking temperature, respiratory, and blood pressure readings for patients; bathing patients and helping with personal care; helping patients with eating, walking, and exercise programs; and supporting patients when they are allowed to get out of bed. Employment opportunities exist in hospitals, long-term care facilities, and other health care institutions.

Occupational Therapist. An occupational therapist enters the field with a bachelor's, master's, or doctoral degree. Occupational therapists (OTs) work with clients who are mentally, physically, developmentally, and/or emotionally disabled to help these individuals become more independent and productive. Occupational therapists must have a license to practice in the state where they work.

Occupational Therapy Assistant. An occupational therapy assistant enters the field with a two-year associate's degree. Occupational therapy assistants work under the supervision of licensed occupational therapists.

Ophthalmic Medical Technician/Technologist. Ophthalmic medical technicians and technologists assist ophthalmologists (medical doctors who specialize in diseases and conditions of the eye) by performing such tasks as collecting data, administering diagnostic tests, and administering some treatments ordered by the supervising ophthalmologist. They may also maintain surgical instruments and office equipment. Graduates of accredited programs are eligible to take the national certifying examination at the approved levels offered by the Joint Commission on Allied Health Personnel in Ophthalmology.

Optician. Opticians are licensed specifically to sell and/or construct optical materials.

Optometrist. Optometrists are trained and licensed to examine the eyes in order to determine the presence of vision problems and to prescribe and adapt lenses to preserve or restore maximum efficiency of vision.

*Orthotist and Prosthetist. Orthotists and prosthetists work directly with physicians and others to rehabilitate people with disabilities. The orthotist designs and fits devices (orthoses) for patients with disabling conditions of the limbs and spine. The prosthetist designs and fits devices (prostheses) for patients who have partial or total absence of a limb.

*Perfusionist. A perfusionist operates transfusion equipment when necessary and consults with physicians in selecting the appropriate equipment, techniques, and transfusion media to be used, depending upon the patient's condition.

*Personal Fitness Trainer. Personal fitness trainers work with individual clients or with small groups. They help clients initiate and maintain fitness programs that maximize physical potential and health. They may become certified through the American Fitness Program Associates or through the National Federation of Professional Trainers.

Phlebotomist. Phlebotomists (Figure 2-1) are trained to draw blood from patients or donors

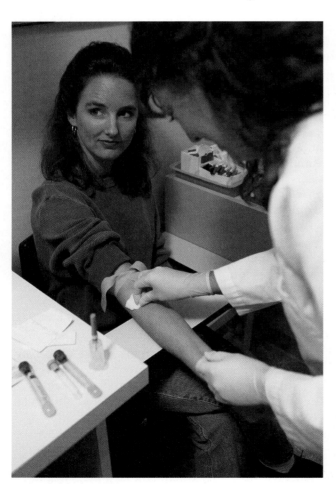

FIGURE 2-1 A phlebotomist drawing blood from a patient.

for diagnostic testing or other medical purposes. They may also perform related tasks, such as preparing stains and reagents and cleaning and sterilizing equipment; taking patients' blood pressure, pulse, and respiration rates; performing ECGs; and billing, performing data entry, and answering telephones.

Physical Therapist. Physical therapists help patients restore function to muscles, nerves, joints, and bones after impairment due to illness or injury. All physical therapy programs are now at the master's or doctoral level.

Physical Therapist Assistant. Physical therapist assistants work under the supervision of licensed physical therapists in implementing treatment programs according to the patient's plan of care. Physical therapist assistants must complete a two-year program, usually offered in a community or junior college.

Physician Assistant. Physicians employ physician assistants (PAs) to perform many of the routine diagnostic and treatment procedures related to patient care. They can legally perform more procedures than registered nurses and can prescribe some medications, but they are not licensed to perform all the duties of a physician. The typical applicant for a physician assistant program already has a bachelor's degree and four years of health care practitioner experience. The average physician assistant program runs about 26 months. Graduates must then pass a national certifying examination. Once certified, PAs must complete 100 hours of continuing education every two years, and they must take the PA recertification examination every six years.

*Polysomnographic Technologist. Polysomnographic technologists work under the supervision of physicians. They perform sleep diagnostics and provide clinical evaluations required for the diagnosis of sleep disorders. Polysomnographic technologists use such equipment as EEG, ECG, electro-occulography (EOG) and electromyography (EMG) monitors.

Radiologic or Medical Imaging Technologist. Radiologic technologists (Figure 2-2) are qualified to position patients for X-rays, operate X-ray equipment, prepare X-ray films for viewing, and maintain records and images for each patient. In addition to X-ray imaging, these technologists may be trained in additional types of imaging, such as ultrasound and magnetic resonance scans. They can prepare and orally administer mixtures for contrast imaging, and in some states they are trained in venipuncture and can inject contrast mediums for imaging. They cannot interpret images. Most states require licensing of radiology technologists.

Registered Nurse. Registered nurses perform a variety of patient care duties, such as administering drugs prescribed by the supervising physician, monitoring the cardiovascular and pulmonary status of the critically ill, caring for newborns and their mothers, and assisting surgeons in the operating room. They also supervise LPNs; LVNs; nursing assistants; and other medical office, clinic, or hospital personnel. In addition, they document patient care for physicians and other health care team members. Nursing education curricula leading to the RN include two-year associate's degree and four-year baccalaureate degree programs.

*Respiratory Therapist (entry level). Entry-level respiratory therapists are employed by hospitals, nursing care facilities, clinics, physicians' offices, pulmonary function laboratories, sleep labs, and home care

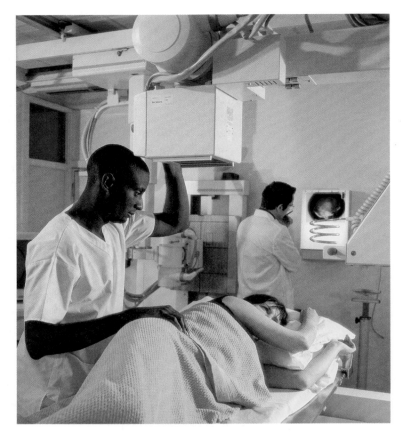

FIGURE 2-2 A radiology technologist prepares a patient for an X-ray.

companies. They perform general respiratory care procedures under the supervision of an advanced-level respiratory therapist and/or a physician.

***Respiratory Therapist** (advanced). Advanced-level respiratory therapists assume primary responsibility for all respiratory patient care procedures to help with breathing disorders. They also supervise entry-level respiratory therapists.

***Specialist in Blood Bank Technology.** These specialists must have a bachelor's degree and certification in medical technology and must have completed the required course of study in blood bank technology. They perform both routine and specialized tests in blood bank immunohematology and perform transfusion services.

***Surgical Assistant.** As defined by the American College of Surgeons, the surgical assistant helps the surgeon carry out a safe operation with optimal results for the patient. In addition to intraoperative duties, the surgical assistant performs preoperative and postoperative duties to better facilitate proper patient care. The surgical assistant works under the direct supervision of the operating surgeon in accordance with hospital policy and appropriate laws and regulations.

***Surgical Technologist.** Surgical technologists work closely with surgeons, anesthesiologists, nurses, and other surgical personnel before, during, and after surgery. They may function as scrub, circulating, or first or second assisting surgical technologist. Duties vary according to assignment.

While a variety of health care practitioners often work together as a team to provide medical care to patients, each individual is legally able to perform only those duties dictated by professional and statutory guidelines. Each health care practitioner is responsible for understanding the laws and rules pertaining to his or her job and for knowing requirements concerning renewal of licenses; recertification; and payment of fees for licensure, certification, and registration.

THE PHYSICIAN'S EDUCATION

Medical Doctor (MD) Degree

Before a person can be licensed to practice medicine, he or she must complete a rigorous course of study. Programs leading to the medical doctor (MD) degree consist of

- Graduation with a bachelor's degree from a four-year, premedicine course, usually with a concentration in the sciences.
- Graduation from a four-year medical school—in the United States, a school accredited by the Liaison Committee on Medical Education. Upon graduation from medical school, students are awarded the doctor of medicine (MD) degree.

After earning the MD degree, the prospective physician must then pass the United States Medical Licensing Examination (USMLE), commonly called "medical boards." Student physicians take Part 1 of the exam after the first year of medical school. They take Part 2 of the exam during the fourth year of medical school, and Part 3 during the first or second year of postgraduate medical training.

The next step in a physician's education is completion of a residency: a period of practical postgraduate training in a hospital. The first year of residency is called an internship.

After completion of the internship and passing the medical boards, the National Board of Medical Examiners (NBME) certifies the physician as an NBME Diplomate.

To specialize, physicians must complete an additional two to six years of residency in the chosen specialty. When the residency is completed, specialists can then apply to the American Board of Medical Specialties (ABMS) to take an exam in their specialty. After passing this exam, physicians are board-certified in their area of specialization. For example, a specialist in oncology becomes a board-certified oncologist, and so on.

Doctor of Osteopathy (DO) Degree

All 50 states also license physicians who have obtained a Doctor of Osteopathy (DO) Degree from an accredited medical school, have successfully completed a licensing examination governed by the National Board of Osteopathic Medical Examiners, and have successfully completed the required internship and residency.

MDs and DOs spend 12 years or more training to become physicians.

Both medical and osteopathic physicians prescribe drugs and practice surgery. The difference between the two is in their approach to medical

allopathic Means "different suffering" and refers to the medical philosophy that dictates training physicians to intervene in the disease process, through the use of drugs and surgery.

treatment. Osteopathic doctors are trained to emphasize the musculoskeletal system of the body and the correction of joint and tissue problems. Medical doctors are trained in **allopathic** medicine, which means, literally, "different suffering" and emphasizes intervention in the form of drugs and/or surgery to alleviate symptoms.

Osteopathic and medical doctors can practice as generalists or primary care physicians—a designation which includes primary care specialties in family medicine/general practice, general internal medicine, and general pediatrics—or they can specialize in a specific type of medicine, such as obstetrics/gynecology, oncology, geriatrics, surgery, orthopedics, or a host of other specialties. Medical and osteopathic physicians may also further specialize in subspecialties, such as abnormalities of the hand within orthopedics, or diseases of the gastrointestinal system within internal medicine.

Recent U.S. government statistics show that in the United States, medical students are three times more likely to specialize than to remain generalists or primary care physicians. This has led to a ratio in the United States of 37.4 percent primary care physicians to 62.6 percent specialists. According to the American Medical Student Association (AMSA), reasons for the preference among medical students to specialize include these:

tertiary care settings Those care settings providing highly specialized services.

- Higher financial compensation for specialists (studies have found that a surgeon can earn up to seven times more than a primary care physician, per time spent with the patient).
- Decreased prestige for generalists.
- Medical training is most often provided in **tertiary care settings**—those providing highly specialized services.
- Decreased exposure to generalist role models.
- Lack of attractiveness of general practices in, for example, rural and underserved areas, because of relative isolation from technology and peer support.

A person educated in a foreign medical school who wants to practice in the United States must serve a residency and must take the Clinical Skills Assessment Exam (CSAE) before being licensed. The CSAE evaluates a candidate's ability to use the English language, to take medical histories, and to interact with patients and treat a case.

THE PHYSICIAN'S LICENSE AND RESPONSIBILITIES

After physicians have finished their education and obtained licenses to practice medicine, their continued licensure falls under the jurisdiction of state medical boards. Each state's medical board has the authority to grant or to revoke a physician's license. The federal government has no medical licensing authority except for the permit issued by the Drug Enforcement Administration (DEA) for any physician who dispenses, prescribes, or administers controlled substances, including narcotics and non-narcotics. (See Chapter 8, "Physicians' Public Duties and Responsibilities.")

The following criteria must be met before a physician can be granted a state license to practice medicine. He or she

- Must have reached the age of majority, generally 21.
- Must be of good moral character.

- Must have completed required preliminary education, including graduation from an approved medical school.
- Must have completed an approved residency program.
- Must be a U.S. citizen or have filed a declaration of intent to become a citizen. (Some states have dropped this requirement.)
- Must be a state resident.
- Must have passed all examinations administered by the state board of medical examiners or the board of registration.

When these conditions are satisfied and a license is granted, the physician who moves out of the licensing state may obtain a license in his or her new state of residence by

- Reciprocity—the process by which a valid license from out of state is accepted as the basis for issuing a license in a second state if prior agreement to grant reciprocity has been reached between those states.
- **Endorsement**—the process by which a license may be awarded based on individual credentials judged to meet licensing requirements in the new state of residence.

In some situations, physicians do not need a valid license to practice medicine in a specific state. These situations include the following:

- When responding to emergencies.
- While establishing state residency requirements in order to obtain a license.
- When employed by the U.S. Armed Forces, Public Health Service, Veterans Administration, or other federal facility.
- When engaged solely in research and not treating patients.

Physicians may be licensed in more than one state. Periodic license renewal is necessary; this usually requires simply paying a fee. However, many states require proof of continuing education units for license renewal; the average is 50 hours annually.

License Revocation or Suspension

A physician's license can be revoked (canceled) or suspended (temporarily recalled) for conviction of a felony, unprofessional conduct, or personal or professional incapacity.

A felony is a crime that is punishable by death or a year or more in prison. Conviction of a felony is grounds for revocation or suspension of the license to practice medicine. Felonies include such crimes as murder, rape, larceny, manslaughter, robbery, arson, burglary, violations of narcotic laws, and tax evasion.

Unprofessional conduct is also cause for revoking or suspending a physician's license. Some states substitute the term *gross immorality* for *unprofessional conduct,* but offenses in either category are considered serious breaches of ethics and may also be illegal. Conduct deemed unprofessional includes falsifying records, using unprofessional methods to treat a disease, betrayal of patient confidentiality, fee splitting, and sexual misconduct.

Personal or professional incapacity may be due to senility, injury, illness, chronic alcoholism, drug abuse, or other conditions that impair a physician's ability to practice.

Fraud may, in some states, be considered unprofessional conduct, or it may be separately specified as grounds for revoking a physician's license.

endorsement The process by which a license may be awarded based on individual credentials judged to meet licensing requirements in a new state.

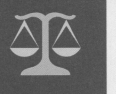
State Board of Nursing Finds Nurse Incompetent

A state board of nursing found that a nurse violated the section of the state code that regulates nursing by repeatedly failing to conform to the minimum standards of practice with regard to the proper maintenance and documentation of controlled substances. Since the finding could have led to revocation of the nurse's license, the nurse filed a petition for judicial review. The district court affirmed the board's decision, and the nurse again appealed. The state court of appeals upheld both the district court and board decisions, clearing the way for temporary or permanent revocation of the nurse's license, or other penalty. (No final decision is available, since the opinion has not yet been published.)

Several times while on duty, the nurse failed to properly document and account for missing controlled substances. In one instance she claimed containers of morphine and other drugs had fallen from her pocket while she was running down a stairwell. On other occasions, she claimed drug ampules had broken in her pocket, or she had misplaced syringes filled with controlled substances. Since her stories could not be corroborated, and she did not properly document losses or destruction of controlled drugs, the state court of appeals upheld the state board of nursing's finding that the nurse was incompetent in violating minimum standards of acceptable nursing practice.

Matthias v. Iowa Board of Nursing, 2-153 / 01-1019, 2002 Iowa App. LEXIS 715.

A physician is considered guilty of fraud if "intent to deceive" can be shown. Acts generally classified as fraud include

- Falsifying medical diplomas, applications for licenses, licenses, or other credentials.
- Billing a governmental agency for services not rendered.
- Falsifying medical reports.
- Falsely advertising or misrepresenting to a patient "secret cures" or special powers to cure an ailment.

Revocations and suspensions of license are never automatic. A physician is always entitled to a written description of charges against him or her and a hearing before the appropriate state agency. If a hearing is held, the physician also has the right to counsel, the right to present evidence in his or her defense, the right to confront and question witnesses, and any other rights granted by state law. Decisions are usually subject to appeal through the state's court system.

An honest mistake or a single incident of alleged incompetence or negligence is not usually sufficient grounds for license revocation.

Respondeat Superior

respondeat superior Literally, "let the master answer." A doctrine under which an employer is legally liable for the acts of his or her employees, if such acts were performed within the scope of the employees' duties.

Under the doctrine of **respondeat superior**, which is Latin for "let the master answer," physicians are legally responsible (liable) for their own acts of negligence and for negligent acts of employees working within the scope of their employment.

The test used to determine whether an employee was or was not acting within the scope of employment when a negligent act was committed is whether or not the employee's behavior serves the interest of the employer or in some way furthers the employer's business.

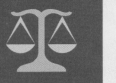
M.D.'s License Revocation Upheld

A New York State Appellate Court upheld a decision by the Hearing Committee of the New York State Board for Professional Medical Conduct revoking a physician's license.

The appellate court agreed that the physician had been grossly incompetent in failing to monitor the various anticoagulant medicines that a hospitalized patient was prescribed, so the patient hemorrhaged to death. In addition, the physician had altered the patient's records in an effort to blame others. Substantial evidence also supported a finding that the physician had lied by failing to disclose a criminal conviction on two applications for hospital privileges. Therefore, the revocation of the physician's license to practice medicine was upheld.

Catsoulis v. New York State Department of Health et al., 2 A.D. 3d 920; 767 N.Y.S.2d 526, 2003 N.Y. App. Div. LEXIS 12787.

For example, after a patient's initial visit for treatment of a hand injury, a physician allows the medical assistant to change the dressings and check the wound over a period of several weeks. The medical assistant fails to recognize early signs of infection, and complications develop that eventually cost the patient the full use of his hand. The patient sues the physician and wins, since the physician/employer is legally responsible for the negligence

CHECK YOUR PROGRESS

9. In the United States, physicians may be licensed to practice medicine as MDs or as DOs. Distinguish between the two.

_____

_____

10. Name three types of unprofessional conduct for which a physician may lose his or her license.

_____

_____

_____

Fill in the blanks to accurately complete the following statements:

11. A physician is licensed by the _____ in which he or she wishes to practice.

12. The federal government's authority regarding medical licensing extends only to _____

_____

13. Revocations and suspensions of medical licenses are never _____

14. Name four situations in which physicians do not need a valid license to practice in a specific state.

_____

_____

_____

_____

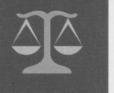
Medical Group Liable Under *Respondeat Superior*

A physician who practiced with a medical group was the on-call obstetrician for the emergency department when a pregnant woman was brought in after a car accident. The woman's baby was stillborn, and she and her husband sued the on-call physician's medical group under the doctrine of *respondeat superior*. A Superior Court found for the defendant medical group, but an appeals court vacated the finding for the defendant, stating that "vicarious liability does not require the employer to have the right or ability to control the specific treatment decisions of a physician-employee. Instead, the plaintiff only has to establish that at the time of the negligence, the physician was an employee of the entity, and that the negligent treatment of the plaintiff occurred within the scope of the physician's employment of the entity."

(Note: This decision would indicate that the case could go back to a lower court for trial, in which case the defendant medical group may have settled out of court. Final results were not published.)

Dias v. Brigham Medical Associates, Inc., 438 Mass. 317 (2002).

of the employee while the employee is acting within the interest of the employer's business.

The physician is vicariously responsible for negligence in the above example, but the medical assistant remains responsible for negligent actions as well. While licensed physicians employ medical assistants, dental assistants, nurses, and other health care practitioners, these individuals are liable for their own acts of negligence and can be sued for malpractice as well.

The law on which the concept of *respondeat superior* is based is the law of agency, which is discussed in further detail in Chapter 3.

MEDICAL PRACTICE MANAGEMENT SYSTEMS

There are four basic types of medical practice:

- Sole proprietorship
- Partnership
- Professional corporation
- Group practice

Laws governing the various types of practices vary, but medical office personnel should be aware of those laws that apply to their employer's practice management system.

Sole Proprietorship

In medicine's bygone days, physicians most often practiced alone, providing all patient services, from receptionist, to medical treatment, to billing, to house calls. They were engaged in a "solo practice," and they took all

sole proprietorship A form of medical practice management in which a physician practices alone, assuming all benefits and liabilities for the business.

associate practice A medical management system in which two or more physicians share office space and employees but practice individually.

partnership A form of medical practice management system whereby two or more parties practice together under a written agreement specifying the rights, obligations, and responsibilities of each partner.

corporation A body formed and authorized by law to act as a single person.

group practice A medical management system in which three or more licensed physicians share the collective income, expenses, facilities, equipment, records, and personnel for the business.

the profits and bore all the risks associated with the **sole proprietorship.** Today, some physicians still practice alone (with the help of employees to perform receptionist, billing, and some patient care tasks), but they are in the minority. A disadvantage to this type of practice is that the physician practicing alone has unlimited personal liability.

Two or more physicians may decide to practice individually but agree to share office space and employees. This arrangement is called an **associate practice** and allows a sharing of expenses, not a sharing of profits and liability.

Partnership

When two or more physicians decide to practice together, they may form a **partnership,** based on a legal written agreement specifying the rights, obligations, and responsibilities of each partner.

Advantages of partnerships include sharing the workload and expenses, and pooling profits and assets. A major disadvantage is that each partner has equal liability for the acts, conduct, losses, and deficits of the partnership, unless specific provisions are made for these contingencies in the initial agreement.

Professional Corporation

A **corporation** is a body formed and authorized by law to act as a single person, although constituted by one or more persons and legally endowed with various rights and duties. State law governs corporations, so requirements for incorporation may vary. The corporation may own, mortgage, or sell property; manage its own business affairs; and sue or be sued.

Physicians who form corporations are shareholders and employees of the organization. There are financial and tax advantages to forming a corporation, and fringe benefits to employees may be more generous than with a sole proprietorship or partnership. Forming a corporation also means that the incorporators and owners have limited liability in case lawsuits are filed.

Group Practice

The **group practice** may function as a corporation or as a partnership. A medical group practice is the provision of health care services by a group of three or more licensed physicians, engaged full time in a formally organized and legally recognized entity. They share the group's income and expenses in a systematic manner and also share facilities, equipment, records, and personnel involved in both patient care and business management.

Physicians in group practice may be engaged in the same specialty, calling themselves, for example, Urology Associates. They may provide care in two or three related specialties, for example, obstetrics-gynecology and pediatrics. Alternatively, they may offer a variety of services, for example, obstetrics-gynecology, pediatrics, family practice, and internal medicine.

For physicians, the advantages of group practice are much the same as those of a corporation, with the added benefit that the legal implications are not so far-reaching or complicated.

managed care A system in which financing, administration, and delivery of health care are combined to provide medical services to subscribers for a prepaid fee.

indemnity A traditional form of health insurance that covers the insured against a potential loss of money from medical expenses resulting from an illness or accident.

Managed care health plans are corporations that pay for and deliver health care to subscribers for a set fee using a network of physicians and other health care providers. The network coordinates and refers patients to its health care providers and hospitals and monitors the amount and patterns of care delivered. The plans usually limit the services subscribers may receive under the plans. Managed care plans make agreed-upon payments to providers (hospitals or physicians) for providing health care services to health care subscribers. The payment from a managed care plan to providers may be one of several types, including contracted fee schedules, percentages of billed charges, capitation, and others. (*Capitation* is a set advance payment made to providers, based on the calculated cost of medical care of a specific population of subscribers.)

Before managed care plans, private health insurance policies were traditionally written as third-party indemnity health insurance. *Third party* means that the insurance company reimburses health care practitioners for medical care provided to policyholders. **Indemnity** is coverage of the insured person against a potential loss of money from medical expenses for an illness or accident. Indemnity insurance benefits are paid in a predetermined amount of money rather than in specific services.

In an attempt to confront increasing health care costs, due in part to increasingly large awards in litigation, an aging population which requires more health care, the expensive technology used in modern day medicine, and the impact of third-party payors for medical care, traditional fee-for-service health insurance companies now incorporate elements of managed care into their plans. (The impact of third-party payors is that there is little incentive to keep health care costs down when health care providers and recipients know that a third party—Medicare, Medicaid, other insurance—will pay.) Consequently, virtually all insured Americans have become familiar with such cost containment/managed care measures as coinsurance, copayment fees, deductibles, formularies, and utilization review.

- *Coinsurance* refers to the amount of money insurance plan members must pay out of pocket, after the insurance plan pays its share. For example, a plan may agree to pay 80 percent of the cost for a surgical procedure, and the subscriber must pay the remaining 20 percent.

- *Copayment* fees are flat fees that insurance plan subscribers pay for certain medical services. For example, a subscriber might be required to make a $20 copayment for each visit to a physician's office.

- *Deductible* amounts are specified by the insurance plan for each subscriber. For instance, the deductible for a single subscriber might be $250 a calendar year. In other words, the plan does not begin to pay benefits until the $250 deductible has been satisfied.

- *Formularies* are a plan's list of approved prescription medications for which it will reimburse subscribers.

- *Utilization review* is the method used by a health plan to measure the amount and appropriateness of health services used by its members.

Health Maintenance Organizations

health maintenance organization (HMO) A health plan that combines coverage of health care costs and delivery of health care for a prepaid premium.

Health maintenance organizations (HMO) are one of several types of managed care organizations providing health care services to subscribers within the United States. HMOs and preferred provider organizations (PPO) are the most common types of managed care plans. Under HMO plans, all

individual (or independent) practice association (IPA) A type of HMO that contracts with groups of physicians who practice in their own offices and receive a per-member payment (capitation) from participating HMOs to provide a full range of health services for members.

preferred provider organization (PPO) A network of independent physicians, hospitals, and other health care providers who contract with an insurance carrier to provide medical care at a discount rate to patients who are part of the insurer's plan. Also called **preferred provider association (PPA)**.

physician-hospital organization (PHO) A health care plan in which physicians join with hospitals to provide a medical care delivery system and then contract for insurance with a commercial carrier or an HMO.

primary care physician (PCP) The physician responsible for directing all of a patient's medical care and determining whether the patient should be referred for specialty care.

gatekeeper physician The primary care physician who directs the medical care of managed care health plan members.

point-of-service (POS) plan A health care plan that allows members to seek health care from non-network physicians but pays the highest benefits for care when it is given by the primary care physician (PCP) or via a referral from the PCP.

health services are delivered and paid for through one organization. The three general types of HMOs are group model HMOs, staff model HMOs, and individual (or independent) practice associations (IPAs).

Group model HMOs contract with independent groups of physicians to provide coordinated care for large numbers of HMO patients for a fixed, per-member fee. They often provide medical care for members of several HMOs. Group model HMOs include prepaid group practices (PGPs). Physicians in PGPs are salaried employees of the HMO, usually practice in facilities provided by the HMO, and share in profits at the end of the year.

Staff model HMOs employ salaried physicians and other allied health professionals who provide care solely for members of one HMO. Subscribers to staff model HMOs can often see their doctors, get laboratory tests and X-rays, have prescriptions filled, and even order eyeglasses or contact lenses all in one location. Staff model HMOs also employ specialists or contract with outside specialists in some cases.

An **individual (or independent) practice association (IPA)** is an association of physicians, hospitals, and other health care providers that contracts with an HMO to provide medical services to subscribers. Health care practitioners who are members of an IPA may usually still see patients outside of the contracting HMO. The providers who contract with an IPA practice in their own offices and receive a per-member payment, or capitation, from participating HMOs to provide a full range of health services for HMO members. These providers often care for members of several HMOs, which gives them a larger patient and income base than staff model HMOs.

Preferred Provider Organizations

Preferred provider organizations (PPO), also called **preferred provider associations (PPA)**, are managed care plans that contract with a network of doctors, hospitals, and other health care providers who provide services for set fees. Subscribers may choose their primary health provider from an approved list and must pay higher out-of-pocket costs for care provided by health care practitioners outside the PPO group.

Physician-Hospital Organizations

Physician-hospital organizations (PHOs) are another type of managed care plan. PHOs are organizations that include physicians, hospitals, surgery centers, nursing homes, laboratories, and other medical service providers that contract with one or more HMOs, insurance plans, or directly with employers to provide health care services.

Other Variations in Managed Care Plans

Managed care plans may also include the following identifying features:

▮ **Gatekeeper or primary care plan.** The insured must designate a **primary care physician (PCP).** Also known as a **gatekeeper physician,** the primary care physician directs all of a patient's medical care and generates any referrals to specialists or other health care practitioners.

▮ **Point-of-service (POS). Point-of-service plans** allow plan members to seek health care from non-network physicians, but the plan pays the highest benefits for care when given by the PCP or via a referral from the PCP. When care is provided without a referral, but still within the network, the plan pays benefits at a reduced level. Members also have out-of-network benefits, but at greatly reduced payment levels.

open access A managed care feature whereby subscribers may see any in-network health care provider without a referral.

■ **Open access.** Under **open access** plans, subscribers may see any in-network health care provider without a referral.

Managed care plans differ from one another in some respects, but all are designed to cut the cost of health care delivery. The impact of cost-cutting measures on the quality of health care remains a major point of contention. Advocates claim that managed care plans can deliver medical services more efficiently and at much less expense than traditional fee-for-service plans. Critics argue that necessary, quality medical services are often sacrificed for profit margins.

The following questions are of special concern to patients enrolled in managed care plans:

■ Will the most knowledgeable and experienced physician treat my medical conditions and those of my family?

■ Is my physician too concerned with saving money?

■ Must I fight to get routine procedures from my HMO?

■ What if my HMO refuses to pay for a procedure I need?

In addition, physicians and other medical professionals, administrators of managed care plans, government officials, and HMO members are concerned with such issues as these:

■ Do managed health care and competition actually drive costs down?

■ Do regulations exist regarding patient rights in managed care plans?

■ Do quality ratings for HMOs help consumers?

■ Does managed health care provide higher-quality care than fee-for-service medicine?

Managed care is a fixture of modern medicine, but health care consumers and practitioners continue to debate its advantages and disadvantages, and may do so for many years to come.

LEGISLATION AFFECTING HEALTH CARE PLANS

Congress has passed legislation intended to improve the quality of health care in the United States, to reduce fraud, and to help assure managed care and other types of health insurance subscribers that they will not be summarily dropped or otherwise be unfairly or unlawfully discriminated against by insurance providers. Two of the most significant health care laws passed in recent years are the Health Care Quality Improvement Act of 1986 (HCQIA) and the Health Insurance Portability and Accountability Act (HIPAA) of 1996.

Health Care Quality Improvement Act of 1986

Health Care Quality Improvement Act of 1986 (HCQIA) A federal statute passed to improve the quality of medical care nationwide. One provision established the National Practitioner Data Bank.

In creating the **Health Care Quality Improvement Act of 1986 (HCQIA),** Congress found that "the increasing occurrence of medical malpractice and the need to improve the quality of medical care have become nationwide problems that warrant greater efforts than those that can be undertaken by any individual state." Accordingly, the act requires that professional peer review action be taken in some cases. It also limits the damages for professional review and protects from liability those who provide information to professional review bodies.

National Practitioner Data Bank (NPDB) A repository of information about health care practitioners, established by the Health Care Quality Improvement Act of 1986.

One of the most important provisions of the HCQIA was the establishment of the **National Practitioner Data Bank (NPDB).** Use of the NPDB was intended to improve the quality of medical care nationwide by encouraging effective professional peer review of physicians and dentists. Information that must be reported to the NPDB includes medical malpractice payments, adverse licensure actions, adverse clinical privilege actions, and adverse professional society membership actions. The NPDB is a resource to assist state licensing boards, hospitals, and other health care entities in investigating the qualifications of physicians, dentists, and other health care practitioners.

National Practitioner Data Bank queries are mandatory for physicians when they apply for privileges at a hospital, and every two years for physicians already on the medical staff who wish to maintain their privileges. They are voluntary for hospitals conducting professional review, other health care entities with formal peer review programs, state licensing boards at any time, those who wish to self-query, and plaintiffs' attorneys under certain circumstances. The NPDB may not disclose information to a medical malpractice insurer, defense attorney, or member of the general public.

CHECK YOUR PROGRESS

15. Define *managed care.*

_____

_____

16. Name and list distinguishing characteristics of three types of managed care plans.

_____

_____

Health Insurance Portability and Accountability Act of 1996 (HIPAA) A federal statute that helps workers keep continuous health insurance coverage for themselves and their dependents when they change jobs, protects confidential medical information from unauthorized disclosure or use, and helps curb the rising cost of fraud and abuse.

Health Insurance Portability and Accountability Act

The **Health Insurance Portability and Accountability Act of 1996 (HIPAA)** was an ambitious attempt by Congress to reform the American health care system. The HIPAA helps workers keep continuous health insurance coverage for themselves and their dependents when they change jobs, but its many provisions go far beyond this mandate. The primary objectives of the law were to

1. Improve the efficiency and effectiveness of the health care industry by
   - accelerating billing processes and reducing paperwork.
   - reducing health care billing fraud.
   - facilitating tracking of health information.
   - improving accuracy and reliability of shared data.
   - increasing access to computer networks within health care facilities.

2. Help employees keep their health insurance coverage when transferring to another job.

3. Protect confidential medical information that identifies patients from unauthorized disclosure or use.

Healthcare Integrity and Protection Data Bank (HIPDB) A national health care fraud and abuse data collection program established by HIPAA for the reporting and disclosure of certain adverse actions taken against health care providers, suppliers, or practitioners.

Federal False Claims Act A law that allows for individuals to bring civil actions on behalf of the United States government for false claims made to the federal government, under a provision of the law called *qui tam* (from Latin meaning "to bring an action for the king and for oneself").

The privacy provisions of HIPAA have had such a sweeping effect on the health care industry that the act is discussed in its entirety in Chapter 7, "Privacy Law and HIPAA."

HIPAA also led to the creation of the **Healthcare Integrity and Protection Data Bank (HIPDB).** The HIPDB is a national health care fraud and abuse data collection program for the reporting and disclosure of certain adverse actions taken against health care providers, suppliers, or practitioners. Data from the HIPDB is available to federal and state government agencies and to health plans, but is not available to the general public.

Controlling Health Care Fraud and Abuse

Partly because of the rising costs of health care, fraud and abuse within the industry have become major issues. As a result, laws have been passed to control three types of illegal conduct:

1. False claims in billing.
2. Kickbacks.
3. Self-referrals.

Several federal and state statutes prohibit false claims. The HIPAA and the federal False Claims Act are two laws that prohibit false claims and detail the penalties that can be levied against violators.

The **Federal False Claims Act** allows for individuals to bring civil actions on behalf of the United States government for false claims made to the federal government, under a provision of the law called *qui tam* (from Latin meaning "to bring an action for the king and for oneself"). These individuals, commonly known as whistleblowers, are referred to as *qui tam relators* and can share in any court-awarded damages.

Suits brought under the False Claims Act are most often related to the health care and defense industries. The act prohibits

▌ Making a false record or statement to get a false or fraudulent claim paid by the government.

▌ Conspiring to have a false or fraudulent claim paid by the government.

▌ Withholding property of the government with the intent to defraud the government or to willfully conceal it from the government.

▌ Making or delivering a receipt for government property that is false or fraudulent.

▌ Buying government property from someone who is not authorized to sell the property.

▌ Making a false statement to avoid or deceive an obligation to pay money or property to the government.

▌ Causing someone else to submit a false claim by submitting false information.

Providing kickbacks, or giving financial incentives to a health care provider for referring patients or for recommending services or products, are prohibited under the federal Anti-Kickback Law and by state laws.

Self-referrals, or referring patients to any service or facility where the health provider has a financial interest, are prohibited by the federal Ethics in Patient Referral Act, as well as other federal and state laws.

Violations of laws against health care fraud and abuse can result in imprisonment and fines, loss of professional license, loss of health care facility staff privileges, and exclusion from participation in federal health care programs.

Court Case

Nurse Sues Under False Claims Act

A registered nurse employed by a medical center from 1979 to 2002 was chair of her state nurses' association, the exclusive bargaining unit for the registered nurses at her employing medical center. In this capacity, she complained to her state Department of Public Health about the inadequacy of nurse staffing at her place of employment. The nurse alleged that staffing inadequacies were affecting patient care and delays in patient treatment. She said she had learned that delays in patient care could affect the medical center's right to participate in and receive reimbursement for Medicare- or Medicaid-related services.

Nurses at the plaintiff's medical center filed hundreds of complaints to appropriate authorities, reporting unsafe, unethical, or illegal care practices or conditions at their medical center during 2001–2002. The plaintiff and several other complaining nurses were fired in 2002. The plaintiff subsequently sued the medical center under the False Claims Act, claiming her conduct was protected under the whistleblower provisions of the act.

The court granted the medical center's motion to dismiss, stating that nothing indicated that the employee threatened a *qui tam* action, nor had she notified the employer that she was investigating fraud. Thus, the plaintiff had no grounds to sufficiently allege a retaliation claim under the FCA.

Robbins v. Provena St. Joseph Medical Center (2004) U.S. Dist. LEXIS 3878.

Patients' Bill of Rights Acts of 1999, 2001, and 2004

Concerns about the quality of medical care patients receive under managed care plans prompted Congress to first consider a Patients' Bill of Rights Act in 1999. The act contained provisions applicable to managed care plans for access to care, quality assurance, patient information and securing privacy, grievances and appeals procedures, protecting the doctor-patient relationship, and promoting good medical practice. Congress failed to act on the bill in 1999, and it was revived in 2001 as H.R. 2563, "The Bipartisan Patient Protection Act of 2001." The House of Representatives passed the act in August 2001 by a narrow margin, and it was sent to the Senate. The Senate passed a revised version of the bill and sent it back to the House for reconsideration, but the bill died there. Major points of contention among lawmakers were the rights of patients to file lawsuits against managed care plans in federal or state courts and whether or not awards in such lawsuits should be limited by law to certain amounts.

The Bipartisan Patient Protection Act was revived in 2004, when S. 2083 was proposed to amend the Public Health Service Act and the Employee Retirement Income Security Act of 1974. The purpose of the bill was to protect consumers in managed care health plans and other health coverage. The bill did not become law.

TELEMEDICINE

telemedicine Remote consultation by patients with physicians or other health professionals via telephone, closed-circuit television, or the Internet.

Telemedicine refers to remote consultation with physicians or other health care professionals via telephone, closed-circuit television, fax machine, or the Internet. When telemedicine was first used, it generally involved transmission of X-rays, sonograms, or other medical data between two distant points. In some cases, usually through closed-circuit television, a physician could examine a patient in a distant location, thus allowing patients in rural

cybermedicine A form of telemedicine that involves direct contact between patients and physicians over the Internet, usually for a fee.

e-health Term for the use of the Internet as a source of consumer information about health and medicine.

areas more complete access to medical care. Today, transmitted medical data includes video, audio, and written or computerized patient data. In fact, increasing use of the Internet has made telemedicine an important component of the health care system.

Two additional aspects of telemedicine are cybermedicine and e-health. **Cybermedicine** involves direct online contact between physician and patient. There are many Web sites on the Internet that allow patients to consult directly with a physician, usually for a fee. The physician may offer medical advice and even prescribe medication.

E-health is the term used for the increasing use of the Internet as a source of consumer information about health and medicine. E-health has become a popular aspect of telemedicine, as increasing numbers of patients query their doctors and other health care providers about where to find health information on the Internet and how to evaluate such information.

Health-related Internet sites included under the category "e-health" most often provide

- Consumer information services.
- Support groups.
- Prescription and nonprescription drug sales.
- Medical advice and diagnosis.
- Contract health services as part of insurance plans for covered subscribers.
- Health business support services for health professionals and health care organizations.

States are responding to the proliferation in telemedicine services with laws that address issues of reimbursement, licensure, funding, and confidentiality. Telemedicine legislation covers various health care providers, including physicians, dentists, chiropractors, nurses, and other health professionals. Since new laws regulating telemedicine are passed every year, health care practitioners who are involved in telemedicine or who plan to be involved will need to research state telemedicine laws.

Consumer Precautions Regarding Telemedicine

Individuals using the Internet for health care and medical information should evaluate Web sites for reliability. Users should ask such questions as these:

- Who is sponsoring the site? Sites sponsored by or linked with major medical centers and groups, government agencies, and medical professionals or major medical publications are most likely to present reliable information.
- Are several reliable Web sites offering similar information? If so, the information is most likely to be reliable.
- Does the site tout miracle cures or peculiar therapies? Users should discuss any claims made with a trusted health care practitioner before sending for materials or "cures" or otherwise following such advice.

Advances in technology have improved our ability to record, store, transfer, and share medical data electronically. They have also magnified privacy, security, and confidentiality concerns that pertain to patient medical records. Privacy issues are discussed at length in Chapter 7, "Privacy Law and HIPAA."

Court Case

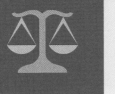

Illegal Telemedicine Drug Sale

A Washington state medical doctor dispensed Viagra through a Web site. He did not perform physical examinations or have direct contact with any of the Web site visitors who purchased the drug. Kansas investigators conducted a "sting" operation to document that individuals, including minors, could purchase Viagra from the Web site operated by the medical doctor. The Kansas attorney general subsequently brought suit against the doctor under the Kansas Consumer Protection Act (KCPA).

The physician was barred from prescribing and dispensing drugs in Kansas via his Web site, since to do so was in violation of that state's pharmacy and medical practice acts. The state sought civil penalties under the KCPA, which resulted in the cited lawsuit. To state a claim under the KCPA, the state had to establish that the transaction was deceptive. The state claimed that since the transaction was illegal, it was necessarily deceptive. The trial court disagreed, finding that the Web site information was correct and that in order for the minor to purchase the drug, he had to falsify information on a site form. The "medical evaluation" included a specific disclaimer explaining its limitations and that it was not a substitute for a proper medical examination by a physician. The court found that the drug that was shipped was what was represented and that charges for the drug were also as represented. The trial court concluded that the transaction was not deceptive, and this ruling was affirmed by the Kansas Supreme Court.

While the state was not able to impose civil penalties, the physician was no longer allowed to sell the drug in Kansas.

State ex rel. Stovall v. Confimed.com, L.L.C., 38 P.3d 707 (Kansas, 2002).

Ethics Issues

Working in Health Care

ETHICS ISSUE 1: The "Code of Ethical Business and Professional Behavior" for the Cleveland Clinic Health System states under the heading "Conflicts of Interest" that "No employee or member of administration or professional staff shall accept gifts, favors, entertainment, or other items of value that might compromise their independent decision making abilities."

DISCUSSION QUESTION

1. Assume you are an audiologist working under the above ethical guidelines. If no state law prohibits the practice, could you agree to accept commissions for recommending a certain brand of hearing aid to patients, if the hearing aid is appropriate to their needs? Explain your answer.

_____

_____

ETHICS ISSUE 2: A physician who owns a health care facility is prohibited by the federal Ethics in Patient Referral Act, as well as other federal and state laws, from referring patients to his facility.

1. Is the practice also unethical? Explain your answer.

_____

_____

ETHICS ISSUE 3: By law, health care practitioners can only perform those duties that are within their *scope of practice*—that is, those duties for which they are duly licensed, certified, registered, and competent.

DISCUSSION QUESTIONS

1. A nurse notices that a physician has prescribed two doses of a medication for a hospitalized patient, one dose at 6 AM and a second one dose at 9 AM. Since the nurse knows that the medication prescribed should be administered after a meal to prevent nausea and other side effects, and breakfast is not served on the nurse's floor until 7 or 7:30 AM, what should the nurse do?

_____

_____

2. A certified nursing assistant takes a job assisting a special education teacher within a school district with a small class of severely mentally challenged students. The CNA has had experience working with mentally challenged individuals, and will assist the teacher in keeping charges clean, feeding them, adjusting wheelchairs, and so on. A month into her employment, a student accidentally dislodges her urinary catheter, and the teacher asks the CNA to reinsert it. This duty is beyond the CNA's scope of practice. What should she do?

_____

_____

ETHICS ISSUE 4: A licensed practical nurse (LPN) working the night shift in a hospital is told by her RN supervisor to administer a "push" IV (intravenous) medication to a patient. This duty assignment is not within the LPN's scope of practice, since state medical practice acts in the state where the LPN is employed specify that only RNs, nurse practitioners, physician assistants, or physicians can administer push IV medications. The LPN objects to her RN supervisor, but the supervisor replies, "This is the night shift and we're short-handed. Just don't tell anyone on the day shift that you did it."

DISCUSSION QUESTION

1. What should the LPN do?

_____

_____

 Go to www.mhhe.com/judson5e to practice your case review skills. Then read on for more information.

Applying Knowledge

Write "L" for licensure, "C" for certification, "R" for registration and "A" for accreditation in the space provided to indicate which is applicable in the following descriptions.

_____1. Involves a mandatory credentialing process established by law, usually at the state level.

_____2. Involves simply paying a fee.

_____3. Involves a voluntary credentialing process, usually national in scope, most often sponsored by a private-sector group.

_____4. Required of all physicians, dentists, and nurses in every state.

_____5. Consists simply of an entry in an official record.

_____6. A process that implies that health care facilities or HMOs have met certain standards.

Circle the correct answer from the choices provided.

7. The legal principle that says that the physician is responsible for the negligent acts of those employees under his/her supervision is called:

   a. Certification

   b. Reciprocity

   c. *Respondeat superior*

   d. *Res ipsa loquitur*

8. A copayment is:

   a. A percentage of the fee for services provided

   b. A set amount that each patient pays for each office visit

   c. The portion of the fee the physician must write off

   d. The portion of the fee that the insurance company pays

9. Under this type of plan, insured patients must designate a primary care physician (PCP):

   a. Point-of-service plan

   b. Preferred provider plan

   c. Independent practice plan

   d. Health maintenance plan

10. When physicians, hospitals, and other health care providers contract with one or more HMOs or directly with employers to provide care, this is called:

    a. A physician-hospital organization

    b. A preferred provider plan

    c. A health maintenance organization

    d. A fee-for-service plan

11. Under this type of plan, a patient may see providers outside the plan, but the patient pays a higher portion of the fees:

   a. Health maintenance plan

   b. Independent practitioner plan

   c. Preferred provider plan

   d. Primary care plan

12. Which of the following is mandatory for certain health professionals to practice in their field?

   a. Endorsement

   b. Reciprocity

   c. Licensure

   d. Certification

13. The National Practitioner Data Bank:

   a. Is accessible to everyone

   b. Is accessible to other providers on a routine basis

   c. Is accessible only to hospitals and health care plans

   d. Is accessible only to the government agencies monitoring health care

14. Licensure to practice medicine is done by:

   a. Each individual state

   b. The federal government

   c. Local and state governments together

   d. The federal government and the local government

15. Physicians today practice primarily:

   a. At the hospital

   b. In sole proprietorships

   c. In group practices

   d. In large corporations

16. The Patients' Bill of Rights:

   a. Is a state statue

   b. Is now law in 30 of the 50 states

   c. Has still not become law

   d. Is a federal law

Answer the following questions in the spaces provided.

17. What is the purpose of medical practice acts?

_____

_____

18. List four requirements that must be met before a physician can be granted a license to practice medicine.

_____

_____

19. List four instances in which a physician might not need a license.

_____

_____

_____

_____

20. Name three circumstances under which a physician's license may be revoked.

_____

_____

_____

21. Who has the authority to revoke a physician's license?

_____

_____

22. Give one advantage and one disadvantage for each of the following practice management systems:

Sole proprietorship

Advantage: _____

Disadvantage: _____

Partnership

Advantage: _____

Disadvantage: _____

Corporation

Advantage: _____

Disadvantage: _____

23. List two types of managed care health care plans.

_____

_____

24. Name the "whistleblower" statute that deals with fraud and abuse in health care.

_____

_____

25. Define _managed care plan_.

_____

_____

26. Distinguish among the terms _telemedicine, cybermedicine,_ and _e-health_.

_____

_____

27. What telemedicine issues must state laws address?

_____

_____

28. What is the sole authority granted the federal government concerning the licensing of physicians?

_____

_____

Case Study

Use your critical-thinking skills to answer the questions that follow the case studies.

A patient complained to the state medical board that her health care plan physician turned her away from a scheduled office visit because she did not have her checkbook with her and thus could not make the required $20 advance copayment. She complained that, because she was ill, it was unfeeling and unrealistic of the physician to expect her to go home and get her checkbook. She pointed out that the physician's office had a record of her insurance coverage and her payment record was good. The physician refused to make an exception to the "copayment in advance" rule, and the woman went home without seeing him.

29. In your opinion, should the physician have made an exception to the copayment rule? Why or why not?

_____

_____

Physician assistants (PA) are employed in physician's offices throughout the United States. Although the PA provides direct patient care, he or she is always under the supervision of a licensed physician. Duties include taking patients' medical histories, performing physical examinations, ordering diagnostic and therapeutic procedures, providing follow-up care, and teaching and counseling patients. In most states PAs may write prescriptions. The PA may be the only health care practitioner a patient sees during his or her visit to the physician's office. Therefore, patients often refer to a PA as "the doctor." Ned, a physician assistant for five years, says the patients he sees often address him as "Doctor."

Similarly, Marie, a long-time employee of a physician in private practice, is often called "the doctor's nurse." Although Marie has never had the training necessary to become a certified medical assistant or a registered nurse, she sometimes refers to herself as the "office nurse."

30. What legal and ethical considerations are evident in these situations?

_____

_____

31. Should Ned allow his patients to call him "doctor"? Explain your answer.

_____

_____

32. Should Marie use the title "nurse" or allow others to call her the doctor's nurse? Explain.

_____

_____

33. What would you do in either Ned's or Marie's situation?

_____

_____

Note: A health care practitioner is held to the standard of care practiced by a reasonably competent person of the same profession. A physician assistant using the title "Doctor" and a medical assistant using the title "Nurse" may be held to the standard of care of a physician and a nurse, respectively, and may be accused of practicing without the appropriate license.

A new source of potential problems for health care practitioners is a surprising one: advertising. Buying print ads, creating a radio spot, or sponsoring a Web site was not something most physicians and other health care practitioners did a few years ago. It is more commonplace today, however, and two New Jersey patients took their physician to court over the Web site ads she ran for LASIK eye surgery. The patients did not make any traditional medical malpractice claims. Instead, they claimed the doctor made false or misleading statements on her Web site, leading them to believe that she would provide all of their treatment. Instead, the patients said a physician who was not fully licensed provided their follow-up care. (This practice is generally medically acceptable.) The two patients sued the physician under their state's Consumer Fraud Act, an area of law from which physicians have traditionally been exempt. A trial court allowed the suit to go forward, but the state supreme court reversed that decision, and the patients could not sue the physician for advertising fraud.

34. In your opinion, should the two patients have been allowed to sue? Explain your answer.

_____

_____

_____

35. What is your opinion regarding health care practitioners who advertise their services?

_____

_____

36. Should laws be passed to specifically exempt doctors from advertising liability? Explain your answer.

_____

_____

Internet Activities

Complete the activities and answer the questions.

37. Conduct a Web search for "Patient's Bill of Rights." Is such a bill currently before Congress? If so, what is its status? (If current status is not available online, you can telephone the federal Bill Status Office at (202) 225-1772 to find out the status of any bill before Congress, but you must have the bill's number, such as S.2083, "The Bipartisan Patient Protection Act of 2004.")

_____

_____

38. Visit the Web site for the National Practitioner Data Bank–Healthcare Integrity and Protection Data Bank (www.npdb-hipdb.com). How does one obtain information from either data bank?

_____

_____

39. Visit the telemedicine Web site for the National Conference of State Legislatures at www.ncsl.org/ programs/health/teleleg.htm. (If this Web site is no longer active, conduct a Web search for "telemedicine" AND "state laws" OR "state legislation.") Does your state have laws governing telemedicine? If so, briefly summarize them. If not, what laws would you recommend be enacted for your state?

_____

_____

CHAPTER 3

Law, the Courts, and Contracts

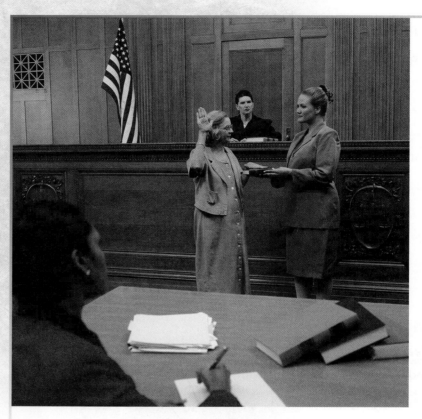

Learning Outcomes

After studying this chapter, you should be able to:

1. Discuss the three primary sources of law.

2. Differentiate between criminal law and civil law.

3. Define the concept of torts and discuss how the tort of negligence affects health care.

4. List and discuss the four essential elements of a contract.

5. Differentiate between expressed contracts and implied contracts.

6. Discuss the contractual rights and responsibilities of both physicians and patients.

7. Relate how the law of agency and the doctrine of *respondeat superior* apply to health care contracts.

Key Terms

administrative law
agent
breach of contract
case law
checks and balances
civil law
common law
constitutional law
contract
criminal law
defendant
executive order
expressed contract
Fair Debt Collection Practices Act (FDCPA)
felony
implied contract
jurisdiction

law of agency
legal precedent
mentally incompetent
minor
misdemeanor
negligence
plaintiff
procedural law
prosecution
respondeat superior
Statute of Frauds
statutory law
substantive law
third party payor contract
tort
tortfeasor
void
voidable

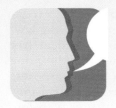

Voice of Experience

No Fraud When Insurance Won't Pay

"Sometimes patients don't understand that what they are asking us to do is insurance fraud," says Christine, a patient billing specialist who works for a hospital in the Pacific Northwest. When Babs, a hospital patient, was treated for breast cancer, her physician obtained her informed consent to use a new treatment that he had helped develop. A drug was injected into her breast that targeted for destruction just the small malignant tumor;

no healthy tissue was destroyed. Babs's medical insurance company refused to pay for the procedure, claiming it was "experimental." The procedure was new, but Babs's physician had used it many times with success. "Can't you just say I had a traditional lumpectomy," Babs asked Christine, "so my insurance company will pay for it?"

"We had to explain to Babs that this would constitute insurance fraud, and we couldn't do it," Christine explains.

THE BASIS OF LAW

The Federal Government

Federal laws governing the administration of health care and all other national matters derive from powers and responsibilities delegated to the three branches of government by the United States Constitution. As you probably recall from basic government classes, the three branches of government are legislative, executive, and judicial. Here is a quick review of the three branches' composition and responsibilities.

The two houses of Congress—the Senate and the House of Representatives—make up the *legislative branch*. Each member of Congress is elected by the people of his or her state. The House of Representatives, with membership based on state populations, has 435 seats, while the Senate, with two members from each state, has 100 seats. Members of the House of Representatives are elected for two-year terms, and Senators are elected for six-year terms. The primary duty of Congress is to write, debate, and pass bills, which are then passed on to the president for approval.

Other powers of Congress include:

- Making laws controlling trade between states and between the United States and other countries.
- Making laws about taxes and borrowing money.
- Approving the making of money.
- Declaring war on other countries.

Functions specific to the House of Representatives include the following. Members of the House can:

- Introduce legislation that compels people to pay taxes.
- Decide if a government official should be put on trial before the Senate if he or she commits a crime against the country. (Such a trial is called *impeachment*.)

Functions specific to the Senate include the following. Senators can:

- Approve and disapprove any treaties the president makes.
- Approve or disapprove any people the president recommends for jobs, such as cabinet officers, Supreme Court justices, and ambassadors.
- Hold an impeachment trial for a government official who commits a crime against the country.

executive order A rule or regulation issued by the President of the United States that becomes law without the prior approval of Congress.

checks and balances The system established by the U.S. Constitution that keeps any one branch of government from assuming too much power over the other branches.

The President of the United States is the chief executive of the *executive branch* of government, which is responsible for administering the law. Through his or her ability to issue **executive orders,** the president has limited legislative powers. Executive orders become law without the prior approval of Congress. They are usually issued for one of three purposes: to create administrative agencies or change the practices of an existing agency, to enforce laws passed by Congress, or to make treaties with foreign powers.

The United States Supreme Court heads the *judicial branch* of government, which also includes federal judges and courts in every state. The judicial branch interprets the law and oversees the enforcement of laws.

The division of powers and responsibilities among three branches of government ensures that a system of **checks and balances** will keep any one branch from assuming too much power. See Figure 3-1.

State Governments

State governments also have three branches: *legislative, executive,* and *judicial.* The number of state legislators a state may elect is based upon the number of political districts in each state, since citizens elect legislators from the various districts. Therefore, the numbers of members of state legislatures are not the same as the number of members in the United States Congress.

State legislative branches also consist of two chambers: the Senate and the House of Representatives. In some states, the House of Representatives is called the Assembly or General Assembly. Terms served may be the same as in the federal government—six years for senators and two years for representatives or assembly members—or they may differ.

The governor is the head of the state's executive branch. Each state has its own constitution, but state constitutions cannot conflict with the United States Constitution. Those responsibilities not delegated by the federal constitution are left to the states. (See Table 3-1.)

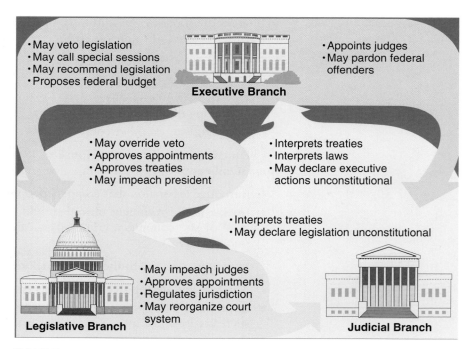

FIGURE 3-1 System of Checks and Balances

TABLE 3-1 Exclusive Powers of the National Government and State Governments

National Government	State Governments
Print money	Issue licenses
Regulate interstate (between states) and international trade	Regulate intrastate (within the state) businesses
Make treaties and conduct foreign policy	Conduct elections
Declare war	Establish local governments
Provide an army and navy	Ratify amendments to the Constitution
Establish post offices	Take measures for public health and safety
Make laws necessary and proper to carry out the above powers	May exert powers the Constitution does not delegate to the national government or prohibit the states from using

SOURCES OF LAW

constitutional law Law that derives from federal and state constitutions.

case law Law established through common law and legal precedent.

common law The body of unwritten law developed in England, primarily from judicial decisions based on custom and tradition.

There are four types of law, distinguished according to their origin:

1. **Constitutional law** is based on a formal document that defines broad governmental powers. Federal constitutional law is based on the United States Constitution (Figure 3-2). State constitutional law derives from each state's constitution.

2. **Case law** is law set by legal precedent. Case law began with **common law.** In the early days in America, laws derived from those originating in

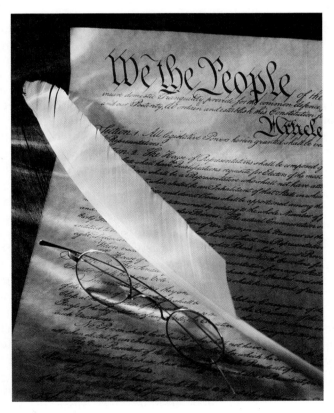

FIGURE 3-2 The United States Constitution.

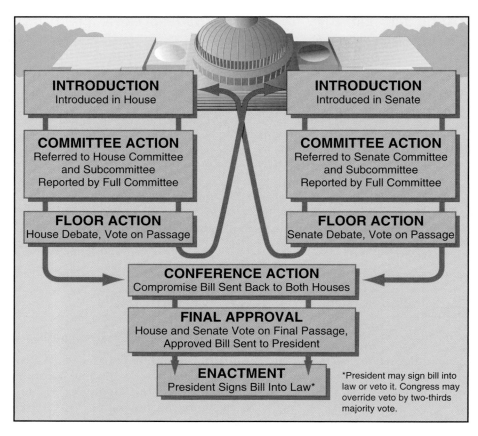

FIGURE 3-3 How a Federal Bill Becomes a Law

England, and they were often not written down. Matters of law were decided based on the customs and traditions of the people. Judges shared their decisions with other judges, and these decisions became common law.

Later, court decisions were written down, and judges could then refer to past cases to help them make current decisions. These written cases were then used as **legal precedents.** When deciding cases with similar circumstances, judges were required to follow these earlier cases or legal precedents. Today, legal precedents are the rule of law, applying to future cases, even though they were not enacted by legislation. Precedents can be changed only by the court that originally decided a case or by a higher court.

3. **Statutory law** refers to laws enacted by state or federal legislatures. Individual laws in this body of law are called statutes. (Laws passed by city governments are called municipal ordinances.) Statutes begin as bills at the federal or state levels. The bills may become laws, or presidents or governors may veto them. Once passed, the laws may be amended, repealed, revised, or superseded by legislatures. The courts can review statutes for constitutionality, application, interpretation, and other legal questions. (See Figure 3-3.)

4. **Administrative law** includes statutes enacted to define specific powers and procedures when agencies are created. Administrative agencies are created by Congress, by the president, or by individual state legislatures. Regulations may be passed that pertain specifically to the functions of one agency, such as the Internal Revenue Service (IRS), Social Security Administration, or Occupational Safety and Health Administration (OSHA).

legal precedents Decisions made by judges in various courts that become rule of law and apply to future cases, even though they were not enacted by legislation.

statutory law Law passed by the U.S. Congress or state legislatures.

administrative law Enabling statutes enacted to define powers and procedures when an agency is created.

Fill in the blanks below to answer the questions.

1. Number the following two types of constitutions in the order in which they must be observed:
   state constitutions _____ federal constitution _____

2. Who has exclusive authority to declare war on another country?

   _____

3. Which chamber of the United States Congress has exclusive authority to hold an impeachment trial?

   _____

4. What are the four types of law, based upon their origin?

   _____

   _____

   _____

5. Which of the above types of law began with common law?

   _____

6. Briefly define *administrative law*.

   _____

CLASSIFICATIONS OF LAW

substantive law The statutory or written law that defines and regulates legal rights and obligations.

procedural law Law that defines the rules used to enforce substantive law.

After laws are created through constitutional, case, statutory, or administrative law, they are classified by type. Two broad types of law are substantive and procedural. **Substantive law** is the statutory or written law that defines and regulates legal rights and obligations. It defines the legal relationships between people or between people and the state, and is further classified as criminal, civil, military, and international law. **Procedural law** defines the rules used to enforce substantive law.

Since criminal and civil laws are most likely to pertain to health care practitioners, they are discussed in more detail below.

CRIMINAL LAW

criminal law Law that involves crimes against the state.

A crime is an offense against the state or sovereignty, committed or omitted, in violation of a public law forbidding or commanding it. Therefore, the body of **criminal law** involves crimes against the state. When a state or federal criminal law is violated, the government brings criminal charges against the alleged offender (for example, *New York v. John Doe*).

State criminal laws prohibit such crimes as murder, burglary, robbery, arson, rape, sodomy, larceny, mayhem (needless or willful damage or violence), and practicing medicine without a license. Federal criminal offenses include matters affecting national security (treason); crimes involving the country's borders; and illegal activities that cross state lines, such as kidnapping or hijacking.

felony An offense punishable by death or by imprisonment in a state or federal prison for more than one year.

A criminal act may be classified as a felony or a misdemeanor. A **felony** is a crime punishable by death or by imprisonment in a state or federal prison for more than one year. Felonies include abuse (child abuse, elder abuse, or domestic violence), arson, burglary, conspiracy, embezzlement, fraud, illegal drug

misdemeanor A crime punishable by fine or by imprisonment in a facility other than a prison for less than one year.

dealing, grand larceny, manslaughter, mayhem, murder or attempted murder, rape, robbery, sodomy, tax evasion, and practicing medicine without a license.

Misdemeanors are less serious crimes than felonies. They are punishable by fines or by imprisonment in a facility other than a prison for one year or less. Examples of misdemeanors include some traffic violations, thefts under a certain dollar amount, attempted burglary, and disturbing the peace.

Can Knowledge of a Crime Make You Guilty?

Persons who commit crimes are, of course, the principals in criminal proceedings. However, those individuals who have knowledge of a crime may, in certain circumstances, also be subject to prosecution. An *accessory* is one who contributes to or aids in the commission of a crime—by a direct act, by an indirect act (such as encouragement), by watching and not giving aid, or by concealing the criminal's crime. For example, the person in charge of billing for health care services in a medical office may be an accessory to insurance fraud if he or she takes no action, even though he or she knows that some health care practitioners are billing for services not rendered.

Players in the Court Scene

plaintiff The person bringing charges in a lawsuit.

prosecution The government as plaintiff in a criminal case.

defendant The person or party against whom charges are brought in a criminal or civil lawsuit.

When criminal and civil cases go to court, a complaining party—the **plaintiff**—must show that he or she was wronged or injured. The government—the **prosecution**—is the plaintiff in criminal cases. A private individual is the plaintiff in civil cases. The **defendant,** who is charged with an offense, must dispute the complaint.

Officers of the court are responsible for carrying out courtroom duties:

▌ *Judges* are elected or appointed to preside over the court and in most states must be licensed attorneys. They rule on points of law about trial procedure, presentation of evidence, and all laws that apply to the case. If there is no jury, the judge determines the facts in the case. Judges hand down sentences after a verdict is rendered.

▌ *Attorneys* represent plaintiffs and defendants, presenting evidence so that the jury or the judge can reach a verdict.

▌ *Court clerks* keep court records and seals, enter court orders and judgments into the record, and keep the papers of the court.

▌ *Bailiffs* keep order in the courtroom and may remove disruptive persons from the court at the judge's request.

▌ *Court reporters* make a running account of all court proceedings, using a stenotype machine that types shorthand symbols onto a tape.

▌ *Juries* are most often selected from lists of registered voters. Six or twelve jurors are chosen to hear the evidence presented in court and render a verdict.

CIVIL LAW

civil law Law that involves wrongful acts against persons.

Criminal law involves crimes against the state; **civil law** does not involve crimes, but, instead, involves wrongful acts against persons. Under civil law, a person can sue another person, a business, or the government. Civil disputes often arise over issues of contract violation, slander, libel, trespassing, product liability, or automobile accidents. Many civil suits involve family matters such as divorce, child support, and child custody. Court judgments in civil cases often require the payment of a sum of money to the injured party.

TORT LIABILITY

tort A civil wrong committed against a person or property, excluding breach of contract.

Civil law includes a general category of law known as torts. A **tort** is broadly defined as a civil wrong committed against a person or property, excluding breach of contract. The act, committed without just cause, may have caused physical injury, resulted in damage to someone's property, or deprived someone of his or her personal liberty and freedom. Torts may be intentional (willful) or unintentional (accidental).

Intentional Torts

tortfeasor The person guilty of committing a tort.

Some torts involve intentional misconduct. When one person intentionally harms another, the law allows the injured party to seek a remedy in a civil suit. The injured party can be financially compensated for any harm done by the **tortfeasor** (person guilty of committing a tort). If the conduct is judged to be malicious, punitive damages may also be awarded. Examples of intentional torts include the following:

Assault. The open threat of bodily harm to another, or acting in such a way as to put another in the "reasonable apprehension of bodily harm."

Battery. An action that causes bodily harm to another. It is broadly defined as any bodily contact made without permission. Battery may or may not result from the threat of assault. In health care delivery, battery may be charged for any unauthorized touching of a patient, including such actions as suturing a wound, administering an injection, or performing a physical examination.

Defamation of Character. Involves damaging a person's reputation by making public statements that are both false and malicious. Defamation can take the form of libel or slander. Libel is expressing in published print, writing, pictures, or signed statements content that injure the reputation of another. Libel also includes reading statements aloud or broadcasting for the public to hear. Slander is speaking defamatory or damaging words intended to prejudice others against an individual in a manner that jeopardizes his or her reputation or means of livelihood.

False Imprisonment. The intentional, unlawful restraint or confinement of one person by another. The offense is treated as a crime in some states. Refusing to dismiss a patient from a health care facility upon his or her request, or preventing an employee or patient from leaving the facility might be seen as false imprisonment.

Fraud. Deceitful practices in depriving or attempting to deprive another of his or her rights. Health care practitioners might be accused of fraud for promising patients "miracle cures" or for accepting fees from patients for using mystical or spiritual powers to heal.

Invasion of Privacy. An intrusion into a person's seclusion or private affairs, public disclosure of private facts about a person, false publicity about a person, or use of a person's name or likeness without permission. Improper use of or breaching the confidentiality of medical records may be seen as invasion of privacy.

Intentional torts may also be crimes. Therefore, some civil wrongs may also be prosecuted as criminal acts in separate court actions. See Table 3-2 for a summary of intentional torts.

Unintentional Torts

The more common torts within the health care delivery system are those committed unintentionally. Unintentional torts are acts that are not intended

TABLE 3-2 Intentional Torts

Tort	Description
Assault	Threatening to strike or harm with a weapon or physical movement, resulting in fear
Battery	Unlawful, unprivileged touching of another person
Trespass	Wrongful injury to or interference with the property of another
Nuisance	Anything that interferes with the enjoyment of life or property
Interference with contractual relations	Intentionally causing one person not to enter into or to break a contract with another
Deceit	False statement or deceptive practice done with intent to injure another
Conversion	Unauthorized taking or borrowing of personal property of another for the use of the taker
False imprisonment (false arrest)	Unlawful restraint of a person, whether in prison or otherwise
Defamation	Wrongful act of injuring another's reputation by making false statements
Invasion of privacy	Interference with a person's right to be left alone
Misuse of legal procedure	Bringing legal action with malice and without probable cause
Infliction of emotional distress	Intentionally or recklessly causing emotional or mental suffering to another
Fraud	Dishonest or deceitful practices in depriving, or attempting to deprive, another of his or her rights

Court Case

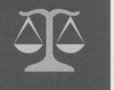

Chiropractor's Outrageous Conduct Results in Trial

A chiropractor had two patients who became his employees. The two patients/ employees sued the chiropractor for outrageous conduct and invasion of privacy, based on the fact that each plaintiff had a sexual relationship with the chiropractor, and when the two plaintiffs told the chiropractor they wanted to end their sexual relationships with him, he threatened to stop their medical treatment and to fire them. He also exposed himself to the two plaintiffs in his office, and allegedly otherwise harassed them sexually.

A trial court found for the two plaintiffs, and the chiropractor appealed. The appellate court concluded that the trial court did not err in determining that "reasonable people could find the chiropractor's conduct so outrageous in character, and so extreme in degree, as to go beyond all possible bounds of decency and be regarded as atrocious and utterly intolerable." The judgment of the trial court was affirmed. A total of $537,685 in damages was awarded to the two plaintiffs.

Note: Whether or not the chiropractor lost his license to practice was not decided by this court but was a matter for his state licensing board to decide.

Pearson and Faby v. Kancilla, 70 P.3d 594; 2003 Colo. App. LEXIS 407.

Court Case

Physician Sued for Negligence

A physician sterilized a female patient who had sought such a procedure to avoid having more children. The woman later became pregnant and delivered a healthy child. She sued her physician, alleging that the doctor's performance of a sterilization procedure had been negligent and seeking damages for the future expenses of raising a child. The physician filed a motion for preliminary determination. A trial court denied the motion, permitting the plaintiff to seek damages for raising the child. The physician appealed.

The appellate court held that the parents were not "injured" by delivering a healthy child, and, therefore, could not receive an award for damages. The court reversed the trial court's order denying the physician's motion for preliminary determination and remanded the case for "further proceedings consistent with this opinion."

Note: Further action on this case was not published. Because of the appellate court's decision, however, it seems unlikely that further proceedings would favor the plaintiff.

Chaffee v. Seslar, 786 N.E.2d 705; 2003 Ind. Lexis 331.

negligence An unintentional tort alleged when one may have performed or failed to perform an act that a reasonable person would or would not have done in similar circumstances.

to cause harm but are committed unreasonably or with a disregard for the consequences. In legal terms, this constitutes **negligence.**

Negligence is charged when a health care practitioner fails to exercise ordinary care, and a patient is injured. The accused may have performed an act or failed to perform an act that a reasonable person, in similar circumstances, would or would not have performed. "Didn't intend to do it" or "should have known better" best describe a negligent act. Under principles of negligence, civil liability exists only in cases in which the act is judicially determined to be wrongful. A health care practitioner, for example, is not necessarily liable for a poor-quality outcome in delivering health care. He or she becomes liable only when his or her conduct is determined to be malpractice, the negligent delivery of professional services.

Negligence and defenses to liability suits are discussed in detail in Chapters 4 and 5, respectively.

Negligence is often alleged in lawsuits against health care practitioners, as in the case at the top of this page.

As illustrated in the court case on page 70, hospitals are not immune to charges of negligence.

THE COURT SYSTEM

The type of court that tries a case depends upon the state law or federal law that was allegedly violated. The federal court system, with some exceptions, hears cases involving federal matters. State court systems are independent of one another, and each system has its own rules and regulations. Generally, state courts decide cases involving matters occurring within their own state borders.

jurisdiction The power and authority given to a court to hear a case and to make a judgment.

Federal Courts

Jurisdiction is the power and authority given to a court to hear a case and to make a judgment. Examples of cases over which federal courts have jurisdiction include federal crimes, federal antitrust law, bankruptcy, patents,

Court Case

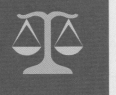

Hospital Sued for Negligence

A home health care and dialysis nurse was injured when she tried to prevent a patient who was being rolled from one hospital bed to another from falling to the floor. On the day she was injured, the nurse visited one of her home health patients and found him in a weakened state. She took the patient to a hospital emergency room, and after several hours, he was admitted to the hospital. The nurse followed an emergency room technician to assist in transferring the patient. The technician's duties included transferring patients from gurneys to beds. The first step in such a transfer is to lock the two beds together. If there is no one aiding in the patient transfer, the bed railing on the opposite side must be in the upright position to prevent the patient from rolling off the bed during the transfer.

The technician positioned the gurney next to the hospital bed to facilitate a rolling transfer, but did not place the bed railing on the opposite side in the upright position. The nurse stood at the foot of the gurney while the patient was asked to roll from the gurney onto the hospital bed. The nurse thought the patient was about to roll off the far side of the bed, and she jumped across the bed to grab him. When the nurse grabbed the patient, she felt pain across her lower back, and severe pain radiating into her left leg.

The nurse filed a two-count complaint against the hospital, alleging negligence and medical negligence. She claimed the hospital had failed to properly train and supervise the emergency room technician and that her patient had received negligent medical services from the hospital. A trial court granted summary judgment to the hospital on both counts. An appellate court reversed the trial court's granting of summary judgment on the negligence count, agreeing with the plaintiff that the hospital was negligent because the emergency room technician failed to take any action to prevent the type of injury reasonably expected from the zone of risk he created (in other words, to prevent the patient from rolling off the far side of the bed). It referred this matter for trial. However, the appellate court affirmed summary judgment for the medical negligence count, stating that the injured nurse received no medical services from the hospital that required the use of professional judgment or skill.

Note: Final disposition was not published. Perhaps the parties settled out of court, or perhaps a trial was scheduled for a date still in the future.

Reeves v. North Broward Hospital District, 821 So.2d 319; 2002 Fla. App. LEXIS 7375.

CHECK YOUR PROGRESS

Complete each of the following statements by filling in the blanks.

7. A civil law that says one person may sue another for a specific reason is broadly classified as _____ law.

8. The laws that determine the rules for one person's suing of another are broadly classified as _____ law.

9. _____ law involves crimes against the state.

10. _____ law involves wrongful acts against persons.

11. Torts are wrongs committed against _____.

12. The two broad types of torts include _____ and _____.

13. The type of torts most likely to concern health care practitioners is _____.

copyrights, trademarks, suits against the United States, and areas of admiralty law (pertaining to the sea).

State Courts

Each state has its own court system, but the general structure is the same in all states. The bottom tier consists of local courts. The next highest tier is trial courts, followed by appellate courts, and then the state supreme court. As with the federal court system, there are also special state courts with jurisdiction in certain kinds of cases.

Figure 3-4 shows the various federal and state court systems in the United States.

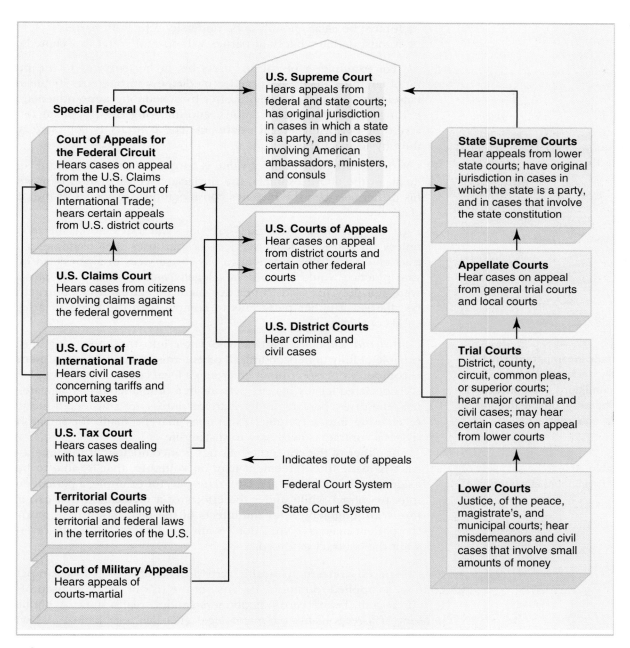

FIGURE 3-4   Court Systems in the United States

CONTRACTS

contract A voluntary agreement between two parties in which specific promises are made for a consideration.

A **contract** is a voluntary agreement between two parties in which specific promises are made for a consideration. The elements of a contract are important to health care practitioners because health care delivery takes place under various types of contracts. To be legally binding, four elements must be present in a contract.

1. *Agreement.* One party makes an offer, and another party accepts it. Certain conditions pertain to the offer:

   ▌ It can relate to the present or the future.
   ▌ It must be communicated.
   ▌ It must be made in good faith and not under duress or as a joke.
   ▌ It must be clear enough to be understood by both parties.
   ▌ It must define what both parties will do if the offer is accepted.

   For example, a physician offers his or her services to the public by obtaining a license to practice medicine and opening for business. Patients accept the physician's offer by scheduling appointments, submitting to physical examinations, and allowing the physician to prescribe or perform medical treatment. The contract is complete when the physician's fee is paid.

2. *Consideration.* Something of value is bargained for as part of the agreement. In the above example, the physician's consideration is providing his or her services; the patient's consideration is payment of the physician's fee.

3. *Legal Subject Matter.* Contracts are not valid and enforceable in court unless they are for legal services or purposes. For example, a contract entered into by a patient to pay for services of a physician in private practice would be **void** (not legally enforceable) if the physician were not duly licensed to practice medicine. **Breach of contract** may be charged if either party fails to comply with the terms of a legally valid contract.

mentally incompetent Unable to fully understand all the terms and conditions of a transaction, and therefore unable to enter into a legal contract.

voidable Able to be set aside or to be revalidated at a later date.

4. *Contractual capacity.* Parties who enter into the agreement must be capable of fully understanding all of its terms and conditions. A **mentally incompetent** person cannot enter into a legal contract. For example, persons declared legally insane, persons in a drug-altered mental state, and in some cases, persons under extreme duress are considered incapable of entering into a contract. Exceptions may be made for situations in which a contract is necessary to sustain life.

   If either of the concerned parties is incompetent at the time a contract is made, the agreement may be **voidable,** that is, able to be set aside or to be validated at a later date. Say, for example, a patient enters into a contract while under the effects of a medication that can interfere with judgment. After the effects of the medication have worn off, the patient may say, "No, I don't want the contract enforced" or "Yes, I want the contract enforced."

Of special concern to health care providers is the physician-patient contract as applied to minors. Because of the risk of being accused of battery or assault, health care practitioners cannot treat a minor without the consent of a responsible parent or legal guardian, except in cases where minors suffer a life-threatening emergency, or have been legally determined

minor Anyone under the age of majority: 18 years in most states, 21 years in some jurisdictions.

to be mature. A **minor** is defined as anyone under the age of majority, which is 18 in most states, and 21 in some jurisdictions. See Chapter 10 for a more extensive discussion of minors and the administration of medical services.

Abortion laws differ considerably across states, but the following court case illustrates how the Texas Supreme Court interpreted the state's abortion law in one case.

Court Case

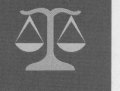

Minor Appeals for Judicial Bypass to Obtain an Abortion

Texas state law says that minors seeking abortions must notify their parents. Exceptions may be made for a minor who can show that

1. She is mature and sufficiently well-informed to make the decision to obtain an abortion without notifying a parent.
2. Notifying a parent would not be in her best interest.
3. Notifying a parent may lead to physical, sexual, or emotional abuse of the minor.

A minor petitioned a Texas court for authorization to consent to an abortion without notifying her parents. An appeals court denied the minor's petition, and she appealed to the Texas Supreme Court. The supreme court overturned the appellate court's decision and authorized the minor to consent to an abortion without notifying a parent. The court determined that the evidence the petitioner presented conclusively established that she was mature and sufficiently well-informed to consent to an abortion without parental notification.

In Re Jane Doe, 19 S.W.3d 346; 2000 Tex. LEXIS 67, 43 Tex. Sup. J. 910.

Sometimes breach of contract becomes an additional issue in medical negligence lawsuits.

Court Case

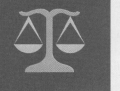

Breach of Contract Also Charged in Medical Negligence Lawsuit

A nurse treated an inmate at the county jail with an injection of 200 mg of Prolixin Decanoate that resulted in the inmate's permanent impotence. He filed an action against the nurse, the hospital, and the health care organization for negligence and breach of contract. A jury found for the plaintiff and awarded him damages in the amount of $450,500. The defendants appealed the decision and the award. An appeals court upheld the trial court's decision and award, except for $100,000 awarded as part of the breach of contract claim. The appeals court held that since the plaintiff was not part of the contract between the nurse and her employer, he was not entitled to damages on that claim.

Dempsey v. Pease, Mercy Health Services, St. Joseph Mercy Hospital (Court of Appeals of Michigan, 2001). Mich. App. LEXIS 273.

TYPES OF CONTRACTS

expressed contract A written or oral agreement in which all terms are explicitly stated.

implied contract An unwritten and unspoken agreement whose terms result from the actions of the parties involved.

Statute of Frauds State legislation governing written contracts.

third party payor contract A written agreement signed by a party other than the patient who promises to pay the patient's bill.

The two main types of contracts are expressed contracts and implied contracts. **Expressed contracts** are explicitly stated in written or spoken words. **Implied contracts** are unspoken. Their terms result from actions of the involved parties.

Expressed Contracts

An expressed contract may be written or oral, but all terms of the contract are explicitly stated. In the medical office, some contracts, in order to be legally valid, must be in writing. In each state the **Statute of Frauds,** derived from the Statute for the Prevention of Frauds and Perjuries formulated in England in 1677, states which contracts must be in writing to be enforced.

A type of contract often used in the medical office that falls under the Statute of Frauds is the **third party payor contract.** Insurance policies are also third party payor contracts, but as used here, the term means agreements by a third party to pay for services rendered to another. Such contracts must be in writing to be enforced and should be signed before health care services are rendered. For example, suppose Susan becomes ill while visiting her aunt in a distant city, and the aunt makes an appointment for Susan to see her physician. The aunt tells the medical office assistant, "I will pay Susan's bill." The medical office assistant may ask Susan's aunt to sign a third party payor contract.

Not all financial arrangements that require written contracts fall under the Statute of Frauds. Others are governed by Regulation Z or Regulation M of the Consumer Protection Act of 1968, also known as the Truth-in-Lending Act. Regulation Z applies to each individual or business that offers or extends consumer credit if four conditions are met:

1. The credit is offered to consumers.
2. Credit is offered on a regular basis.
3. The credit is subject to a finance charge (interest) or must be paid in more than four installments according to a written agreement.
4. The credit is primarily for personal, family, or household purposes. Regulation M applies only if credit is extended to businesses, or for commercial or agricultural purposes.

For example, Regulation Z of the Consumer Protection Act applies in a health care setting such as the following: A patient and a physician make a bilateral payment agreement (one in which both parties are mutually affected) that medical fees will be paid in four or more installments or will include finance charges. (It is legal and ethical for physicians to levy finance charges, as long as this is made clear to the patient before the charges are incurred.) This agreement must be in writing and must contain the following information:

- Fees for services.
- Amount of any down payment.
- The date each payment is due.
- The date of the final payment.
- The amount of each payment.
- Any interest charges to be made.

The patient signs the agreement and is given a copy. A second copy is filed with the patient's records.

For agreements falling under Regulation Z of the Truth-in-Lending Act, the medical office must supply the patient with a written disclosure statement. (See Figure 3-5.) The primary purpose of this legislation is to protect

Bruce Whiting, MD
310 Madison Avenue
Anderson, Indiana 46027

I agree to pay $_____ per week/month on my account balance of $_____.

Payments are due by the_____ of each _____ and will begin _____.
(week/month)   (date)

Interest will/will not be charged on the outstanding balance (see Truth-in-Lending form below for rate of interest).

I agree that if payments are not made in the full amount stated above or if payments are not received on time, the entire account balance will be considered delinquent and will be due and payable immediately.

I agree to be responsible for any reasonable collection costs or attorney fees incurred in collecting a delinquent account.

_____   _____

Date   Signature

This disclosure is in compliance with the Truth-in-Lending Act.

_____   _____

Patient's Name   Address

_____   _____

Responsible Party (if other than patient)   City, State, Zip Code

1. Cash Price (Medical and/or Surgical Fee)   _____
    Less Cash Down Payment (Advance)   _____
2. Unpaid Balance of Cash Price   _____
3. Amount Financed   _____
4. FINANCE CHARGE   _____
5. Total of Payments (3 + 4)   _____
6. Deferred Payment Price (1 + 4)   _____
7. ANNUAL PERCENTAGE RATE   _____

The "Total of Payments" shown above is payable to Bruce Whiting, MD, at the address shown above in _____ monthly installments of $_____, the first installment being payable _____ and all subsequent installments are due on the same day of
            (date)
each consecutive month until paid in full.

_____   _____

Date   Signature

FIGURE 3-5 Truth-in-Lending Payment Agreement

Fair Debt Collection Practices Act A federal statute prohibiting certain unfair and illegal practices by debt collectors and creditors. It prohibits certain methods of debt collection, including harassment, misrepresentation, threats, disseminating false information about the debtor, and engaging in unfair or illegal practices in attempting to collect a debt.

consumers from fraudulent or deceptive hidden finance charges levied by creditors, but creditors can also use it to collect outstanding debts.

The federal **Fair Debt Collection Practices Act (FDCPA)** of 1996 requires debt collectors and creditors to treat debtors fairly. It ensures fair treatment by prohibiting certain methods of debt collection. Debt collections practices prohibited by the act include harassment, misrepresentation, threats, disseminating false information about the debtor, and engaging in unfair or illegal practices in attempting to collect a debt. Personal, family, and household debts are covered under the act. This includes money owed for the purchase of an automobile, medical care, and charge accounts.

In the court case on the facing page, a patient sued a radiologist for breach of an expressed warranty (contract), alleging that the radiologist had told him he would not suffer any ill effects from an arteriogram procedure. What are the implications for health care practitioners who tell patients, "This procedure won't cause any damage"?

Implied Contracts

Implied contracts are those in which the conduct of the parties, rather than expressed words, creates the contract. Most contracts in the medical office are implied. For example, suppose a patient comes to a clinic complaining of a sore throat and asks to see a physician. The physician does not literally say, "I offer to treat your condition," to the patient, but by making his or her services available, he or she has made an offer to treat. A patient does not state to the physician, "I accept your offer to provide medical care." Acceptance is implied by the patient's actions in allowing the physician to examine him or her and prescribe treatment (see Figure 3-6). The physician's consideration is providing services. The patient's consideration is payment of the physician's fee. The contract is valid if both parties understand the offer, both are competent, and the services provided are legal.

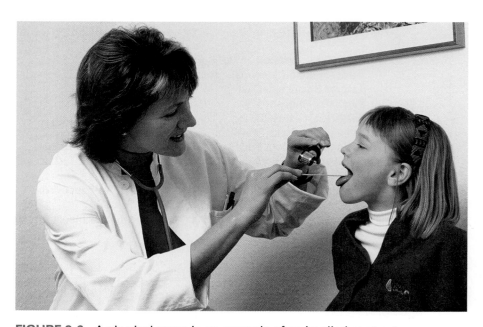

FIGURE 3-6 A physical exam is an example of an implied contract.

Court Case

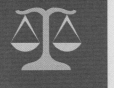

No Breach of Contract by Radiologist

A Georgia appellate court ruled that a patient's claim that a radiologist breached an expressed warranty had been properly dismissed by a lower court.

The radiologist performed an arteriogram procedure, which allegedly caused permanent injuries to the patient. The patient sued the radiologist for medical malpractice and breach of an expressed contract that he would not suffer any ill effects. The patient argued that the radiologist had stated the procedure would be routine and that he had nothing to worry about.

Affirming dismissal of the claim based on breach of contract, the appellate court said the radiologist had not expressly warranted that the patient would suffer no ill effects.

Servias v. Philbrick, 380 S.E.2d 496 (Ga. Ct. of App., March 10, 1989, rehearing denied, March 22, 1989, cert. Denied, Ga. Sup. Ct., May 4, 1989).

A physician who provides emergency treatment to a patient in a situation not covered by a special arrangement, such as in an emergency room, is limited to providing treatment at the site of the emergency. In such a situation, an implied limited contract between the physician and the patient is created, based upon the patient's implied request for and consent to emergency treatment. The patient's promise to pay for the physician's services is also implied. In this case, the physician's obligation for care does not extend to treatment after the emergency situation has been resolved.

CHECK YOUR PROGRESS

14. Tell whether each of the following examples involves an expressed or an implied contract:

_____ A man agrees to buy his friend's car and seals the deal with a handshake.

_____ A medical center outpatient agrees to undergo a colonoscopy.

_____ A patient in a physician's office agrees to a physical examination.

_____ A physician treats a patient for a broken leg in a hospital emergency room.

15. List the four elements present in a legally valid contract and give an example of each.

_____

_____

_____

_____

16. List three federal laws governing collections in the medical office.

_____

_____

_____

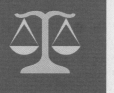
Although the previous court case was decided in 1989, it remains relevant in today's world, where printed or electronic images of patients are likely to be widely circulated.

THE PHYSICIAN-PATIENT CONTRACT AND MANAGED CARE

Managed care plans have added a third element to the physician-patient contract. Physicians still have contracts with their patients, but they may also have contracted with managed care programs to deliver medical services. If a physician terminates his or her contractual relationship with a managed care plan, this does not mean he or she cannot continue to see patients insured with the plan. It simply means the managed care plan will no longer pay for the subscriber's visits to this physician.

All insurance providers, including managed care plans, have access to patients' medical records for purposes of utilization review, inpatient stay review, case management review, and quality management. Insurance providers also check enrollees' medical records to monitor care and to identify ways of preventing illness and disease.

THE PHYSICIAN'S RIGHTS AND RESPONSIBILITIES

A physician has the right, after agreeing to accept an individual as his or her patient, to make reasonable limitations on the relationship. The physician is under no legal obligation to treat patients who may wish to exceed those limitations. Under the provisions of the physician-patient contract, both parties have certain rights and responsibilities. A physician has the right to:

▌ Set up practice within the boundaries of his or her license to practice medicine. A specialist, for instance, does not have to practice outside the area of specialty and, in fact, would be severely criticized for doing so, except in an emergency in which no other physician were available.

- Set up an office wherever he or she chooses and establish office hours.
- Specialize.
- Decide which services he or she will provide and how those services will be provided.

While practicing within the context of an implied contract with the patient, the physician is not bound to:

- Treat every patient who seeks medical care. The physician is free to use his or her own discretion—with one exception. If a physician is hired specifically to treat patients in one area or locale, such as a hospital emergency room, he or she must treat every patient who comes to that locale.
- Restore the patient to his or her original state of health. The fact that a patient grows progressively worse while under a physician's care and shows improvement when care is withdrawn does not necessarily constitute liability.
- Possess the highest skills possible within the profession or the maximum education attainable.
- Effect a recovery with every patient. The physician who fails to heal a patient cannot be condemned for lack of skill.
- Be familiar with the various reactions of patients to anesthetics or drugs of any kind. However, the physician is bound to note any allergic or adverse reactions to medications reported by the patient before treatment is administered.
- Be as skilled as a specialist if he or she is a general practitioner.
- Make a correct diagnosis in every case.
- Be free from mistakes of judgment in difficult cases.
- Display infallibility of judgment.
- Continue services after being discharged by the patient or by some responsible person, even if harm should come to the patient.
- Guarantee the successful result of any treatment or operation. In fact, guarantees of "cures" may constitute fraud on the part of the physician.

Under an implied contract with the patient, the physician has the obligation to:

- Use due care, skill, judgment, and diligence in treating patients, which other physicians of the same practice usually exercise in similar locations and under similar circumstances.
- Stay informed about the best methods of diagnosis and treatment.
- Perform to the best of his or her ability, whether or not he or she is to receive a fee.
- Exercise his or her best professional judgment in all cases, particularly those in which considerable doubt is involved.
- Consider the established, customary treatment administered by members of the medical profession in similar cases.
- Abstain from performing experiments on a patient without first securing the patient's complete understanding and approval.
- Provide proper instructions for a patient's care to the person responsible for such care, so that proper treatment will be administered to the patient in the doctor's absence.

- Furnish complete information and instructions to the patient about diagnosis, options and methods of treatment, and fees for services.
- Take every precaution to prevent the spread of contagious disease.
- Advise patients against needless or unwise operations.

THE PATIENT'S RIGHTS AND RESPONSIBILITIES

In the United States, patients generally have the right to choose the physician they will see, although some managed care plans may limit choices. They also have the right to terminate a physician's services if they wish. Most states have adopted a version of the American Hospital Association's Patients' Bill of Rights, created in 1973 and revised in 1992, to be used as a list of standards patients can rightfully expect in health care. The Joint Commission on Accreditation of Healthcare Organizations (JCAHO) requires hospitals to post a copy of the AHA's Patients' Bill of Rights, and most managed care organizations also require contracted physicians to post a copy of the bill. This document is *not law* and is separate and distinct from the Patient Bill of Rights the U.S. Congress has considered enacting into law but, to date, has failed to pass.

CHECK YOUR PROGRESS

Cross out the incorrect responses to complete the statements below that pertain to implied contracts between physicians and patients:

17. A physician is/is not obligated to effect a recovery with every patient.

18. A physician is/is not obligated to use due care, skill, and diligence in treating each patient.

19. A physician is/is not obligated to note allergic or adverse reactions to medications reported by a specific patient.

20. A physician is/is not obligated to be as skilled as a specialist if he or she is a general practitioner.

21. A physician is/is not obligated to consider established, customary treatment (standard of care) when treating a patient.

The AHA claims the patient has a right to:

- Receive considerate and respectful care.
- Receive complete current information concerning his or her diagnosis, treatment, and prognosis.
- Receive information necessary to give informed consent prior to the start of any procedure and/or treatment.
- Refuse treatment to the extent permitted by law.
- Receive every consideration of his or her privacy.
- Be assured of confidentiality.
- Obtain reasonable responses to requests for services.
- Obtain information about his or her health care.
- Know whether treatment is experimental and be free to refuse to participate in research projects.

- Expect reasonable continuity of care.
- Examine his or her bill and have it explained.
- Know which hospital rules and regulations apply to patient conduct.

The patient also has certain implied duties to:

- Follow any instructions given by the physician and cooperate as much as possible.
- Give all relevant information to the physician in order to reach a correct diagnosis. If an incorrect diagnosis is made because the patient fails to give the physician the proper information, the physician is not liable.
- Follow the physician's orders for treatment, provided the treatment is similar to that administered by members of the system or school of medicine to which the physician belongs. If a patient willfully or negligently fails to follow the physician's instructions, that patient has little legal recourse.
- Pay the fees charged for services rendered.

TERMINATION OF CONTRACTS

The contract between a physician and a patient is usually terminated (ended) when all treatment has been completed and the bill has been paid. Situations may arise, however, in which premature termination of the contract takes place, as in the following situations:

Failure to Pay for Services. A physician may stop treatment of a patient and end the physician-patient relationship if the patient habitually does not pay or fails to make satisfactory arrangements to pay for medical services, but only if adequate notice is given to the patient.

Failure to Keep Scheduled Appointments. To protect the physician from charges of abandonment, all missed appointments should be noted on the patient's chart.

Failure to Follow the Physician's Instructions. It makes no difference whether the failure is due to a patient's willfulness or negligence.

A Patient Seeks the Services of Another Physician. Whenever a patient acknowledges, orally or in writing, that he or she will seek medical care from another physician, the medical office employee should document this on the patient's chart, and then send a letter to the patient verifying the termination. A copy of the letter should be filed with the patient's records. Seeking a second opinion, however, does not necessarily terminate the physician-patient relationship.

A patient may terminate a physician-patient relationship at any time. After a physician agrees to treat a patient, however, his or her responsibilities to the patient continue until the relationship is properly terminated. If a physician suddenly withdraws from treatment while the patient is still in need of medical care, fails to visit a hospitalized patient, or otherwise abandons the patient without arranging for substitute care, he or she may be charged with abandonment. Depending upon the circumstances, the physician may also be charged with breach of contract and/or negligence.

To properly terminate the physician-patient relationship, the physician must give the patient formal written notice that he or she is withdrawing from the case. The physician should also note any need for the patient to

Lane Medical Center
310 Lane Road
Bedford, Idaho 83210

October 10, 2012

Ted Rowe
Box 1041A
Bedford, Idaho 83210

Dear Mr. Rowe:

This is to inform you of our intent to discontinue medical care to you and the members of your family, due to habitual and continued nonpayment of medical bills. This will go into effect 30 days from the date of this letter, to allow you sufficient time to locate another physician. During this 30-day period, we will require you to pay cash for any care extended to your family. This includes our satellite offices.

We will be happy to forward your medical records to the physician of your choice. There is also 24-hour medical care available to you at the hospital.

If you need assistance in locating a new physician, please contact the Idaho Medical Society at 1-800-666-7777.

Sincerely,

P. White

Patricia White, M.D.

FIGURE 3-7   Physician's Letter of Dismissal for Nonpayment

receive continued medical care. In addition, the patient must be given time to find another physician. The notice of discharge of withdrawal should be sent by certified mail, return receipt requested, and a copy should be filed with the patient's records. Figure 3-7 illustrates a notice of termination.

Managed care plans *may* restrict a physician from terminating patient care without the approval of the managed care plan.

LAW OF AGENCY

law of agency The law that governs the relationship between a principal and his or her agent.

agent One who acts for or represents another. In performing workplace duties, the employee acts as the agent, or authorized representative, of the employer.

By law, employers are liable for the actions of their employees when employees perform said actions as part of their work under the supervision of the employer. This is called the **law of agency.** In performing workplace duties, the employee acts as the **agent** of the employer.

Agency may be expressed or implied. In the medical office, it is most often implied. Medical office employees act as the physician's agent when they schedule appointments, speak with patients and other individuals, order supplies for the office, or otherwise perform duties ordered by and supervised by the employing physician in the conduct of his or her business.

respondeat superior
Literally, "Let the master answer." A doctrine under which an employer is legally liable for the acts of his or her employees, if such acts were performed within the scope of the employees' duties.

Under the doctrine of ***respondeat superior,*** or "Let the master answer," physicians are liable for the acts of their employees performed "within the course and scope" of employment. Therefore, health care practitioners must avoid making promises their employers cannot keep.

Ethics Issues

Law, the Courts, and Contracts

ETHICS ISSUE 1: Advertising by health care providers used to be considered inappropriate and unprofessional. However, now advertising by health care providers is commonplace and accepted by the various professional organizations, as long as there are no false or misleading statements.

DISCUSSION QUESTIONS

1. A dentist advertises that he specializes in creating "dazzling smiles." In your opinion, is this an ethical advertisement? Explain your answer.

_____

_____

_____

2. A chiropractor advertises "miracle" treatments to alleviate back pain. In your opinion, is this an ethical advertisement? Explain your answer.

_____

_____

3. Check your local newspaper for advertising by health care providers. Listen carefully to television ads by health care providers. Bring to class at least two ads from the newspaper and notes from the ads you listened to on television. Be sure to sort out ads that are for providers and those that are for prescription or nonprescription drugs. Are those ads misleading? Do they make promises that cannot be kept? Explain your answer.

_____

_____

4. Study the print ads and notes from television ads you collected for the above exercise. Choose two as examples. What advantages and disadvantages for consumers can you see to the ads?

_____

_____

_____

5. What advantages and disadvantages for health care practitioners can you see to the ads?

_____

_____

_____

ETHICS ISSUE 2: The patient-physician relationship is contractual in nature. That means that either the physician or the patient may terminate the relationship. The physician must abide by certain rules when terminating an established relationship, but the patient is free to terminate the relationship at any time. Physicians may decline to undertake the care of a patient whose medical condition is not within the physician's current competence. Physicians may not decline to accept patients because of race, color, religion, national origin, or sexual orientation, or on any other basis that would constitute individual discrimination.

DISCUSSION QUESTION

1. A dental hygienist refuses to work on a patient because he has revealed that he is HIV positive. Is her decision ethical? Explain your answer.

_____

_____

_____

ETHICS ISSUE 3: While in private practice, physicians may determine that they will not accept certain new patients because of their inability to pay or because they have an insurance plan with a poor reimbursement policy.

DISCUSSION QUESTION

1. Should all physicians be required to accept a certain number of patients that cannot pay their bills? In other words, should physicians be required to do a certain amount of charity care? Explain your answer.

_____

_____

_____

ETHICS ISSUE 4: The first objective and the primary goal of every code of ethics and ethics guideline for health care practitioners is the *welfare of the patient*.

DISCUSSION QUESTION

1. A nursing assistant working under the supervision of an RN in a hospital has witnessed several occasions when the RN behaves abusively to elderly patients. What should the nursing assistant do?

_____

_____

_____

Go to www.mhhe.com/judson5e to practice your case review skills. Then read on for more information.

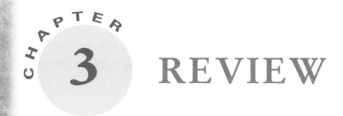
Applying Knowledge

Answer the following questions in the spaces provided.

1. List and define three functions a state government *can* assume.

_____

_____

_____

2. Which governmental functions are reserved strictly for the federal government?

_____

_____

_____

3. Define *common law.*

_____

_____

4. Define *administrative law.*

_____

_____

5. Decisions made by judges in the various courts and used as a guide for future decisions are called

_____

6. Distinguish between substantive and procedural law.

_____

_____

7. Distinguish between criminal and civil law.

_____

_____

8. May a civil offense also be a crime? Explain your answer, giving one example.

_____

_____

9. Define *jurisdiction.*

_____

_____

10. Define *tort.*

_____

_____

11. Define *tortfeasor.*

_____

_____

12. Distinguish between intentional and unintentional torts.

_____

_____

_____

13. An unintentional tort alleging that a health care practitioner has failed to exercise ordinary care is called

_____

14. If a physician examines a patient without consent, can he or she be charged with an offense? Explain your answer.

_____

_____

15. Are health care practitioners legally liable for all unsatisfactory medical outcomes? Explain your answer.

_____

_____

16. Define *contract.*

_____

_____

17. List and briefly define the four essential elements of a contract.

_____

_____

_____

_____

18. List those situations in which a contract may be voidable.

_____

_____

19. Under what circumstances may breach of contract be charged?

_____

_____

20. Briefly explain the purpose of the Statute of Frauds.

_____

_____

21. Define *third party payor contract.*

_____

_____

22. Regulation Z of the Consumer Protection Act of 1968 requires that certain financial arrangements be in writing and include

_____

23. What is the Fair Debt Collection Practices Act?

_____

_____

_____

24. Give an example of an implied limited contract.

_____

_____

25. List ten items to which a physician is *not* bound contractually in the context of an implied physician-patient contract.

_____   _____

_____   _____

_____   _____

_____   _____

_____   _____

26. List ten items to which a physician is obligated in an implied physician-patient contract.

_____   _____

_____   _____

_____   _____

_____   _____

_____   _____

27. List five responsibilities borne by the patient in an implied contract.

_____

_____

_____

_____

_____

28. Name four situations in which premature termination of the physician-patient contract may occur.

_____

_____

_____

_____

29. Why must a physician give the patient ample notice when withdrawing from a case?

_____

_____

30. Briefly explain how the law of agency applies to health care practitioners.

_____

_____

31. How does the doctrine of *respondeat superior* relate to the law of agency?

_____

_____

Case Study

Use your critical-thinking skills to answer the questions that follow each of the case studies.
Dan, a medical office assistant in a busy clinic, is a sympathetic and understanding employee. Therefore, when an elderly patient complained to him that she "felt terrible most of the time," Dan consoled her. "Don't worry, Mrs. Smith," he told the woman. "Dr. Jones will make you feel better in no time."

32. Has Dan, acting as Dr. Jones's agent, created an implied contract with Mrs. Smith? Explain your answer.

_____

_____

33. If so, can Mrs. Smith sue Dr. Jones if he fails to fulfill the "terms" of the contract? Explain your answer.

_____

_____

34. How might you respond to a patient under similar circumstances?

_____

_____

35. A physician was notified that the extension he had built on his house to serve as his office violated the town's zoning law. Has he committed a crime? If so, what kind?

_____

_____

36. Does a patient have the legal right to leave the hospital, even though his or her physician believes treatment is incomplete? Explain your answer.

_____

_____

37. Does a patient have the right to know if medical treatment is experimental and to refuse to participate in such treatment? Explain your answer.

_____

_____

An internist had a 54-year-old obese patient who smoked and had a stressful job. After he died of a heart attack, an autopsy revealed that the overweight man had coronary artery disease. The patient's family sued the physician for negligence and won a $3.5 million judgment against the internist. During jury deliberations, some jurors who heard testimony in the case argued that the physician did everything possible to try to help the patient, but others maintained that he could have done more.

38. In your opinion, was the internist negligent for not referring this patient to a cardiologist, as the patient's wife claimed in court? Why or why not?

_____

_____

_____

39. In your opinion, does this case show that people need to take more personal responsibility for what they do to their bodies? Explain your answer.

_____

_____

_____

Internet Activities

Visit the recommended Web sites and answer the questions that follow.

40. Find a Web site that defines the term *affidavit*. Briefly explain the term and describe a situation in which a health care professional may have to give an affidavit.

_____

_____

_____

41. Visit the Web site for the U.S. House of Representatives. List any health care legislation currently pending before the House that you believe is relevant to the health care profession you will practice.

_____

_____

_____

42. List two additional Web sites where information about health care legislation can be found.

_____

_____

_____

2

Legal Issues for Working Health Care Practitioners

Professional Liability and Medical Malpractice

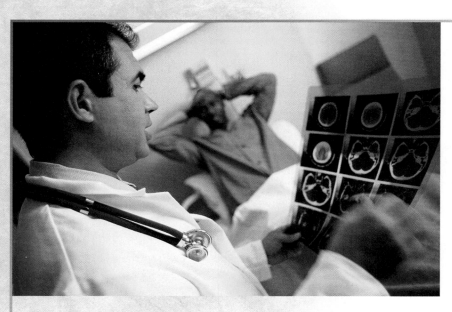

Learning Outcomes

After studying this chapter, you should be able to:

1. Identify three areas of general liability for which a physician/employer is responsible.

2. Describe the reasonable person standard, standard of care, and duty of care.

3. Briefly outline the responsibilities of health care practitioners concerning privacy, confidentiality, and privileged communication. (More detail is provided in Chapter 7.)

4. List the four elements necessary to prove negligence (the four Ds), and explain them.

5. Outline the phases of a lawsuit.

6. Name two advantages to alternative dispute resolution.

Key Terms

alternative dispute resolution (ADR)

confidentiality

damages

deposition

duty of care

interrogatory

liable

malfeasance

misfeasance

nonfeasance

privileged communication

res ipsa loquitur

standard of care

subpoena

subpoena *duces tecum*

summons

testimony

wrongful death statutes

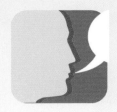

Voice of Experience
Talking Outside of Work Can Result in Lawsuits

Tina, a medical records supervisor in a small-town medical clinic, always spends a lot of time with new employees reviewing the importance of confidentiality. One of her real-life lessons is about the new employee, Samantha, who accidentally and innocently violated confidentiality, causing the clinic where she worked to be sued.

Samantha saw one of her high school friends in the hallway of the clinic. The friend told Samantha that she was pregnant. A week later, Samantha saw her friend's mother in the local grocery store and congratulated her on becoming a grandmother. What Samantha did not know was that her friend was not planning to continue the pregnancy and had told no one that she was pregnant. The clinic was sued for violating confidentiality. Tina's strong advice to all employees has since become: "What you learn in this clinic **stays** in this clinic."

LIABILITY

liable Accountable under the law.

All competent adults are **liable,** or legally responsible, for their own acts, both on the job and in their private lives. As homeowners and operators of automobiles, we carry liability insurance in case someone is injured in our homes or we are involved in a car accident. In the workplace, employers carry liability insurance to cover situations in which employees, or anyone else on the premises, may be injured or harmed.

As employers, physicians have general liability for

The Practice's Building and Grounds. Adequate upkeep will help ensure that employees and patients are not injured on the premises. Employers must provide protection against theft, fire, and burglary in the building and must take all precautions to ensure that patients' records are protected. Theft, fire, and liability insurance to cover the workplace is a must for the physician/employer.

Automobiles. If employees must use their own or the physician's automobile in the performance of their daily work (for example, to drop off or pick up mail or supplies), the employer must be adequately insured for liability in the event of an accident.

Employee Safety. Employers must provide a reasonably comfortable and safe work environment for employees. State (and, in some instances, federal) regulations apply, but they vary from state to state. Employers should check with the state agency governing safety in the workplace, with workers' compensation laws, and with state medical societies to determine safety rules, rights, and responsibilities. A general safety procedure book for medical office workers should include guidelines for the handling of hazardous laboratory wastes and materials.

Might the outcome of the following court case have been different if the employing physician practice group had owned the parking lot where the employee fell?

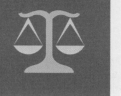
STANDARD OF CARE AND DUTY OF CARE

Standard of care The level of performance expected of a health care practitioner in carrying out his or her professional duties.

Duty of care The legal obligation of health care workers to patients and, sometimes, nonpatients.

Standard of care refers to the level of performance expected of a health care practitioner in carrying out his or her professional duties. **Duty of care** is the obligation of health care workers to patients and, in some case, nonpatients. Physicians have a duty of care to patients with whom they have established a doctor-patient relationship, but they may also be held to a duty of care toward people who are not patients, such as the patient's family members, former patients, and even office personnel. Generally, if actions or omissions within the scope of a health care practitioner's job could cause harm to someone, that person is owed a duty of care.

For example, medical facility custodians are nonpatients to whom a duty of care is owed. Various drugs, equipment, and supplies are used and discarded daily in a medical facility. Procedures for the proper disposal of drugs and potentially hazardous materials should be detailed in a facility's safety manual (Figure 4-1), so that employees who handle these materials do not accidentally prick themselves with used needles or otherwise injure themselves.

In some instances, depending on the situation and state law, physicians may have a duty under standard of care to warn nonpatients of danger, as in the case of a psychiatric patient who threatens harm to others or in the case of a patient with a communicable disease. The following court case illustrates that state law must be followed when courts make decisions.

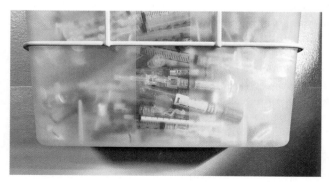

FIGURE 4-1 Proper disposal of hazardous and medical wastes helps protect all medical facility employees.

Court Case

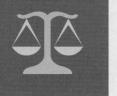

Father Sues Son's Psychiatrist

A psychiatrist evaluated a man and found his condition did not meet the legal requirements for involuntary commitment to a mental institution. The man was released from temporary confinement in a mental hospital, and he killed his wife and then killed himself. The man's father filed a medical negligence action on behalf of his son's and his daughter-in-law's estates alleging that the defendant psychiatrist negligently evaluated the son, failed to adequately assess the son, and failed to commit the son to a mental institution.

The jury in the trial court found for the psychiatrist. The father appealed and the psychiatrist cross-appealed.

Since the state in which the psychiatrist practiced did not recognize a psychiatrist's duty to warn third persons, the related involuntary commitment statutes were not public safety statutes and thus, any violation thereof could not be considered negligence per se. The father was denied a new trial.

Estates of Gregory and Gregory v. Kilbride, 150 N.C. App. 601; 565 S.E.2d 685; 2002 N.C. App. LEXIS 685, June 18, 2002.

As explained in Chapter 3, we are responsible for our actions (or our failure to act) under the reasonable person standard. That is, we may be charged with negligence if someone is injured because we failed to perform an act that a reasonable person, in similar circumstances, would perform or if we committed an act that a reasonable person would not commit. Professionals—those individuals who are specially trained to perform specific tasks—are held to a higher standard of care than nonprofessionals (laypersons). If a patient is injured because a health care professional failed to exercise the care and expertise that under the circumstances could reasonably be expected of a professional with similar experience and training, then that professional may be liable for negligence.

Court Case

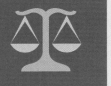

Perfusionist and Hospital Liable

When a couple's two-month-old baby experienced respiratory distress, they took him to the hospital. The baby had a heart murmur, and surgery was recommended. During surgery, the perfusionist, a technician responsible for oxygenation of the patient's blood, made critical mistakes while operating a heart-lung machine. As a result, the flow of oxygen to the patient's brain was stopped, causing brain damage. The child, six years old when this case was finally settled, suffered from cerebral palsy, clinical blindness, loss of speech, and mental retardation.

A trial court ruled that although the perfusionist was the employee of a subcontractor at the time of the child's injuries, the hospital was not absolved of vicarious liability for the technician's negligence.

The case went back to a trial court, and a jury handed down a $10.8 million verdict against the hospital. The family settled with the perfusionist out of court for $2 million.

Shands Teaching Hospital and Clinic, Inc. v. Juliana, Case # 1002-1530, Ct. of App. Of Florida, 1st Dist., 2003 Fla. App. LEXIS 10157.

Physicians

A physician in general practice is expected to conform to the standards of other general practitioners in his or her own or a comparable community. A specialist is held to a higher standard of care than that expected of a general practitioner. The standard of care for a specialist is generally the same as those for like specialists, wherever they practice. Similarly, any health care practitioner—nurse, phlebotomist, dental assistant, physician assistant—is expected to conform to the standards of like practitioners in his or her own or a comparable community.

Direct patient contact is not always necessary for establishing a duty, as the following case illustrates.

Courts have generally held that informal consultations among physicians do not create a doctor-patient relationship and thus do not create a duty of care, as in the classic case discussed below.

Court Case

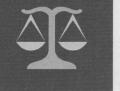

Duty Established by Referral

A plastic surgeon examined a patient in a hospital emergency department. An X-ray of the patient's knee revealed a possible malignant neoplasm, so the plastic surgeon referred the patient to an orthopedist, but did not tell the patient why. The patient did not keep any of the three appointments he scheduled with the orthopedist, and the orthopedist refused to reschedule him.

The patient died of cancer, and his estate sued the two physicians. A lower court granted summary judgment to the orthopedist, but an appeals court reversed, holding that a doctor-patient relationship began when the orthopedist accepted the referral and scheduled the patient for an appointment. The court also said that "a letter to plaintiff advising him of his condition and to consult with another physician without delay might well have been sufficient" to discharge the duty to the patient.

Davis v. Weiskopf, 108 Ill; App. 3rd 505, 439 N.E.2nd 60, (ILL. App. Ct. 2nd Dist. 1982).

CLASSIC
Court Case

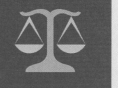

Consultation Did Not Establish a Duty of Care

The doctrine that informal physician consultations do not create a doctor-patient relationship was established in 1973 in the California decision *Ranier v. Grossman.* Morton Grossman was a professor of gastroenterology who often lectured physicians at their hospitals, then offered to review their cases with them. After one such lecture, a physician presented the X-rays and medical history for a patient who suffered from ulcerative colitis. Grossman advised surgery without examining the patient. The surgery was subsequently performed, and the patient sued, claiming that the surgery had been unnecessary. Grossman was cited as a codefendant in the patient's lawsuit. An appeals court upheld summary judgment in Grossman's favor, holding that he had no duty to the patient because he had no direct contact with her and had no control over her treating physicians.

Ranier v. Grossman, Ct. of App. 2nd Dist., 31 Cal. App. 3rd 539, April 11, 1973.

Guidelines for Physicians and Other Health Care Practitioners

The following guidelines can help all health care practitioners to stay within the scope of their practices and operate within the law and the policy of any employing health care facility. All are addressed at length throughout the text.

- Practice within the scope of your training and capabilities.
- Use the professional title commensurate with your education and experience.
- Maintain confidentiality.
- Prepare and maintain health records.
- Document accurately.
- Use appropriate legal and ethical guidelines when releasing information.
- Follow an employer's established policies dealing with the health care contract.
- Follow legal guidelines and maintain awareness of health care legislation and regulations.
- Maintain and dispose of regulated substances in compliance with government guidelines.
- Follow established risk-management and safety procedures.
- Meet the requirements for professional credentialing.
- Help to develop and maintain personnel, policy, and procedure manuals.

Laws clearly dictate what a member of a heath care profession can and cannot do on the job. However, in addition to knowing the law, a health care practitioner should know what policies and procedures apply specifically to his or her place of employment. Policy and procedure manuals that clearly define a health care practitioner's responsibilities can serve as a valuable guide and as evidence that policies and procedures are in writing if legal suits should arise.

CHECK YOUR PROGRESS

1. As employers, physicians have general liability for

_____

_____

Write "T" or "F" in the blank to indicate whether you think the statement is true or false.

_____ 2. *Standard of care* refers to the level of performance expected of a health care practitioner in carrying out his or her professional duties.

_____ 3. *Duty of care* is the obligation of health care practitioners to patients but never applies to nonpatients.

_____ 4. An obstetrician who helps deliver a baby to a woman who happens to be riding with him in a taxicab would be held to the reasonable person standard.

_____ 5. Policies and procedures of the employing medical facility, as well as the law, should be considered when a health care practitioner performs his or her duties.

PRIVACY, CONFIDENTIALITY, AND PRIVILEGED COMMUNICATION

confidentiality The act of holding information in confidence, not to be released to unauthorized individuals.

privileged communication Information held confidential within a protected relationship.

Not only do physicians and other health care professionals owe a duty of care to patients, but it is also their ethical and legal duty to safeguard a patient's privacy and maintain **confidentiality.**

Privileged communication refers to information held confidential within a protected relationship. Attorney-client and physician-patient are examples of relationships in which the law, under certain circumstances, protects the holder of information from forced disclosure on the witness stand. Privileged communication statutes vary from state to state, but in most states, patients may sue a physician or any other health care practitioner for breach of confidence if the holder released protected information and damage to the patient resulted. In many states, breach of confidence is grounds for revocation of a physician's license.

Since health care procedures and facilities present numerous opportunities for a breach of confidentiality, health care practitioners must make every effort to safeguard each patient's privacy. Privacy, confidentiality, and privileged communication are such important subjects for health care practitioners that they are discussed separately, in Chapter 7, "Privacy Law and HIPAA." Chapter 7 also includes a discussion of the many requirements of the Health Insurance Portability and Accountability Act (HIPAA).

The following suggestions for maintaining confidentiality of patient health care records can serve as a guide for all health care practitioners who may be asked to provide or release patient information:

- Do not disclose any information about a patient to a third party without signed consent. This extends to insurance companies, attorneys, and curious neighbors, and it includes acknowledging whether or not the person in question is a patient.

- Do not decide confidentiality on the basis of whether or not you approve of or agree with the views or morals of the patient.

- Do not reveal financial information about a patient, since this is also confidential. For instance, be discreet when revealing a patient's account balance so that others in the vicinity do not overhear.

- When talking on the telephone with a patient, do not use the patient's name if others in the room might overhear.

- Use caution in giving the results of medical tests to patients over the telephone to prevent others in the medical office from overhearing. Furthermore, when leaving a message on a home answering machine or at a patient's place of employment, simply ask the patient to return a call regarding a recent visit or appointment on a specific date. No mention should be made of the nature of the call. It is inadvisable to leave a message with a receptionist or coworker on an answering machine for the patient to call an oncologist, an obstetrician/gynecologist, and so forth. If test results are abnormal, usually the physician speaks directly to the patient, and an appointment is made to discuss the results.

- Do not leave medical charts or insurance reports out where patients or office visitors can see them. See that confidentiality protocol is duly noted in the office procedures manual, and make sure new employees learn it.

- If a patient is unwilling to release privileged information, the information should not be released. Exceptions include legally required disclosures, such as those ordered by subpoena; those dictated by statute to protect public health or welfare; or those considered necessary to protect the welfare of a patient or a third party.

Confidentiality may be waived under the following circumstances:

- Sometimes when a third party requests a medical examination, such as for employment, and that party pays the physician's fee.
- Generally when a patient sues a physician for malpractice and patient records are subpoenaed.
- When a waiver has been signed by the patient allowing the release of information (see Figure 4-2).

The issue of confidentiality is not always clear-cut. For example, are autopsy records protected as medical records, or are they considered public record and, therefore, subject to release upon demand? The following court case shows how one court decision answered that question.

Court Case

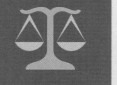

Newspaper Cannot Get Autopsy Photos

On February 18, 2001, while he was driving the last lap of the Daytona 500 race at the Daytona International Speedway, NASCAR driver Dale Earnhardt's car struck the wall, and he was killed instantly. An autopsy was performed the following day.

Since the *Orlando Sentinel* had been running a series of articles about NASCAR safety, the newspaper requested copies of Earnhardt's autopsy photos so that a medical examiner it had hired could determine if wearing the HANS device for head stabilization might have saved the race car driver's life. Upon learning of the *Sentinel's* request, Dale Earnhardt's widow, Teresa, filed suit in Volusia County Circuit Court seeking an injunction to prevent the *Sentinel's* representative from examining the photos. Mrs. Earnhardt claimed that releasing the photos would violate the Earnhardt family's privacy. The Circuit Court judge granted a temporary injunction, stating that the family's privacy interest outweighed the public interest in seeing the photographs.

Before the case was settled, the Florida legislature passed a law, known as the Earnhardt Family Protection Act, that allows autopsy photographs or recordings of the autopsy to be examined only by a surviving spouse, parent, or child. Anyone else must obtain a court order and examine the materials under the "direct supervision of the custodian." Exceptions were made for some service providers, such as the medical examiner and state or federal agencies performing official duties. The law restricted access to such information by journalists and others.

Mrs. Earnhardt settled her suit against the *Orlando Sentinel* on March 16, 2001. An independent medical expert could examine Earnhardt's autopsy photos; then the photos would be permanently sealed.

Several news organizations challenged the constitutionality of the Earnhardt Family Protection Act, but the law has been upheld in Florida as constitutional.

Earnhardt v. Volusia County Office of the Medical Examiner, Case No. 2001-30373-C1C1 (Fla.Cir.Ct.).

I authorize: Name of person or institution _____

                                                                                (Provider of information)

                   Street address _____

                   City, state, Zip Code _____

To release medical information to:

                   Name of person or institution: _____

                                                                                (Recipient of information)

                   Street address _____

                   City, state, Zip Code _____

                   Attention: _____

Nature of information to be disclosed:

                   ☐ Clinical notes pertaining to evaluation and treatment
                   ☐ Other, please specify _____

Purpose of disclosure:

                   ☐ Continuing medical care
                   ☐ Second opinion
                   ☐ Other, please specify _____

This authorization will automatically expire one year from the date of signature, unless specified otherwise _____

This consent may be revoked at any time by sending written notice to the above-named provider of information. Any release of information made prior to the revocation of this compliant authorization is not a breach of confidentiality. Disclosed information may be reviewed by contacting the provider of information.

Patient's name _____

Signature of patient or legal guardian _____ Date _____

Complete address _____

Relationship, if not the patient _____ Patient's date of birth _____

SPECIFIC CONSENT FOR RELEASE OF INFORMATION
PROTECTED BY STATE OR FEDERAL LAW

Iowa law (and in some cases federal law) provides special confidentiality protection to information relating to substance abuse, mental health, and HIV-related testing. In order for information to be released on this subject matter, this specific authorization and the above authorization must be signed:

I authorize release of information relating to:

☐ Substance abuse (alcohol/drug abuse)
   Signature of patient or legal guardian

   _____ Date _____

☐ Mental health (includes psychological testing and mental health counseling)
   Signature of patient or legal guardian

   _____ Date _____

☐ HIV-related information (AIDS-related testing)
   Signature of patient or legal guardian

   _____ Date _____

Date information is sent _____ Sent by (name) _____

To the recipient of this information: This information has been disclosed to you from records protected by federal confidentiality rules. The federal rules prohibit you from making further disclosure without additional consent.

FIGURE 4-2   Consent to Release Information

THE TORT OF NEGLIGENCE

The unintentional tort of negligence is the basis for professional malpractice claims and is the most common liability in medicine. When health care practitioners are sued for medical malpractice, the term generally means any deviation from the accepted medical standard of care that causes injury to a patient.

In a court case decided in 1965 (see the Classic Court Case below), for the first time a hospital was found guilty of negligence. Since then, under the theory of corporate liability, hospitals have been found to have an independent duty to patients, including a duty to grant privileges only to competent doctors, to supervise the overall medical treatment of patients, and to review the competence of staff physicians.

All medical professional liability claims are classified in one of three ways, based upon the root word *feasance,* which means "the performance of an act."

malfeasance The performance of a totally wrongful and unlawful act.

Malfeasance. The performance of a totally wrongful and unlawful act. For example, in the absence of the employing physician, a medical assistant determines that a patient needs a prescription drug and dispenses the wrong drug from the physician's supply. Medical assistants are not licensed to practice medicine, and the wrong drug was dispensed, so the act was totally wrongful and unlawful and could be called malfeasance.

misfeasance The performance of a lawful act in an illegal or improper manner.

Misfeasance. The performance of a lawful act in an illegal or improper manner. Suppose a physician orders his or her nurse-employee to change a sterile dressing on a patient's burned hand. The nurse changes the dressing but does not use sterile technique, and the patient's burn becomes infected. The nurse is legally authorized to carry out the physician's instructions in dressing the patient's hand, but violated proper procedure in carrying out the physician's order.

nonfeasance The failure to act when one should.

Nonfeasance. The failure to act when one should. For example, a newly certified emergency medical technician is first upon the scene of a traffic accident. An injured motorist stops breathing and appears to be in cardiac arrest. The EMT, though trained in cardiopulmonary resuscitation, "freezes" and does nothing. The patient dies. In failing to act, the EMT could be guilty of nonfeasance.

There are four elements that must be present in a given situation to prove that a health care professional is guilty of negligence. Sometimes called the "four Ds of negligence," these elements include

- *Duty*—The person charged with negligence owed a duty of care to the accuser.
- *Dereliction*—The health care provider breached the duty of care to the patient.
- *Direct Cause*—The breach of the duty of care to the patient was a direct cause of the patient's injury.
- *Damages*—There is a legally recognizable injury to the patient.

When a plaintiff sues a health care practitioner (defendant) for negligence, the burden of proof is on the plaintiff. That is, it is up to the accuser's attorney to present evidence of the four Ds.

State statutes must be consulted for restrictions that apply to actions against health care providers. Some states limit damage awards or mandate procedural rules that must be followed in medical malpractice claims. In some states, for example, medical review panels must screen claims before

Court Case

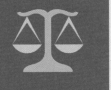

Hospital Found Negligent

A patient was admitted to a small hospital's emergency room in southern Illinois with a broken leg. The treating doctor was not an orthopedic specialist, and complications developed. The patient developed gangrene in the injured leg, and it was amputated.

In a lawsuit the patient brought against the hospital, the hospital was required to pay damages when the court decided that the facility was negligent in permitting the treating doctor to do orthopedic work and in not requiring him to review his operative procedures to be sure they were current. The hospital was also found negligent in failing to exercise adequate supervision in the case and in not requiring consultation, especially after complications developed.

Darling v. Charleston Community Hospital, 211 N.E.2d 253 (Ill., 1965).

they are brought to court. The panel examines the facts and then issues a finding of "malpractice" or "no malpractice." Such panels are generally composed of physicians with expertise in the medical specialty in question and sometimes include a neutral attorney.

Court Case

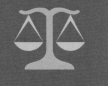

Patient Falls and Sues Hospital

A woman attempted suicide by overdosing on medication. She was taken to the emergency room of a local hospital. The medical staff there determined that she posed a danger to herself and placed her on a 72-hour hold. Hospital authorities also contacted the woman's primary care physician, who requested that she be admitted to the hospital for treatment related to her overdose. During the 72-hour hold, a nurse following a physician's order assisted the patient as she walked down a hospital corridor. The woman was wearing a rubber slipper that caught on the floor, causing her to fall and fracture a bone in her leg. The patient sued the hospital for negligence and premises liability. Her negligence claim alleged that the hospital "negligently and carelessly failed to supervise and monitor her while she was making a doctor-ordered walk down the hospital corridor." She also alleged that the defendants "knew, . . . or should have known, that she was likely to fall . . . as a result of her physical and mental condition, and that a substance on the floor caused her to fall."

The trial court granted the hospital's motion for summary judgment on the ground that the patient's causes of action were barred by the state's hospital immunity law, which granted the hospital immunity from liability . . . provided in connection with a lawfully initiated 72-hour hold. The woman appealed the court's judgment.

The state Court of Appeal reversed the judgment of the lower court. The court held that the patient's allegation that the hospital's negligence during the 72-hour hold caused her injuries was not related to the hospital's immunity under the "hold" law.

Note: A final disposition of this case has not been published. Either the hospital settled with the plaintiff out of court, or the case was scheduled to be heard again in a lower court and that action has not been published.

Jacobs v. Grossmont Hospital, 433 Cal.2d.9, CA (2003).

JCAHO Standards on Medical Mistakes and Patient Safety

Avoiding medical mistakes and safeguarding patients while they are being examined or treated are vital issues for health care practitioners, both to ensure excellent patient care and to avoid issues of medical malpractice liability.

While conscientious health care practitioners do their best to avoid making mistakes, they are human, and mistakes do occur. The legal and ethical response when health care mistakes are made is to report the mistake to attending physicians and supervisors and on the patient's medical record, and to tell the patient he or she has been harmed. In fact, health care practitioners and health care facilities that try to cover up mistakes are most likely to be sued, and hospitals and other facilities that fail to disclose mistakes could lose their Joint Commission on Accreditation of Healthcare Organizations (JCAHO) accreditation.

To further address patient safety, as of January 1, 2004, all JCAHO accredited health care organizations are surveyed for implementation of the following requirements:

1. Improve the accuracy of patient identification.

   ▪ Use at least two patient identifiers whenever taking blood samples or administering medications or blood products. Do not use a hospital patient's room number as an identifier.
   ▪ Prior to the start of any surgical or invasive procedure, confirm the correct patient, procedure and site, using active—not passive—communication.

2. Improve the effectiveness of communication among caregivers (Figure 4-3).

   ▪ Use a process for taking verbal or telephone orders or critical test results that requires a verification read-back by the person receiving the information.
   ▪ Standardize abbreviations, acronyms, and symbols used throughout the organization, including a list of all such terms that are *not* to be used.

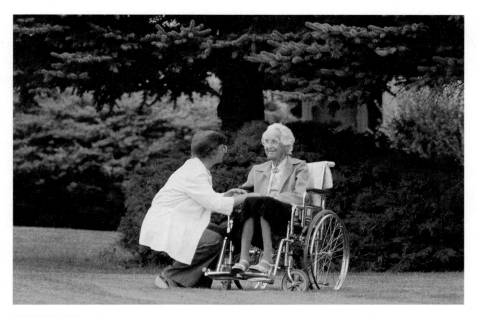

FIGURE 4-3 Listening to a patient's concerns is vital in maintaining a desirable doctor-patient relationship.

3. Improve the safety of using high-alert medications.
   ▌ Remove concentrated electrolytes (including, but not limited to, potassium chloride, potassium phosphate, and sodium chloride) from patient care units.
   ▌ Standardize and limit the number of drug concentrations available in the organization.
4. Eliminate wrong-site, wrong-patient, wrong-procedure surgery.
   ▌ Create and use a preoperative verification process, such as a checklist, to confirm that appropriate documents, such as medical records and imaging studies, are available.
   ▌ Use procedures to mark the surgical site and involve the patient in the marking process.
5. Improve the safety of using infusion pumps.
   ▌ Ensure free-flow protection on all general-use and patient-controlled analgesia intravenous infusion pumps.
6. Improve the effectiveness of clinical alarm systems.
   ▌ Use regular preventative maintenance and testing of alarm systems.
   ▌ Be sure that alarms are activated with appropriate settings and can be heard over distances and competing noise within a care unit.
7. Reduce the risk of health care–acquired infections.
   ▌ Comply with current Centers for Disease Control and Prevention (CDC) hand hygiene guidelines.
   ▌ Manage as sentinel events all identified cases of unanticipated death or major permanent loss of function associated with a health care–acquired infection.

JCAHO established these requirements to help accredited health care organizations address issues of patient safety that can lead to adverse events that, in turn, can result in lawsuits.

CHECK YOUR PROGRESS

6. Define *privileged communication*.

_____

_____

7. Is a breach of confidentiality an offense for which a health care practitioner can be sued? Explain your answer.

_____

_____

8. Distinguish among *malfeasance, misfeasance,* and *nonfeasance*.

_____

_____

_____

9. Name the four Ds of negligence.

_____

_____

_____

_____

res ipsa loquitur "The thing speaks for itself"; also known as the doctrine of common knowledge. A situation that is so obviously negligent that no expert witnesses need be called.

Res Ipsa Loquitur

Res ipsa loquitur is Latin for "the thing speaks for itself." It is also known as the doctrine of common knowledge. It means that the mistake is so obvious—such as leaving a sponge or surgical instrument inside a patient after surgery or operating on the wrong body part—that negligence is obvious. Because the fact that a mistake was made is not debatable, expert witnesses need not be called to testify in a medical malpractice lawsuit alleging *res ipsa loquitur*. However, for this doctrine to apply, three conditions must exist:

1. The act of negligence must obviously be under the defendant's control.
2. The patient must not have contributed to the act.
3. It must be apparent that the patient would not have been injured if reasonable care had been used.

Cases that fall under the doctrine of *res ipsa loquitur* include

- Unintentionally leaving foreign bodies, such as sponges or instruments, inside a patient's body during surgery.
- Accidentally burning or otherwise injuring a patient while he or she is anesthetized.
- Damaging healthy tissue during an operation.
- Causing an infection by the use of unsterilized instruments.

Damage Awards and Medical Malpractice Insurance

When a defendant is found guilty of a tort—such as negligence, breach of contract, libel, or slander—the plaintiff is awarded compensation based upon the extent of his or her injuries, loss of income, damage to reputation, or other harm that can be proved. This monetary compensation is called **damages.** Table 4-1 explains the various types of damages and how the court determines them.

damages Monetary awards sought by plaintiffs in lawsuits.

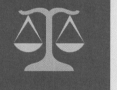

Court Case

Res Ipsa Loquitur Applied

A plaintiff had a total right knee replacement (arthroplasty) at a Missouri hospital under general anesthesia. Upon awakening from anesthesia, the patient immediately experienced pain in her right hand, arm, and shoulder. She sued the hospital and her physician for medical malpractice. Because the patient was under anesthesia during the event, and therefore unable to identify specific acts of negligence, she sued under the doctrine of *res ipsa loquitur*. Defendants moved for summary judgment, which the trial court granted because there was no expert testimony to show the specific injury-causing act. Plaintiff appealed. The appellate court concluded that the trial court erred in granting summary judgment for the defendants, holding that the plaintiff had established the three elements of *res ipsa loquitur*, therefore inferring the defendants' negligence.

The appellate court sent the matter back to the trial court for further proceedings consistent with a *res ipsa loquitur* filing.

Note: To date, no final disposition has been published. An out-of-court settlement could have occurred, or the new trial could have been scheduled for a future date, not yet reached.

Zumwalt v. Koreckij, 24 S.W.3d 166 (Mo. Ct. App., 2000).

10. Expert witnesses do not need to testify in order for a plaintiff to establish

_____

_____

11. _Res ipsa loquitur_ means

_____

_____

12. Name two types of cases that fall under the doctrine of _res ipsa loquitur._

_____

_____

Physicians and many other professional health care providers carry liability insurance, which pays damage awards in the event of a negligence or malpractice suit up to the limits of the policy.

Medical groups maintain that high damage awards in tort cases have led to a malpractice insurance crisis for physicians, especially those in high-risk specialties, such as obstetrics-gynecology, orthopedic surgery, and general surgery. Recent studies and news articles have reported that doctors in some states are participating in walkouts and demonstrations, relocating to states where caps have been legislated on medical malpractice damage awards, limiting procedures, performing additional patient tests

TABLE 4-1 Damage Awards

Types of Damages	Purpose	Considered by Court	Award
General compensatory	To compensate for injuries or losses due to violation of patient's rights.	Physical disability? Loss of earnings? Mental anguish? Loss of service of spouse or child? Losses to date? Future losses?	Specified by court. Dollar value need not be proved; loss must be proved.
Special compensatory	To compensate for losses not directly caused by the wrong.	Additional medical expenses?	Specified by court. Dollar value and loss must be proved.
Consequential	To compensate for losses caused indirectly by a product defect.	Loss covered by product warranty? Personal injury?	No limit on damages if personal injuries.
Punitive	To punish the offender.	How serious was the breach of conduct? How much can the defendant afford to pay?	In some cases, amount of damages is set by law.
Nominal	To recognize that rights of the patient were violated, though no actual loss was proved.	Legal rights of the patient violated? Actual loss proved?	Token award, usually $1.

to cover all liability bases, and even leaving the profession. Furthermore, some hospitals have shut down or threatened to shut down trauma centers, and long-term care facilities have closed.

In an attempt to address rapidly rising premiums for medical malpractice insurance, some states have placed caps on damage awards in medical malpractice cases. Attorney organizations, however, insist that damage caps are unfair to injured patients.

The issue is an important one for both health care practitioners and patients and is not likely to be settled uniformly across the country. As a future or present health care practitioner, you should stay informed on the issues of medical malpractice insurance and tort reform and form your own opinion.

Wrongful Death Statutes

wrongful death statutes State statutes that allow a person's beneficiaries to collect for loss to the estate of the deceased for future earnings when a death is judged to have been due to negligence.

Most states have enacted **wrongful death statutes** which allow a patient's beneficiaries to collect from a health care practitioner for loss to the patient's estate of future earnings when a patient's death is judged to have been due to negligence of health care practitioners. In most states, a cap has been placed on the amount of damages that can be recovered in a civil action for wrongful death.

The state may also prosecute a health care practitioner under criminal statutes for the wrongful death of a patient.

The following court cases illustrate a wrongful death action and the issue of contributory negligence, which is discussed in Chapter 5.

Court Case

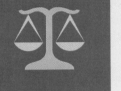

Wrongful Death and Physician-Patient Relationship Both at Issue in Lawsuit

Nichelle, a 22-year-old woman who lived with her parents, was eight weeks pregnant. The woman's mother returned home from work to find her daughter in bed, complaining of abdominal pain. That evening the mother spoke over the telephone with the family physician. The physician had not examined Nichelle, but learned that she was pregnant and experiencing pain and shortness of breath. The physician later claimed that Nichelle's mother did not express urgency or serious concern during their telephone conversation. He told the mother to take Nichelle to the emergency room if the pain got worse and to have Nichelle see a doctor the next day.

At midnight Nichelle was admitted to the hospital emergency room. She rapidly went into cardiac arrest and was rushed to surgery, but she died later after a period of time on life support. Doctors who treated Nichelle diagnosed a ruptured ectopic pregnancy. There was evidence that Nichelle might have lived if she had received medical care earlier in the evening. Nichelle's parents sued the hospital where Nichelle was treated and the family physician for wrongful death.

The hospital settled out of court with Nichelle's parents for $170,000. The claim against the family physician proceeded to trial. The defendant claimed that a physician-patient relationship did not exist with Nichelle, since he had not seen, talked to, or treated her for approximately four years prior to his telephone call with her mother, and he did not speak directly with Nichelle when her mother called him. The trial court jury found that a physician-patient relationship existed, based on the judge's instructions:

"The physician-patient relationship is a consensual one in which the patient knowingly seeks the physician's assistance and the physician knowingly accepts the patient as a patient.

(continued)

"The relationship is contractual and wholly voluntary, and is created by agreement expressed or implied.

"A physician-patient relationship may be created in any number of ways, including the act of a physician agreeing to give or giving advice to a patient in person or by telephone."

The trial court returned a wrongful death verdict in favor of Nichelle's parents and awarded $1.8 million in damages.

Note: The jury correctly held that if the defendant wanted to avoid forming a physician-patient relationship or liability for his advice, he should have told Nichelle's mother to take her to the emergency room at once, instead of telling her to take her if Nichelle's condition got worse. The case is important because it deals directly with the formation of the physician-patient relationship through a telephone conversation.

Albert & Forestean Adams v. Via Christi Regional Medical Center, 19 P.3d 132 (Kan., 2001).

Court Case

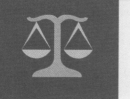

Doctor Sued for Wrongful Death Caused by Inadequate Hospital Discharge Instructions

A patient had chronic kidney failure that required continual dialysis treatment. Hemodialysis catheters, also called access grafts, were surgically inserted in the patient's arms so that he could receive the dialysis treatments. When the access grafts caused problems, a vascular surgeon removed them. While the patient was hospitalized after the grafts in his arms were removed, he suffered two incidents during which he bled copiously from a surgery site in his left arm. Bleeding was stopped with pressure dressings, and the patient received a blood transfusion.

The patient remained hospitalized for observation for four days. He had no other bleeding episodes, received his dialysis treatment successfully, ate well, and had normal vital signs, so he was dismissed from the hospital. The physician noted in his discharge summary that the patient had been instructed on how to apply pressure if his arm should bleed and was told to call his physician if problems occurred.

On the evening of his return home, the patient had two bleeding incidents. Pressure was applied, and the site was wrapped with gauze. No one called the physician to report the two bleeding incidents. The next day the patient was left alone while his wife took their daughter to school and filled a prescription. When she returned home about 30 minutes later, she found her husband dead, lying in a pool of blood.

The patient died from loss of blood caused by hemorrhaging from the incision in his left arm. His wife filed a wrongful death suit against the physician and his vascular surgery corporation. The trial judge found that the physician had not erred in treating the patient's bleeding incidents in the hospital and had not discharged the patient too soon. The judge found, however, that the physician had issued inadequate discharge instructions to the patient, and this constituted a breach of care. The discharge instructions were inadequate, according to the judge's ruling, in that the patient had not been warned about the seriousness of a potential bleeding episode and was not told to have someone at home with him at all times.

The patient was found to be 50 percent responsible for causing his own death, in that he failed to call the physician as instructed when he had two bleeding episodes after discharge from the hospital.

An appeals court upheld the trial judge's ruling.

Note: A final disposition was not published. Perhaps the parties settled out of court.

Samuel v. Baton Rouge General Medical Center, 2000 La.App. Lexis 321 (Court of Appeal of Louisiana, First Circuit, February 18, 2000).

As indicated in Chapter 3, the type of court that hears a case depends upon the offense or complaint. In civil malpractice or negligence cases, the party bringing the action must prove the case by presenting to a judge or jury evidence that is more convincing than that of the opposing side.

Phases of a Lawsuit

The typical malpractice or negligence lawsuit proceeds as follows:

1. A patient feels he or she has been injured.
2. The patient seeks the advice of an attorney.
3. If the attorney believes the case has merit, he or she then requests copies of the patient's medical records. The attorney reviews the medical records and the appropriate standard of care to ascertain merits of the case. In some states, before proceeding to a lawsuit, the attorney must obtain an expert witness report stating that the standard of care has been violated. An affidavit to that effect must then be submitted. An affidavit is a sworn statement in writing made under oath. It may also be a declaration before an authorized officer of the court.

Pleading Phase

4. The plaintiff's (injured patient's) attorney files a complaint with the clerk of the court. In this document, the plaintiff states his or her version of the situation and the amount of money sought from the defendant (the practitioner being sued) for the plaintiff's injury.
5. A **summons** is issued by the clerk of the court and is delivered with a copy of the complaint to the defendant, directing him or her to respond to the charges. If the defendant does not respond within the specified time limit, he or she can lose the case by default.
6. The defendant's attorney files an answer to the summons, and a copy of it is sent to the plaintiff. In this document, the defendant presents his or her version of the case, either admitting or denying the charges. The defendant may also file a counterclaim or a cross-complaint.
7. If a cross-complaint is made, the plaintiff files a reply.

Interrogatory or Pretrial Discovery Phase

8. The court sets a trial date.
9. Pretrial motions may be made and decided. For example, the defendant may request that the lawsuit be dismissed, the plaintiff may amend the original complaint, or either side may request a change of venue (ask that the trial be held in another place).
10. Discovery procedures may be used to uncover evidence that will support the charges when the case comes to court. A court order called a **subpoena** may be issued commanding the presence of the physician or a medical facility employee in court or requiring that a **deposition** be taken. A deposition is sworn testimony given and recorded outside the courtroom during the pretrial phase of a case. (See the following section, entitled "Witness Testimony.")

    An **interrogatory** may be requested instead of or in addition to a deposition. This is a written set of questions requiring written answers from a plaintiff or defendant under oath.

    The subpoena commanding a witness to appear in court and to bring certain medical records is called a **subpoena** *duces tecum.* Failure

summons A written notification issued by the clerk of the court and delivered with a copy of the complaint to the defendant in a lawsuit, directing him or her to respond to the charges brought in a court of law.

subpoena A legal document requiring the recipient to appear as a witness in court or to give a deposition.

deposition Sworn testimony given and recorded outside the courtroom during the pretrial phase of a case.

interrogatory A written set of questions requiring written answers from a plaintiff or defendant under oath.

subpoena *duces tecum* A legal document requiring the recipient to bring certain written records to court to be used as evidence in a lawsuit.

to obey a subpoena may result in contempt-of-court charges. Contempt of court is willful disobedience to or open disrespect of a court, judge, or legislative body. It is punishable by fines or imprisonment.

11. A pretrial conference may be called by the judge scheduled to hear the case. During this conference, the judge discusses the issues in the case with the opposing attorneys. This helps avoid surprises and delays after the trial starts and may lead to an out-of-court settlement. (Note: At any point after the complaint is filed before the case comes to trial, an out-of-court settlement may be reached.)

Trial Phase

12. The jury is selected (if one is to be used), and the trial begins.
13. Opening *statements* are made by the lawyers for the plaintiff and the defendant, summarizing what each will prove during the trial.
14. Witnesses are called to testify for both sides. They may be cross-examined by opposing attorneys.
15. Each attorney makes closing *arguments* that the evidence presented supports his or her version of the case. No new evidence may be presented during summation.
16. The judge gives instructions to the jury (if one was chosen), and the jury retires to deliberate.
17. The jury reaches a verdict.
18. The final judgment is handed down by the court. The judge bases his or her decision for judgment upon the jury's verdict.

Appeals Phase

19. Posttrial motions may be filed.
20. An appeal may be made for the case to be reviewed by a higher court if the evidence indicates that errors may have been made or if there was injustice or impropriety in the trial court proceedings. A judgment is final only when all options for appeal have been exercised.

Witness Testimony

An estimated nine out of ten lawsuits are settled out of court, but health care practitioners are often asked to give testimony. Testimony may be given in court on the witness stand, or it may be given in an attorney's conference room in a pretrial proceeding called a deposition. (See the earlier section entitled "Interrogatory or Pretrial Discovery Phase.") Depositions are of two types:

1. Discovery depositions.
2. Depositions in lieu of trial.

Discovery depositions cover material that will most likely be examined again when the witness testifies in court. Since there will be an opportunity for the opposing attorney to question the witness a second time in court, the deposition need not cover every possible question.

Both before a deposition and before in-court testimony, the witness is sworn to tell the truth and then is questioned by attorneys representing both sides. During courtroom testimony, however, a judge is present to rule on objections raised by the attorneys. When an objection is raised, the witness should stop speaking until the judge either *sustains* or *overrules* the objection. If the objection is sustained, the witness need not answer the question. If the objection is overruled, the witness must answer. If in doubt about whether an objection to a question was sustained or overruled, the witness may ask the judge whether a question should be answered. During a deposition, witnesses should take the attorney's advice regarding questions that should be answered.

Depositions in lieu of trial are used instead of the witness's in-person testimony in court. Since the opposing attorney has one opportunity to question the witness, questions are thorough, and the witness should carefully consider his or her answers.

Sometimes depositions in lieu of trial are videotaped, to be played in the courtroom during the trial. Witnesses whose depositions will be videotaped should be informed in advance, so they can dress as though they were appearing in court in person.

Witnesses may offer two kinds of **testimony:** fact and expert. Health care practitioners or laypersons may offer *fact testimony,* and this type of testimony concerns only those facts the witness has observed. For example, regarding testimony in a medical malpractice case, medical assistants, LPNs/LVNs, and registered nurses may testify about how many times a patient saw the physician, the patient's appearance during a particular visit, or similar observations. If asked to give fact testimony, a health care practitioner's powers of observation and memory are more important than his or her professional qualifications. A health care practitioner giving fact testimony is not allowed to give his or her opinion on the facts.

testimony Statements sworn to under oath by witnesses testifying in court and giving depositions.

CHECK YOUR PROGRESS

13. Name the four phases of a typical medical professional liability lawsuit, and describe how a medical assistant might be involved in each trial phase.

_____

_____

_____

_____

14. A subpoena *duces tecum* is issued during which trial phase?

_____

15. The complaint is filed during which trial phase?

_____

_____

16. During which trial phase is the court's judgment handed down?

_____

_____

17. A judgment is final only when

_____

_____

18. Distinguish between *deposition* and *interrogatory.*

_____

_____

Only experts in a particular field have the education, skills, knowledge, and experience to give *expert testimony*. In medical negligence lawsuits, physicians are usually called as expert witnesses to testify to the standard of care regarding the matter in question. Expert witnesses may, and usually do, give their opinions on the facts. If the defendant/physician is a specialist, the expert witness generally practices or teaches in the same specialty. Acceptable expert witnesses are not coworkers, friends, or acquaintances of the defendant. It is ethical and acceptable for expert witnesses to set and accept a fee commensurate with time taken from regular employment and time spent preparing their expert testimony.

Courtroom Conduct

Most health care practitioners will never have to appear in court. If you should be asked to appear, however, the following suggestions can help:

- Attend court proceedings as required. If you were subpoenaed but fail to appear, you could be charged with contempt of court. (If either the plaintiff or the defendant fails to appear, that person forfeits the case.)
- Find out in advance when and where you are to appear, and do not be late for scheduled hearings.
- Bring the required documents to court and present them only when requested to do so.
- Before testifying, refresh your memory concerning all the facts observed about the matter in question, such as dates, times, words spoken, and circumstances.
- When testifying, speak slowly, use layperson's terms instead of medical terms whenever possible, and do not lose your temper or attempt to be humorous.
- Answer all questions in a straightforward manner, even if the answers appear to help the opposing side.
- Answer only the question asked, no more and no less.
- Because you are testifying about what you recall, be careful of broad generalizations, such as, "That is all that took place." A better answer might be, "As I recall, that is what took place."
- Your attorney may help you prepare your testimony, but do not discuss your testimony with other witnesses or others outside the courtroom. Answer truthfully if asked whether you discussed your testimony with counsel.
- Appear well groomed, and dress in clean, conservative clothing.

ALTERNATIVE DISPUTE RESOLUTION

alternative dispute resolution (ADR) Settlement of civil disputes between parties using neutral mediators or arbitrators without going to court.

Alternative dispute resolution (ADR), also known as appropriate dispute resolution, consists of techniques for resolving civil disputes without going to court. As court calendars have become overcrowded in recent years, ADR has become increasingly popular. Several alternative methods of settling legal disputes are possible, including mediation, arbitration, and a combination of the two methods called med-arb.

Some states require mediation and/or arbitration for certain civil cases, while in other states alternative dispute resolution methods are voluntary. *Mediation* is an ADR method in which a neutral third party listens to both sides of the argument and then helps resolve the dispute. The mediator does not have the authority to impose a solution on the parties involved.

ARTICLE 1: It is understood that any dispute as to medical malpractice, that is as to whether any medical services rendered under this contract were unnecessary or unauthorized or were improperly, negligently, or incompetently rendered, will be determined by submission to arbitration as provided by California law, and not by a lawsuit or resort to court process except as California law provides for judicial review of arbitration proceedings. Both parties to this contract, by entering into it, are giving up their constitutional right to have such dispute decided in a court of law before a jury, and instead are accepting the use of arbitration.

ARTICLE 2: I understand and agree that this arbitration agreement binds me and anyone else who may have a claim arising out of or related to all treatment or services provided by the physician, including any spouse or heirs of the patient and any children, whether born or unborn at the time of the occurrence giving rise to any claim. This includes, but is not limited to, all claims for monetary damages exceeding the jurisdictional limit of the small claims court, including, without limitation, suits for loss of consortium, wrongful death, emotional distress or punitive damages. I further understand and agree that if I sign this agreement on behalf of some other person for whom I have responsibility, then, in addition to myself, such person(s) will also be bound, along with anyone else who may have a claim arising out of the treatment or services rendered to that person. I also understand and agree that this agreement relates to claims against the physician and any consenting substitute physician, as well as the physician's partners, associates, association, corporation or partnership, and the employees, agents, and estates of any of them. I also hereby consent to the intervention or joinder in the arbitration proceeding of all parties relevant to a full and complete settlement of any dispute arbitrated under this Agreement, as set forth in the CAHHS/CMA Medical Arbitration Rules.

ARTICLE 3: I understand and agree that I will be bound by this arbitration agreement and that this agreement will be valid and enforceable for any and all treatment provided by the physician in the future regardless of the length of time since my last visit to this physician, and regardless of the fact that the patient-physician relationship between myself and the physician may be interrupted for any reason and then recommenced.

ARTICLE 4: I UNDERSTAND THAT I DO NOT HAVE TO SIGN THIS AGREEMENT TO RECEIVE THE PHYSICIAN'S SERVICES, AND THAT IF I DO SIGN THE AGREEMENT AND CHANGE MY MIND WITHIN 30 DAYS OF TODAY, THEN I MAY CANCEL THIS AGREEMENT BY GIVING WRITTEN NOTICE TO THE UNDERSIGNED PHYSICIAN WITHIN THAT TIME STATING THAT I WANT TO WITHDRAW FROM THIS ARBITRATION AGREEMENT.

ARTICLE 5: On behalf of myself and all others bound by this agreement as set forth in Article 2, agreement is hereby given to be bound by the Medical Arbitration Rules of the California Association of Hospitals and Health Systems (CAHHS) and the California Medical Association (CMA), as they may be amended from time to time, which are hereby incorporated into this agreement. A copy of these Rules is included in the pamphlet in which this agreement is found. Additional copies of the Rules are available from the California Medical Association, P.O. Box 7690, San Francisco, Ca. 94120-7690, Attention: Arbitration Rules. I understand that disputes covered by this Agreement will be covered by California law applicable to actions against health care providers, including the Medical Injury Compensation Reform Act of 1975 (including any amendments thereto).

ARTICLE 6: OPTIONAL: RETROACTIVE EFFECT
If I intend this agreement to cover services rendered before the date it is signed (for example, emergency treatment), I have indicated the earlier date I intend this agreement to be effective from and initialed below.

Earlier effective date: _____ Patient's Initials: _____

ARTICLE 7: I have read and understood all the information in this pamphlet, including the explanation of the Patient-Physician Arbitration Agreement, this Agreement, and the Rules. I understand that in the case of any pregnant woman, the term "patient" as used herein means both the mother and the mother's expected child or children.

If any provision of this arbitration agreement is held invalid or unenforceable, the remaining provisions shall remain in full force and shall not be affected by the invalidity of any other provision.

NOTICE: BY SIGNING THIS CONTRACT YOU ARE AGREEING TO HAVE ANY ISSUE OF MEDICAL MALPRACTICE DECIDED BY NEUTRAL ARBITRATION AND YOU ARE GIVING UP YOUR RIGHT TO A JURY OR COURT TRIAL. SEE ARTICLE 1 OF THIS CONTRACT.

_____ Dated: _____, _____
(Patient, Parent, Guardian or Legally Authorized Representative of Patient)

If signed by other than patient, indicate relationship: _____

PHYSICIAN'S AGREEMENT TO ARBITRATE
In consideration of the foregoing execution of this Patient-Physician Arbitration Agreement, I likewise agree to be bound by the terms set forth in this agreement and in the rules specified in Article 5 above.

_____ Dated: _____, _____
(Physician or Duly-Authorized Representative)

_____
Title — e.g., Partner, President, etc.   Print name of Physician, Medical Group, Partnership or Association
©California Medical Association, 1998

FIGURE 4-4 Sample Patient-Physician Arbitration Agreement

Arbitration is a method of settling disputes in which the opposing parties agree to abide by the decision of an arbitrator. An arbitrator is either selected directly by the disputing parties or chosen in one of the following two ways:

1. Under the terms of a written contract, an arbitrator is chosen by the court or by the American Arbitration Association.

2. If no contract exists, each of the two involved parties selects an arbitrator, and the two arbitrators select a third.

In an informal proceeding, each side presents evidence and witnesses. In the alternative dispute resolution method called med-arb, the mediator resolves the dispute if the two parties are unable to reach agreement after mediation.

Advocates of alternative dispute resolution claim that these methods are faster and less costly than court adjudication. Critics claim that medical malpractice cases are best decided when all the factual information is brought out, as in pretrial judicial discovery procedures. Critics also argue that selecting arbitrators acceptable to both parties can take weeks, months, even years, and that attorneys' fees and damage awards can be as costly as in court-tried cases. Figure 4-4 illustrates a sample arbitration agreement to be signed by the patient and physician involved in a dispute.

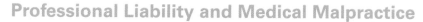

Ethics Issues

Professional Liability and Medical Malpractice

ETHICS ISSUE 1: As citizens and as professionals with special training and experience, health care practitioners are ethically obligated to assist in the administration of justice. If a patient who has a legal claim requests a health care practitioner's assistance, he or she should furnish medical evidence, with the patient's consent, in order to secure the patient's legal rights.

Medical experts should have recent and substantive experience in the area in which they testify and should limit testimony to their sphere of medical expertise.

DISCUSSION QUESTIONS

1. An orthopedic surgeon who has been retired from practice for 15 years and is a friend of the plaintiff's has been called to testify in the plaintiff's suit alleging damage to his hip joint sustained in a car accident. In your opinion, is it ethical for the physician described above to testify? Explain your answer.

_____

_____

_____

2. In your opinion, is it ever ethical for a health care practitioner to testify against another health care practitioner in a medical malpractice lawsuit? Explain your answer.

_____

_____

3. As a health care practitioner, do you consider it ethical to charge for your services to testify as an expert witness? Explain your answer.

_____

_____

4. Are there circumstances when you might consider it unethical to charge for your services as an expert witness? Explain your answer.

_____

_____

ETHICS ISSUE 2: Health care practitioners are ethically bound to respect the patient's dignity and to make a positive effort to secure a comfortable and considerate atmosphere for the patient, in such ways as providing appropriate gowns and drapes, private facilities for undressing, and clear explanations for procedures.

DISCUSSION QUESTIONS

1. An adolescent male patient is visibly uncomfortable as a female physician begins a physical examination. What actions might the physician and/or her attending certified medical assistant take to make the patient more comfortable?

_____

_____

2. A mentally disturbed hospital patient becomes extremely agitated and violent. She disrobes and runs through the hallways. Nurses and other employees are unable to calm the woman, and security officers arrive. Other patients and employees in the area stand around watching the woman as the officers attempt to subdue her. As a health care practitioner in the immediate vicinity, what, if anything, might you do to protect the woman's privacy?

_____

_____

3. A woman requests a breast exam when, upon self-examination, she detects a small lump. Her male family physician performs the breast examination without a chaperone, and begins massaging the patient's nipple in a suggestive manner. What should the patient do?

_____

_____

4. Are there legal implications in the above example? Explain your answer, detailing any preventative measures that could have been taken to avoid them.

_____

_____

 Go to www.mhhe.com/judson5e to practice your case review skills. Then read on for more information.

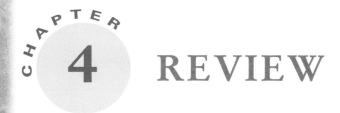

Applying Knowledge

Answer the following questions in the spaces provided.

1. As employers, physicians have general liability in what three areas?

_____

_____

_____

2. According to the reasonable person standard, a person may be charged with negligence if someone is injured because of failure to perform an act that a reasonable person in similar circumstances would perform, or if an act is committed that

_____

_____

3. To whom is a duty of care owed? _____

4. If a custodian sues an employing physician for ordering her to lift a heavy bookcase that injures her back, is the issue of liability standard of care or duty of care?

_____

5. What is the basis for most medical malpractice claims?

_____

_____

6. A patient falls on a hospital's slippery tile floor and injures herself. Assuming that patient safety procedures were lax, what two undesirable occurrences could result for the hospital?

_____

_____

_____

7. List and describe the four Ds of negligence.

_____

_____

_____

_____

_____

_____

8. When a patient sues a physician for negligence, who has the burden of proof, the plaintiff or the defendant? _____

9. In a case in which a patient sues a physician, the patient is called the _____ and the physician is called the _____.

10. Why are expert witnesses often required in a medical negligence lawsuit?

_____

11. When is the doctrine of *res ipsa loquitur* applied? _____

12. Explain the status of expert witnesses in cases in which *res ipsa loquitur* is applied.

_____

_____

13. Monetary compensation awarded by a court of law is called _____.

14. Why might a medical assistant purchase a professional liability insurance policy separate from the employer's policy? _____

15. A court order for an individual to appear in court is called a(n) _____, and an order for bringing certain records is called _____.
An order to appear in court to defend yourself is a(n) _____.

16. What is the difference between a deposition and an interrogatory?

_____

_____

_____

17. Define the two types of depositions that might be taken prior to a medical malpractice lawsuit.

_____

_____

_____

18. As a health care practitioner asked to testify, are you more likely to give factual or expert testimony? Why?

_____

_____

_____

19. Define *alternative dispute resolution*. List and define two commonly used ADR methods.

_____

_____

_____

20. As a health care practitioner, can you legally and ethically use any title you want? Explain your answer.

_____

_____

21. Define *res ipsa loquitur.*

_____

_____

22. Explain what legal action may be taken if you are subpoenaed to appear in court as a witness or to give a deposition and you fail to appear.

_____

_____

23. What is the result if you are the plaintiff or the defendant in a lawsuit and you fail to appear in court?

_____

_____

Circle the correct answer for the following multiple-choice questions.

24. Those damages that recognize the wrong, but award only a token amount are called
    a. general compensatory
    b. punitive
    c. nominal
    d. special compensatory

25. Those damages awarded by the court to punish the defendant are called
    a. general compensatory
    b. punitive
    c. nominal
    d. special compensatory

26. A jury is selected in the _____ phase of a lawsuit.
    a. appeals
    b. pleadings
    c. trial
    d. pretrial discovery

27. A plea is made for the case to be reviewed by the higher court in the _____ phase of a lawsuit.
    a. appeals
    b. pleadings
    c. trial
    d. pretrial discovery

28. The performance of a totally wrongful and unlawful act is a
    a. malfeasance
    b. nonfeasance
    c. misfeasance
    d. tortfeasor

29. *Res ipsa loquitur* is the doctrine of
    a. common sense
    b. common damages
    c. common knowledge
    d. common belief

30. In the _____ phase of a lawsuit, subpoenas are issued.
    a. trial
    b. appeals
    c. pretrial discovery
    d. pleadings

31. The failure to act when one should is called
    a. malfeasance
    b. nonfeasance
    c. misfeasance
    d. tortfeasor

32. A jury is selected in the _____ phase of a lawsuit
    a. trial
    b. appeals
    c. pretrial discovery
    d. pleadings

33. Damages awarded by the court so that the defendant pays for violation of rights where the dollar value need not be proved are called
    a. general compensatory
    b. punitive
    c. nominal
    d. special compensatory

34. To establish a standard of care in a trial, _____ is required.
    a. deposition
    b. subpoena
    c. expert testimony
    d. interrogatories

35. Attorneys make opening and closing statements in the _____ phase of a lawsuit.
    a. trial
    b. appeals
    c. pretrial discovery
    d. pleadings

36. Damages awarded by the court where the dollar value need not be proved but the loss must be proved are called
    a. general compensatory
    b. punitive
    c. nominal
    d. special compensatory

37. Witnesses are called to testify in the _____ phase of a lawsuit.
    a. trial
    b. appeals
    c. pretrial discovery
    d. pleadings

38. A deposition is taken in the _____ phase of a lawsuit.
    a. trial
    b. appeals
    c. pretrial discovery
    d. pleadings

Case Study

Use your critical-thinking skills to answer the questions that follow each of the case studies.

A woman gave birth in the back seat of a taxicab while en route to the hospital. To what standard of care would each of the following individuals be held?

39. The taxicab driver who comforted the mother.

_____

40. A registered nurse, also a passenger in the cab, who assisted the mother.

_____

41. A physician in general practice who was a passenger in the cab with the expectant mother and assisted the birth taking place in the cab.

_____

42. A police officer who stopped the cab for speeding, observed the situation, and assisted the birth.

_____

A trained anesthesiologist ran out of oxygen before an operation was completed, causing the patient to suffer a fatal cardiac arrest.

43. This case was adjudicated (decided legally) as a medical malpractice case, and the plaintiff won. Referring to the four Ds of negligence, explain why.

_____

_____

_____

_____

During an endoscopic retrograde cholangiopancreatography (ERCP) (a gall bladder X-ray that requires injection of a dye), an inexperienced nurse injected the dye too forcefully and caused the patient to develop pancreatitis (inflammation of the pancreas) and suffer other debilitating injuries.

44. The patient sued and won. Refer to the four Ds of negligence to explain the court's decision.

_____

_____

_____

_____

An on-call ophthalmologist, without seeing the patient, diagnosed his eye pain, sensitivity to light, and nausea as sinusitis. In fact, the patient had acute angle closure glaucoma and lost sight in the eye.

45. When this case came to trial, the court found in favor of the patient/plaintiff. Explain the court's decision based on the four Ds of negligence.

_____

_____

_____

_____

A woman trained in cardiopulmonary resuscitation (CPR) worked as the office manager for an insurance business. When her coworker at the next desk had a heart attack and fell to the floor, the office manager began CPR and shouted for others in the room to dial 911. The department supervisor came running and told the office manager to stop CPR. She reluctantly obeyed. Emergency medical technicians arrived, but the heart attack victim died.

46. The victim's husband sued the supervisor, the office manager, and the employees' parent organization for failure to render medical assistance. In a finding for the defendants, an appeals court ruled there was "no duty of care" for the employees to render assistance. Despite this court's ruling, in a similar situation, would you have acted as the CPR-trained office manager did? Explain your answer.

Internet Activities

Complete the activities and answer the questions that follow.

47. Visit the Web site of the American Arbitration Association. Click on "Rules/Procedures," then "Model Standard of Conduct for Mediators." List three major points you find there for standards of conduct for mediators.

48. Find the Web site for the Joint Commission for the Accreditation of Healthcare Organizations. Briefly summarize the most recently recommended standards for health care organizations seeking JCAHO accreditation.

49. Conduct two Web searches: One for "medical malpractice insurance" and a second for "tort reform." Briefly summarize how the two relate. Do all reliable sources advocate tort reform as one solution to high medical malpractice insurance rates? Explain your answer.

5

Defenses to Liability Suits

Learning Outcomes

After studying this chapter, you should be able to:

1. List and define the four Cs of medical malpractice prevention.

2. Describe the various defenses to professional liability suits.

3. Know where to find the statute of limitations for malpractice litigation in your state.

4. Discuss five different types of medical liability insurance.

5. Explain the purpose of quality improvement and risk management within a health care facility.

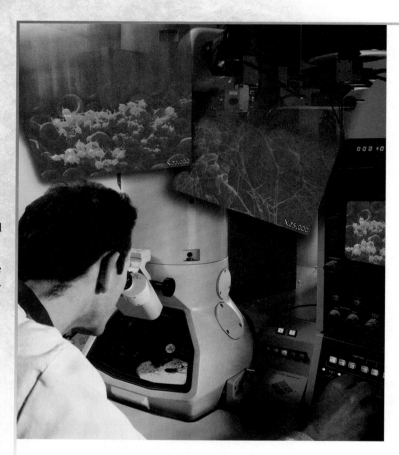

Key Terms

affirmative defenses

assumption of risk

claims-made insurance

comparative negligence

contributory negligence

denial

emergency

liability insurance

occurrence insurance

prior acts insurance coverage

quality assurance

quality improvement (QI)

release of tortfeasor

res judicata

risk management

self-insurance coverage

statute of limitations

tail coverage

technical defenses

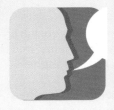

Voice of Experience
Communication Is Key

Carol, an RN Master of Science in Nursing (MSN), who teaches university nursing students, stresses proper communication techniques to help physicians, nurses, and other health care practitioners strengthen their therapeutic relationships with patients and help reduce the possibility of medical malpractice lawsuits. She often uses the following true situation to show students how to communicate with a "difficult" patient:

A 58-year-old man has changed insurance plans, and he is now required to see his primary care physician for a referral to the cardiologist he has been seeing for six years. "I don't see why I had to come here," he tells his primary care physician, anger obvious in his tone and body language. "All I wanted was to see my cardiologist, and it's hard for me to get time off work for an extra doctor's appointment."

"I can understand your frustration," the physician replies. "But since you're here now, can we work together to make the most of your visit? I know you want that referral, but is there anything else you would like to get out of today's visit?"

"Well, I'm a smoker, and I know I should quit," the man admits after a few moments of thought. "And I've been wondering if there might be some other ways I could help improve my health."

The physician then offers to help the patient stop smoking and makes suggestions for reduction of some other cardiac risk factors.

"In terms of communication, this case is a challenge," Carol tells her students, "because the patient was angry before he ever saw the physician. . . .

"The patient interview is an important aspect of medical care, and we all need to address a patient's emotional or mental state before we can effectively address the physical complaint."

PREVENTING LIABILITY SUITS

Malpractice litigation not only adds to the cost of health care, it also takes a psychological toll on both patients and health care practitioners. Both sides would probably agree that prevention is preferable to litigating a malpractice claim. Health care practitioners who use reasonable care in preventing professional liability claims are least likely to be faced with defending themselves against such claims.

THE FOUR Cs OF MEDICAL MALPRACTICE PREVENTION

How can you protect yourself from a medical malpractice lawsuit? By following the four Cs of medical malpractice prevention:

1. *Caring.*
   ▌ There are two important benefits to showing your patients that you care. First is improvement in their medical condition. A secondary benefit is the decreased likelihood that your patients will feel the need to sue if treatment has unsatisfactory results, or if adverse events occur. Of course it is important that you be sincere in your concern, because others often quickly sense insincerity and may distrust you.
   ▌ Avoid destructive and unethical criticism of the work of other physicians and/or other health care practitioners. Do not discuss with a patient his or her former physician. Listen carefully to each patient's complaints and remarks about dissatisfaction with treatment, and see that the comments reach the treating physician.

2. *Communication.*

▮ If you communicate clearly and ask for confirmation that you have been understood, you will be more likely to earn your patients' and your colleagues' trust and respect. If your duties include taking telephone messages, relate them accurately.

▮ Offer to make appointments when appropriate. Remember that when health care practitioners other than physicians, or in some instances physician assistants, diagnose or prescribe, they may be charged with practicing medicine without a license. When adverse events occur, use correct procedures in reporting the event, and never avoid or ignore any patients involved.

3. *Competence.*

▮ Know your professional area well, including your limitations. Follow standards of care and appropriate procedures for medical practitioners in similar practices and in similar communities. Avoid any action which you are not fully trained or equipped to handle.

▮ Maintain and constantly update your knowledge and skills.

▮ Consult with other health care practitioners appropriately, early, and often (Figure 5-1).

▮ Know the requirements of good medical practice in caring for each patient.

▮ If you prepare or administer medications, check each drug three times: once when taking it from the supply cabinet, again when preparing the dosage, and a third time when returning the container to the shelf. All outdated medications should be discarded and promptly replaced. Prescription blanks should not be left on desktops or work areas.

▮ Stay informed about general medical and scientific progress by reading professional journals, attending seminars and professional association meetings, and fulfilling continuing study requirements.

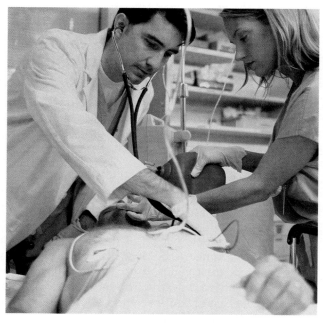

FIGURE 5-1 Caring and competence serve health care practitioners and patients well.

4. *Charting.*

▌ Documentation is proof. For legal purposes, if it isn't in writing and explained completely and accurately, it wasn't done. Medical records should include X-rays, test results, progress notes, and anything else related to the patient's medical treatment.

▌ Document as though the patient will read his or her medical record. Never write something you would not want the patient to see.

EMPLOYING PHYSICIANS AND MEDICAL FACILITIES

The following guidelines for employing physicians and/or medical facilities can help you evaluate the quality of care offered by your employing physician or medical facility and make appropriate suggestions for improving patient care and reducing liability risks in the workplace environment:

▌ Employing physicians should carefully select and supervise all employees and should be careful in delegating duties to them, expecting them to perform only those duties they may reasonably be expected to perform, based on their qualifications, credentials, training, and experience.

▌ Physicians should exhaust all reasonable methods of securing a diagnosis before embarking upon a therapeutic course.

▌ Physicians should use conservative and the least dangerous methods of diagnosis and treatment whenever possible, rather than those that involve highly toxic agents or risky surgical procedures.

▌ As telemedicine has become more commonplace, physicians often diagnose and prescribe medication for new patients and for established patients over the Internet. Physicians also prescribe medication for established patients over the telephone. To avoid malpractice claims, any communication with the patient, whether over the Internet or by telephone, should be properly documented in the patient's medical record. Those health care practitioners who communicate with patients over the Internet should know and conform to state and federal laws regarding the practice of telemedicine.

▌ Except in emergencies, male physicians should not examine female patients and female physicians should not examine male patients unless an assistant, a nurse, or a member of the patient's family is present. In ideal situations, a female medical assistant or female nurse should be present when a male physician examines a female patient, and when a female physician examines a male patient, a male medical assistant or male nurse should be present. Due to shortages of male nurses and male medical assistants, however, this may be impossible. In any case, physicians can protect themselves from unfounded patient charges by having a nurse, physician assistant, or medical assistant of either sex present during examinations.

▌ Employing physicians should check equipment and facilities frequently for safety, including the reception area. All employees should know safe procedures for operating equipment and should remind employing physicians when repair or replacement of equipment is necessary for continued safe operation. Employees should be alert to all hazards in the medical office that might cause injury, such as slippery floors, electric cords in unsafe places, tables with sharp edges, and so forth. The reception area at the health care facility should include a safe area for children, perhaps including such items as child-sized tables and chairs and picture books.

▮ When using toxic agents for diagnosis or treatment, physicians should know customary dosages or usage for such substances, any possible side effects or known toxic reactions, and the proper methods for treating reactions. Medical assistants and other medical office employees should ensure that when supplies are received, they are handled according to office policy and that all relevant literature is readily accessible to physicians. As required by the Occupational Safety and Health Administration (OSHA), employees should have access to Material Safety Data Sheets (MSDS) for each hazardous chemical in use in the medical facility. (See Chapter 9, "Workplace Legalities," for more information about OSHA medical workplace requirements.)

WHY DO PATIENTS SUE?

The following reasons have often been cited by patients and their family members who sue health care practitioners:

Unrealistic expectations. Because of the abundance of available medical information, and recent technological advancements, patients may expect perfection. When the outcome of medical care is not perfect, patients may feel betrayed by the health care system.

Poor rapport and poor communication. Few patients sue health care practitioners they like and trust (see Figure 5-2). If patients perceive health care providers as cold, uncaring, or rude, however, they may be more inclined to sue if something goes wrong, and patients who feel ignored, deserted, or who suspect that there is a medical "cover-up" may also be more inclined to sue.

Greed. While money is seldom the reason for medical malpractice lawsuits, in some cases it may be an influencing factor. Patients read about huge awards made by juries, and some may feel that a lawsuit is worth the potential reward.

Lawyers and our litigious society. Contingency arrangements, where a lawyer does not charge an hourly fee but receives a percentage of a court award if he or she wins the case, are common in the United States, and the loser of a lawsuit does not have to pay the winner's legal expenses. Consequently, lawyers may be more apt to accept a medical malpractice suit.

Poor quality of care. Poor quality *in fact* means that a patient is truly not receiving quality health care. Poor quality *in perception* means that the patient *believes* he or she is not receiving quality health care, even if that is untrue. Either situation can lead to a malpractice lawsuit.

Poor outcome. If medical treatment is unsuccessful or adds to a patient's health problems and a plaintiff can provide evidence of the four Ds of negligence, an attorney will probably accept his or her medical malpractice lawsuit.

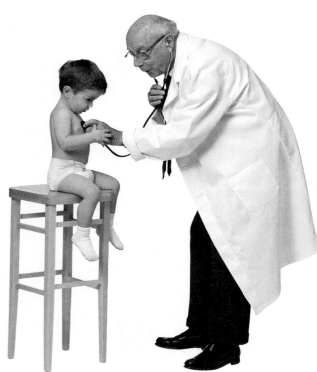

FIGURE 5-2 Age differences disappear with effective communication.

Attorneys can use the *lost chance doctrine* in medical malpractice actions where the injured patient alleges that medical providers negligently deprived him or her of a chance to survive or recover from a health problem.

Failure to understand the patient's and the family's perspective and devaluing their point of view. Health care practitioners who do not return telephone calls or are otherwise unavailable to a patient's family members may be perceived as arrogant, cold, or uncaring. When such perceptions exist, patients and their family members may be more apt to sue if something goes wrong.

Communicating with Patients

Those patients who see the medical office as a friendly place are generally less likely to sue. As a health care practitioner and/or a medical facility employee, you can help prevent medical malpractice lawsuits by:

- Developing good listening skills and nonverbal communication techniques so that patients feel the time spent with them is not rushed. For example, patients will see a health care practitioner as caring and interested if he or she sits rather than stands while interviewing or conversing with the patient. Conversely, lack of eye contact and defensive body postures convey disinterest to a patient. In short, obey the Golden Rule when communicating with patients.

- Setting aside a certain time period during the day for returning patients' telephone calls and advising patients over the phone. Medical facility staff members responsible for answering the telephone should learn to recognize when patients' reported symptoms require the physician's immediate attention and when patients should be advised to seek emergency care.

- Reminding physicians to thoroughly explain illnesses and treatment options, including risks and possible complications, in terms the patient can understand. Patients should be encouraged to ask questions and to participate in the decision-making process. The best way to keep patients' expectations in line is through education. When dealing with accidents and bad results, a straightforward approach is desirable.

- Checking to be sure that all patients or their authorized representatives sign informed-consent forms before they undergo medical and surgical procedures. Next of kin or designated representatives must also sign informed-consent forms to authorize autopsies.

- Avoiding statements that could be construed as an admission of fault on the physician's part. If a lawsuit is filed against a physician, his or her employees should say nothing to anyone except as required by the physician's attorney or the court. However, an employee may be held liable if he or she knowingly remains silent to protect a physician who has performed an illegal act.

- Using tact, good judgment, and professionalism in handling patients. Physicians should insist on a professional consultation if the patient is not doing well, if he or she is unhappy and complaining, or if the patient's family expresses dissatisfaction.

- Refraining from making overly optimistic statements about recovery or prognoses. Health care practitioners who are not physicians or physician assistants generally do not diagnose or prescribe, but their responsibilities may include patient education. For example, nurses and medical assistants often discuss the patient's problems and review treatment options, and this is entirely appropriate. However, such health care practitioners should not make promises on the physician's behalf, such as, "The doctor will have you feeling better soon."

- Advising patients when their physicians intend to be gone for long periods of time and reminding physicians to recommend or make available qualified substitutes. The patient must not be abandoned. If a physician is retiring, moving to another location, leaving the practice of medicine, or otherwise becoming unavailable, patients should be informed, and a copy of a letter of referral, notice of a physician's intended absence from practice, or letter of dismissal should be placed in the patient's record. Notices placed in local newspapers are also appropriate if a physician retires, moves, dies, or leaves the practice of medicine. The name and telephone number of the covering physician should be available for those patients requesting care in the absence of their regular physician.

- Making every effort to reach an understanding about fees with the patient before treatment so that billing does not become a point of contention. When handling fees for the physician, employees should explain all charges to patients, detailing those that are not included in regular fees. They should also follow legal collection procedures.

Documentation

Patient records are often used as evidence in medical malpractice cases, and improper documentation can lose a case (see Chapter 6). In some situations that may arise in medical practice, such as drug testing or the examination of a rape victim, evidence may need to be collected in a certain manner in order to be admissible in court. When in doubt about what documentation to make, you should contact legal authorities for advice.

Physicians should keep records that clearly show what treatment was done and when it was done. It is important that they be able to demonstrate that nothing was neglected and that the care given fully met the standards demanded by law. Physicians should also document all referrals to other physicians, withdrawals from cases, and cases in which patients refuse to follow their advice. Today's health care environment requires complete documentation of actions taken and, in many cases, actions not taken. Medical facility employees should pay particular attention to the following:

Referrals. Make sure the patient understands whether the referring physician's staff will make the appointment and notify the patient or whether the patient must call to set up the appointment. Make notations that the patient has been referred, and follow up with telephone calls to verify that an appointment was scheduled and kept. Note whether or not reports of the consultation were received in your office, and document all recommendations from the referring physician concerning further care of the patient.

Missed Appointments. At the end of each day, a designated person in the medical office should gather all patient records of those who missed or canceled appointments without rescheduling. Charts and electronic or handwritten schedule books should be dated, stamped, and documented "no show" or "canceled, no reschedule," respectively. The treating physician should review these records and note whether

1. Name and briefly define the four Cs of medical malpractice prevention.

_____

_____

_____

_____

2. Briefly describe how practicing effective communication skills can help prevent a medical malpractice lawsuit.

_____

_____

3. If a patient refuses treatment, what legal options remain for the health care practitioner in charge?

_____

_____

4. Name five reasons often cited for the suing of health care practitioners by patients and their families.

_____

_____

_____

_____

_____

or not follow-up is indicated. If follow-up occurs, it should be documented as completed.

Dismissals. To avoid charges of abandonment, the physician must formally withdraw from a case or formally dismiss the patient. Be sure that a letter of withdrawal or dismissal has been filed in the patient's records.

Treatment Refusals. A patient's decision to decline treatment, evaluation, or testing should be documented in the patient record. "Informed refusal" should be obtained with respect to any treatment or procedure which could have either diagnostic or therapeutic consequences. "Informed refusal" should be obtained in writing or, at the very least, noted in the patient's medical record.

All Other Patient Contact. Patients' records should include reports of all tests, procedures, and medications prescribed, including refills. Make sure all necessary informed-consent papers have been duly signed and filed in a patient's record. Keep a record of all telephone conversations with the patient. Remember that correct documentation requires the initials or signature of the person making a notation on the patient's medical record, as well as the date and time. Remember the rule, "If it wasn't documented, it wasn't done."

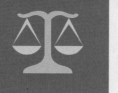
Physician Sued for Malpractice

A gynecologist treated a woman for pelvic pain. The physician eventually performed a hysterectomy, which was successful and relieved the woman's pain. Later, the woman complained of mild incontinence. The woman's physician found that she had a cystocele (herniation of part of the bladder through the wall of her vagina), and this condition progressed to a rectocele, when the rectum also herniated through the wall of the patient's vagina. Since the patient's stress incontinence had also progressed, the gynecologist recommended surgery, but she did not discuss Kegel exercises with the patient. (Kegel exercises are designed to strengthen muscles in a woman's pelvic floor and muscles supporting the urethra.)

Surgery was performed, and it corrected the patient's incontinence and the anatomical defects that caused it. However, shortly after surgery, the patient developed pain in her right leg. A second surgery was performed to release two sutures which the gynecologist believed might be impinging on the patient's obturator nerve and causing the pain. The pain persisted, and a third surgery on the patient's leg was performed. The third surgery and follow-up did not alleviate the patient's pain, despite referrals to and treatments by specialists in physical medicine, pain management, and neurosurgery. The pain and impairment in the patient's right leg was finally diagnosed as due to nerve damage as a result of the hysterectomy.

The patient filed suit alleging the following:

1. The gynecologist negligently failed to offer the nonsurgical option of Kegels exercises.
2. The patient would have chosen and performed the nonsurgical option had it been offered.
3. The Kegel exercises probably would have corrected the patient's incontinence without surgery.
4. The patient's nerve damage would have been avoided if the surgery had not been done.

The trial court found for the patient and named an award. The gynecologist appealed, and the appellate court overturned the trial court's decision, holding that the patient could not prove that the Kegel exercises would have prevented surgery. Since the trial court's decision was overturned, the patient did not receive an award.

Archer v. Warren, 118 S.W. 3d 779, 2003 Tex. App. LEXIS 6011.

TYPES OF DEFENSES

When, in spite of all best efforts to avoid litigation, a medical malpractice lawsuit is filed, the physician or other health care professional must defend himself or herself against the charges.

denial A defense that claims innocence of the charges or that one or more of the four Ds of negligence are lacking.

Denial

Denial of wrongdoing, or the assertion of innocence, may be used as a defense in professional liability suits. If some of the alleged facts are true, defendants may not claim innocence. Instead, they should claim that the charge or charges do not meet all of the elements of the theory of recovery. In other words, the charge may be missing one of the four Ds of negligence.

affirmative defenses Defenses used by defendants in medical professional liability suits that allow the accused to present factual evidence that the patient's condition was caused by some factor other than the defendant's negligence.

Affirmative Defenses

Affirmative defenses that may be used by the defendant in a medical professional liability suit allow the accused to present factual evidence that the patient's condition was caused by some factor other than the defendant's negligence.

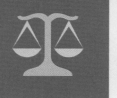

contributory negligence An affirmative defense that alleges that the plaintiff, through a lack of care, caused or contributed to his or her own injury.

comparative negligence An affirmative defense claimed by the defendant, alleging that the plaintiff contributed to the injury by a certain degree.

assumption of risk A legal defense that holds that the defendant is not guilty of a negligent act because the plaintiff knew of and accepted beforehand any risks involved.

Contributory Negligence

When the defense claims **contributory negligence,** this alleges that the patient or complaining party, through a "want of ordinary care," caused or contributed to his or her own injury. The physician may deny that he or she committed a negligent act and claim the patient was totally responsible for the damage or injury. Alternatively, the physician may admit negligence but claim that the patient was also somehow at fault and so contributed to the injury.

In some states, damages are apportioned according to the degree to which a plaintiff contributed to the injury. This is called **comparative negligence.** For instance, if the court decides that a patient, through his or her own negligence, contributed 20 percent toward the injury and the physician contributed 80 percent, the patient's damage award may be reduced by 20 percent.

In hearing cases alleging contributory negligence, the court will consider the patient's ability to comprehend and carry out the physician's instructions. Minors or adults who are unconscious, mentally impaired, insane, or otherwise incompetent may be judged unable to have contributed to a negligent act.

Assumption of Risk

Assumption of risk is a defense based upon the contention that the patient knew of the inherent risks before treatment was performed and agreed to those risks. Informed consent (see Chapter 6) is vital to this defense, since the defendant must show that the patient was fully informed of the risks prior to treatment and that the risks inherent in the treatment were the cause of the patient's injury.

For example, in one lawsuit in which the defendant used the assumption of risk defense, it was held that a physician was not liable for injuries suffered by a chronically ill woman when she fell in the examining room

while attempting to undress without assistance. Because she had refused assistance, the woman had assumed the risk of injury.

In other cases it has been held that individuals submitting to X-ray treatment assume the risk of burns from a proper exposure to X-rays but not the risk of negligence in the application of the treatment.

emergency A type of affirmative defense in which the person who comes to the aid of a victim in an emergency is not held liable under certain circumstances.

Emergency

If services were provided during an **emergency,** this may also be used as an affirmative defense. The health care practitioner who comes to the aid of a victim in an emergency would not be held liable under common law if the defense established that

1. A true emergency situation existed and was not caused by the defendant.

2. The appropriate standard of care was met, given the emergency situation.

Health care professionals who provide assistance in emergencies may also be protected from liability under Good Samaritan Acts, which are discussed in Chapter 6.

While the following court case dates from 1970, the trial court's opinion clearly illustrates the elements required for a health care practitioner to establish an emergency defense.

technical defenses Defenses used in a lawsuit that are based on legal technicalities.

Technical Defenses

When defenses to liability suits are based on legal technicalities, instead of on factual evidence, they are called **technical defenses.** Technical defenses include those that claim the statute of limitations has run out, there is

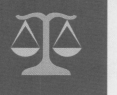

Court Case

Emergency Defense Established

The father of a minor plaintiff sought consequential damages in a malpractice suit against an anesthesiologist. The patient suffered cardiac arrest during a tonsillectomy. Resuscitation was performed, and the patient's heartbeat was restored, but she was left with severe and extensive brain damage.

The defendants used an emergency defense. The plaintiff alleged that cardiac arrest is a complication that is a constant possibility in surgery and, therefore, not to be considered "an emergency within the meaning of the emergency doctrine."

A trial court found for the defendants. The court held that

1. In an emergency a person does not have the time to think in the way that he or she would in ordinary circumstances.
2. When a layperson or a professional is confronted with an emergency, conduct is to be judged according to his or her skill, care, and due diligence with respect to the emergency.

Linhares v. Hall, 257 N.E.2d 429 (1970).

insufficient evidence to support the plaintiff's claim of negligence, and the assertion that the plaintiff has no standing to sue.

Release of Tortfeasor

release of tortfeasor A technical defense that prohibits a lawsuit against the person who caused an injury (the tortfeasor) if he or she was expressly released from further liability in the settlement of a suit.

A tortfeasor is one who is guilty of committing a tort. Suppose a third party causes injury to a person as in an automobile accident, and a physician treats the injured person. In most states, the party who caused the accident (the tortfeasor) is liable both for the victim's injury and for any medical negligence by the physician who treats the injured victim. This is the basis for the **release of tortfeasor** defense.

If the injured party sues the tortfeasor, settles the case, and then releases the tortfeasor from further liability, the injured party cannot also sue the physician unless the victim expressly reserved that right in the release. If the victim's settlement with the tortfeasor provided compensation for all medical expenses, the release of tortfeasor is usually an absolute defense.

Laws governing release of tortfeasor contain many modifiers, which must be applied in individual cases.

Res Judicata

res judicata "The thing has been decided." Legal principle that a claim cannot be retried between the same parties if it has already been legally resolved.

Under the doctrine of *res judicata*, "The thing has been decided," a claim cannot be retried between the same parties if it has already been legally resolved. For example, if a patient sues a physician for negligence and loses, the patient cannot then sue the physician for breach of contract based on evidence presented in the trial for negligence. If a patient refuses to pay a physician's fees on the grounds that the physician was negligent and the physician sues for money owed and wins, the patient cannot then sue the physician for negligence. However, if the patient fails to respond to the suit (defaults) or does not allege negligence in his or her defense, then usually he or she may sue the physician for negligence. If a physician has been sued by a nonpaying patient for negligence and does not file a counterclaim for the fee while defending the suit, the patient cannot be sued later for unpaid bills.

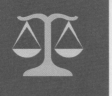

Court Case

Release of Tortfeasor

A driver of an automobile was injured in an accident. A physician subsequently treated the driver's broken arm. The injured party sued the physician for malpractice, alleging that the physician was negligent in that he had severed a nerve in her arm.

Before trial, the plaintiff had signed a release of tortfeasor agreement with the insurer of the other driver involved in the accident, releasing that driver from any further liability.

Both a trial court and a superior court had granted summary judgment in favor of the physician in a medical malpractice action. The plaintiff appealed those decisions, alleging that the release of tortfeasor agreement she had signed did not also release the physician who was allegedly negligent in treating her injury.

The Court of Appeals that heard the final appeal reversed lower court rulings granting summary judgment in favor of the physician, based on the court's agreement that the release of tortfeasor did not include the physician and that the plaintiff had not been allowed to present expert witness testimony in previous hearings. The court remanded the case to the trial court for rehearing.

Note: Final disposition was not published. The parties may have settled out of court, or the trial may have been rescheduled for a future date.

Depew v. Burkle, 786 N.E.2d 1144; 2003 Ind. LEXIS 962 (Ind., Nov. 12, 2003).

Statute of Limitations

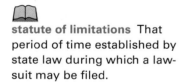

statute of limitations That period of time established by state law during which a lawsuit may be filed.

Since statutes of limitations vary with states, health care practitioners must be familiar with specific laws for their state. Statutory time limits apply to a number of legal actions, including collections, damages for child sexual abuse, retaining medical records, wrongful death claims, medical malpractice, and many other causes of action. The **statute of limitations** for filing professional negligence suits varies with states but generally specifies one to six years, with two years being most common. In other words, patients may not file suit for negligence against physicians if the designated length of time has elapsed.

Establishing when the statute of limitations begins also varies with state law, but the most common dates for marking the beginning of the statutory period are as follows:

- The day the alleged negligent act was committed.
- When the injury resulting from the alleged negligence was actually discovered or should have been discovered by a reasonably alert patient.
- The day the physician-patient relationship ended or the day of the last medical treatment in a series.

In some states, statutory periods may be modified for minors, for the legally insane, or in certain circumstances, such as imprisonment or a situation in which foreign objects were left in the body during surgery.

Since statutes of limitations vary greatly from one state to another, health care practitioners must be familiar with specific laws in their state. Specific statutory time limits may be found in the state code, online, and in most public and university libraries.

The following court case illustrates the importance of statutes of limitations in determining whether or not a medical malpractice complaint can go to trial.

Court Case

Action Dismissed Due to Statute of Limitations

A patient's family sued a physician in Texas for wrongful death for failure to diagnose the patient's cancer. A Texas state law passed in 1977, The Medical Liability and Insurance Improvement Act, established a two-year statute of limitations for medical malpractice claims; therefore, the Supreme Court of Texas barred the action because by the time the lawsuit reached the courts, the statute of limitations had run out.

The patient was first evaluated for anemia in 1986, but test results revealed a lesion in the stomach. A biopsy showed no sign of malignancy in the lesion. A second biopsy performed in 1987 was also negative for cancer, but upon further examination two weeks later, cells from the lesion were found to be consistent with carcinoma.

Follow-up exams and another biopsy performed in 1988 revealed cancer cells in the patient's stomach lesion, which by then had ulcerated. Surgery was recommended, but was not performed because advanced cancer was found in the patient's lung and stomach. The patient died, and her family continued the lawsuit on her behalf.

The appellate court ruled that the statute of limitations period began at the time of the second biopsy in 1987. The claim was not brought until after 1989; therefore, the time limitation had run out.

Bala v. Maxwell, 909 S.W.2d 889 (Texas Sup. Ct., Nov. 2, 1995).

RISK MANAGEMENT

risk management The taking of steps to minimize danger, hazard, and liability.

Since liability is a major factor in health care delivery, and since health care delivery systems and practitioners seek to minimize liability whenever possible, **risk management** has become a necessary practice component. Risk management is one approach to reducing the likelihood of a malpractice lawsuit. Risk management involves identifying problem practices or behaviors, then eliminating or controlling them. Risk management activities that may help avoid litigation include providing written job descriptions for health care practice employees and providing office procedures manuals and employee handbooks that can help avoid misunderstanding and mistakes that lead to liability risks. Other common health care facility activities that may affect the likelihood or course of litigation include medical record charting, patient scheduling, writing prescriptions, and communicating with patients.

quality improvement (QI) (or quality assurance) A program of measures taken by health care providers and practitioners to uphold the quality of patient care.

Methods used to manage risk are part of **quality improvement (QI),** or **quality assurance:** a program of practices performed by health care providers and practitioners to uphold the quality of patient care and to reduce liability risk.

Most health care facilities and plans employ quality improvement and risk managers to oversee risk and quality issues relating to physicians and support staff. Quality improvement and risk managers may also assume responsibility for compliance with federal, state, and other health care regulatory agencies. A compliance plan is developed to help ensure that all governmental regulations are followed. Such a plan is especially beneficial for following coding and billing regulations for Medicare, Medicaid, and other government plans.

Most health care institutions and organizations also employ individuals who are responsible for credentialing. Credentialing may be done by risk management staff or by other departments within a health care organization. Credentialing is the process of verifying a health care provider's credentials. The process may be performed by an insurance company before a provider is admitted to the network, by medical offices prior to granting hospital privileges, or by other groups who routinely employ or contract with health care providers. Credentialing usually consists of the following:

1. A provider fills out an application and attaches copies of his or her medical license, proof of malpractice insurance coverage, and other requested credentials.
2. The listed sources are asked to verify the information.
3. Medicare and Medicaid sanctions and malpractice history are checked via the National Practitioner Data Bank.
4. The findings are presented to a credentialing committee.
5. A peer review process completes the credentialing procedure.

PROFESSIONAL LIABILITY INSURANCE

liability insurance Contract coverage for potential damages incurred as a result of a negligent act.

Since costs for defending a medical malpractice lawsuit can be high, **liability insurance** may be purchased to cover the costs up to the limits of the policy. For example, if a medical professional liability insurance policy covers an insured physician up to $10 million, in the event that he or she loses a malpractice suit and must pay damages, the insurance company will not pay more than that amount.

The cost of liability insurance premiums for a physician is based upon the physician's specialty and the dollar amount covered by the policy. Insurance for those physicians in the least risky insurance risk class (for example, family practitioners and specialists who do not perform surgery) is generally less costly than insurance for those in specialties considered more risky (for example, orthopedic surgeons and obstetricians). States vary regarding those medical specialties considered to carry the highest risk of liability and, therefore, are subject to the highest liability insurance premiums.

Some physicians drop liability insurance coverage when rates become too high. However, this can adversely affect a physician's practice, since most hospitals require proof of coverage up to a predetermined minimum amount in order to grant hospital privileges. In addition, managed care organizations require physicians to provide proof of liability insurance coverage as a prerequisite for entering into a contractual agreement and as a component of their credentialing process.

There are two main types of medical malpractice insurance:

claims-made insurance A type of liability insurance that covers the insured only for those claims made (not for any injury occurring) while the policy is in force.

occurrence insurance A type of liability insurance that covers the insured for any claims arising from an incident that occurred, or is alleged to have occurred, during the time the policy is in force, regardless of when the claim is made.

1. **Claims-made insurance** covers the insured only for those claims made (not for any injury occurring) while the policy is in force. With this kind of insurance, the determining factor is when the claim is made, not when the injury occurs. For example, a policy in force during a previous year would cover only those claims made during that year.
2. **Occurrence insurance** (also known as claims-incurred insurance) covers the insured for any claims arising from an incident that occurred or is alleged to have occurred while the policy is in force, regardless of when the claim is made. For example, suppose an alleged incident of negligence by a physician occurred in September 2003, while the physician's occurrence insurance policy was in effect with XYZ Insurance Company. If a patient files a claim against the physician in January 2005, after the

5. What is the difference between an affirmative defense and a technical defense?

_____

_____

6. Identify the type of defense described in each of the following:

One in which the defendant claims innocence.

_____

One in which the accused is allowed to present factual evidence that the physician's negligence did not cause the patient's condition.

_____

One in which the defendant claims that the patient contributed to his or her own injury.

_____

One in which informed consent is a vital factor.

_____

One that hinges on legal technicalities rather than factual evidence.

_____

7. If a medical malpractice claim is dismissed due to a state's statute of limitations, does this imply that the defendant health care practitioner is exonerated? Explain your answer.

_____

_____

tail coverage An insurance coverage option available for health care practitioners: when a claims-made policy is discontinued, it extends coverage for malpractice claims alleged to have occurred during those dates that claims-made coverage was in effect.

prior acts insurance coverage A supplement to a claims-made insurance policy that can be purchased from a new carrier when health care practitioners change carriers.

policy period has passed, the physician is covered under the terms of the occurrence insurance policy.

There are three types of insurance that health care practitioners can purchase in order to extend coverage of a canceled claims-made policy or for claims-made coverage when the insured switches to a different insurance carrier:

Tail coverage. When a claims-made policy is discontinued, tail coverage (sometimes called a reporting endorsement) is an option available to health care practitioners from their former carriers to continue coverage for those dates that claims-made coverage was in effect. Once a claims-made policy is canceled, coverage does not continue in the future for any claims that might be reported unless tail coverage or prior acts coverage is secured at the time the policy is canceled. If neither is purchased, any future claims that might arise from services performed during the policy period will no longer be covered.

Prior acts insurance coverage. A supplement to a claims-made policy that health care practitioners can purchase from a new carrier when they change carriers. Prior acts coverage, also known as "nose" coverage, covers incidents that occurred prior to the beginning of the new insurance relationship but have not yet been brought to the insured's attention as a claim. Prior acts coverage is an alternative to a

self-insurance coverage An insurance coverage option whereby insured subscribers contribute to a trust fund to be used in paying potential damage awards.

reporting period endorsement (also known as tail coverage), which is purchased from the original carrier when a change in carriers is made. Companies typically require the new insured to purchase either tail or nose coverage to protect against claims arising from prior acts.

Self-insurance coverage. As medical malpractice insurance premiums have continued to rise, self-insurance coverage has become an option for health care practitioners in some states. It works like this: An insurance company writes a policy with a limit of $X, and the insured parties contribute to a trust fund up to a limit of $X to be used in paying potential medical malpractice awards. The insurance company charges fees for managing the fund. One advantage to self-insurance coverage is that premiums are considerably lower than with traditional types of medical malpractice insurance. A disadvantage is that state laws regulating insurance do not always allow such plans, and even in states where such coverage is allowed, hospitals must agree to accept self-insurance plans for those physicians who apply for hospital privileges.

Physicians and other health care practitioners should notify their insurance companies immediately if advised of the possibility of a malpractice lawsuit. Insurance companies almost always provide legal representation for covered physicians, and some insurance contracts require that the insurance company's attorneys represent the insured physician.

Once a lawsuit seems imminent, the health care practitioner and/or his or her employees should not mention the suit on the telephone or in correspondence unless the insurance company's legal counsel approves such a reference.

CHECK YOUR PROGRESS

8. If a health care practitioner covered by medical malpractice insurance receives notice of a lawsuit, he or she should first notify

_____

_____

9. Claims-made insurance pays for

_____

_____

10. Occurrence insurance pays for

_____

_____

11. Name two types of insurance that, in certain circumstances, extend coverage of claims-made insurance.

_____

_____

12. Explain how physicians might insure themselves.

_____

_____

Ethics Issues

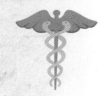

Defenses to Liability Suits

ETHICS ISSUE 1: According to the ethical guidelines for a number of professional organizations, incompetence, corruption, or dishonest or unethical conduct on the part of health care practitioners is never acceptable. In addition to posing a real or potential threat to patients, such conduct undermines the public's confidence in the health care professions.

A medical office employee who routinely enters codes for Medicaid, Medicare, HMO, and private insurance billing visits her physician across town in a different medical office for an examination of a finger she believes is broken. As she is leaving her physician's exam room, she glances at the billing sheet in her hand and sees that her physician has coded for an examination that was not performed. The code the physician has entered means that the patient's insurance carrier will be billed for a more expensive exam than the one that was actually performed.

DISCUSSION QUESTIONS

1. What should the knowledgeable patient in the above situation do?

_____

_____

2. Assume the patient in the above situation confronts her physician and the physician replies, "So? That's no big deal." What should the patient do in this case?

_____

_____

ETHICS ISSUE 2: The American Dental Association's *Principles of Ethics and Code of Professional Conduct* states: "According to the principle of beneficence, dentists have a duty to promote and advance the patient's welfare."

A dentist mistakenly removes three healthy teeth from a patient's mouth, then fits the patient with a fixed bridge that will not stay in place and causes the patient great pain. The patient sees a second dentist who repairs the damage done by the first dentist and remarks about the "shoddy quality" of the first dentist's work. The patient sues the first dentist for medical malpractice, and the defendant is found not guilty.

DISCUSSION QUESTIONS

1. Was the second dentist acting ethically when she criticized the first dentist's work? Explain your answer.

_____

_____

2. Is the dentist who was found not guilty of medical malpractice thereby exonerated of any wrongdoing? Explain your answer.

_____

_____

3. Might the dentist found not guilty in the above scenario be subject to sanctions from the professional organization to which he belongs? Explain your answer.

_____

_____

ETHICS ISSUE 3: The American Medical Association's *Code of Medical Ethics* states that physicians and other health care practitioners should not provide, prescribe, or bill for services they know are unnecessary.

A patient sees his physician for symptoms of viral influenza. After completing his examination, the patient's physician is convinced the patient is, indeed, suffering from the flu, but he seems to be healing. The patient demands a prescription for antibiotics.

DISCUSSION QUESTION

1. Is it ethical for a physician or any other health care practitioner to prescribe or administer a medical treatment just to pacify an anxious or demanding patient? Explain your answer.

_____

_____

Go to www.mhhe.com/judson5e to practice your case review skills. Then read on for more information.

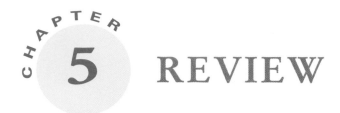

Applying Knowledge

Name the four Cs of medical malpractice prevention, and after each term, list at least one way you can comply.

1. _____

2. _____

3. _____

4. _____

Circle the correct answer for each of the multiple-choice questions below.

5. Under _____ a claim may not be retried between the same two parties if it has been legally resolved.

   a. common law
   b. *res ipsa loquitur*
   c. *res judicata*
   d. arbitration

6. The _____ is the time limit for filing a lawsuit.

   a. affirmative defense
   b. assumption of risk
   c. statue of limitations
   d. technical defense

7. Which of the following is NOT a form of affirmative defense to a professional liability suit?

   a. Contributory negligence
   b. Denial
   c. Assumption of risk
   d. Emergency

8. Under the _____ defense, a health care practitioner who comes to the aid of an accident victim at the scene would not be held liable.

   a. *res judicata*
   b. *res ipsa loquitur*
   c. emergency
   d. denial

9. When the defendant alleges that he or she did no wrong, that defense is called

   a. negligence
   b. contributory negligence
   c. denial
   d. assumption of risk

10. If the patient knew the inherent risk before treatment, the defendant may use _____ as a defense in a lawsuit.
    a. negligence
    b. contributory negligence
    c. denial
    d. assumption of risk

11. Which of the following is an affirmative defense?
    a. Release of tortfeasor
    b. Emergency
    c. *Res judicata*
    d. Statute of limitations

12. Which of the following is a technical defense?
    a. *Res judicata*
    b. Contributory negligence
    c. Comparative negligence
    d. Assumption of risk

13. Risk management is a process
    a. to assess liability insurance
    b. to manage difficult patients
    c. to minimize danger, hazard, and liability
    d. none of the above

14. Medical malpractice insurance that covers the insured only for those claims made while the policy is in force is called
    a. prior acts coverage
    b. self-insurance coverage
    c. claims-made coverage
    d. occurrence insurance

15. Medical malpractice insurance that covers the insured for any claims arising from an incident that occurred, or is alleged to have occurred, during the time the policy was in force, regardless of when the claim is made, is called
    a. prior acts coverage
    b. self-insurance coverage
    c. claims-made coverage
    d. occurrence insurance

16. When damages are apportioned according to the degree a plaintiff contributed to his or her injury, this is called
    a. negligence
    b. contributory negligence
    c. denial
    d. assumption of risk

17. The statue of limitations
    a. is the same in each state
    b. is a federal law
    c. is determined by the courts
    d. is different depending on the state

18. *Res judicata* is Latin for
    a. buyer beware
    b. the judge is in charge
    c. the jury is in charge
    d. the thing has been decided

19. Which of the following is a supplemental insurance to medical liability insurance?

   a. Occurrence coverage

   b. Prior acts coverage

   c. Claims-made coverage

   d. Self-insurance coverage

Name eight guidelines for physicians and other health care practitioners to follow that may help prevent malpractice lawsuits.

20. _____

21. _____

22. _____

23. _____

24. _____

25. _____

26. _____

27. _____

28. Define *risk management*.

   _____

   _____

Case Study

Use your critical-thinking skills to answer the questions that follow each case study.

A patient in her mid-twenties saw an ophthalmologist for a routine eye exam. Due to her young age, a glaucoma test was not performed. She later was diagnosed with glaucoma and sued the ophthalmology group, alleging negligence in failing to perform a glaucoma test.

   The defense argued that the standard of care was to not administer the test to patients younger than 40 because the instance of glaucoma at younger ages was rare.

   Which of the following statements do you think best describes the applicable standard of care in this case? Explain your choice.

29. The defense should prevail because the reasonable, customary, and prudent course of action followed by practitioners in the same or similar circumstances would be the same.

   _____

   _____

30. The plaintiff should prevail because all patients should be protected against glaucoma, regardless of age.

   _____

   _____

You are a phlebotomist for a community laboratory, and you report for work on an extremely busy day. You travel daily from the lab where you work to the hospital to draw blood, and then back to the lab. You have finished drawing blood at the hospital and are on your way back to the lab when you get a cell phone call that the hospital needs a complete blood count (CBC) and electrolytes drawn STAT for a patient that has just come into the emergency room (ER).

31. Would you turn around and go back to the ER or drop off your current blood samples and then go back to the ER? Explain your answer.

_____

_____

_____

32. What does question 31 have to do with preventing medical malpractice lawsuits?

_____

_____

A urologist removed a cancerous prostate from a patient. During surgery the balloon that held a urinary catheter in place burst inside the patient's bladder. After the patient regained consciousness, the urologist told him about the incident. He said he had meticulously removed all fragments of the catheter balloon but cautioned the patient to report any untoward symptoms. The patient recovered without incident.

33. In your opinion, does the patient have a standing to sue either the company that manufactured the urinary catheter or the urologist who operated on him? Why or why not?

_____

_____

_____

Internet Activities

Complete the activities and answer the questions that follow.

34. Do a Web search for "physician malpractice insurance" to find out how malpractice insurance premium rates vary among states. Which states seem to be in crisis regarding the cost of medical malpractice insurance? In states with lower rates, what is credited with keeping costs lower than they are in other states? What is the situation in the state where you plan to practice? Should all health care practitioners carry medical malpractice insurance? Explain your answer.

_____

_____

_____

_____

35. Search the Web site of the American Tort Reform Association (ATRA). Use the site to find out if your state has passed civil justice reform acts that pertain specifically to health care practitioners. If so, briefly describe the acts and how they might affect health care practitioners.

_____

_____

_____

_____

_____

Medical Records and Informed Consent

CHAPTER

6

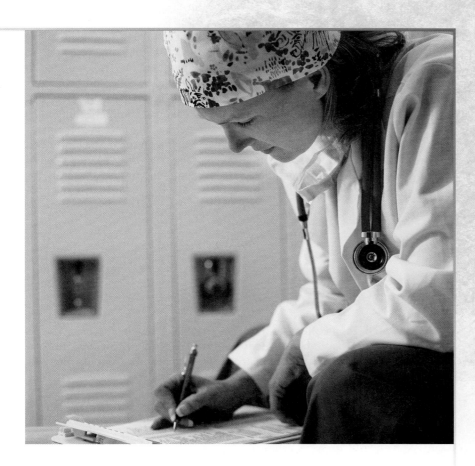

Learning Outcomes

After studying this chapter, you should be able to:

1. Explain the purpose of medical records and the importance of proper documentation for legal protection.

2. Demonstrate the procedure for making a correction in a medical record.

3. Identify ownership of medical records and determine how long a medical record must be kept by the owners.

4. Describe the purpose of obtaining a patient's consent for release of medical information.

5. Explain the doctrine of informed consent.

6. Describe the necessity for electronic medical records and the efforts being made to record all medical records electronically.

Key Terms

Confidentiality of Alcohol and Drug Abuse, Patient Records

consent

doctrine of informed consent

doctrine of professional discretion

fiduciary duty

Good Samaritan acts

health information technology (HIT)

medical record

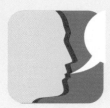
Sally, Michael, and Teresa handle requests for release of patients' medical records for a midwestern hospital serving a five-state area. They emphasize that they can release records only with signed authorization from the patient or upon subpoena, and that they may then release photocopies, but never original medical records. When someone visits the hospital to pick up copies of a patient's records, that person is asked to show identification.

Michael lets experience be his guide and checks out any request for release of records that "doesn't feel right." For example, if a husband brings an authorization form for release of medical records that he says his wife signed, her signature should be checked against the signature on hospital admission forms. It could be that a divorce is in progress in such a situation, and the husband or wife is seeking medical records to prove the spouse an unfit parent.

"Never release medical records because the person making the request has intimidated you," adds Teresa. "The most officious person I've dealt with was an FBI agent who told me, 'I want this record. If you don't give it to me, I'll get it myself.' I said, 'Go for it.' Later the agent called and apologized to me."

Since the employing hospital is located in a city with an air force base, Sally, Michael, and Teresa often receive requests for medical records for active duty military personnel. "We have now been told that the military can get the records they request on any active duty person," adds Sally. "We still ask for an authorization, but it is not required, since the active duty person signs away that right when he or she signs up for the military. This applies to active duty personnel on duty or on leave, but it does not include dependents of the person in the military."

MEDICAL RECORDS

medical record A collection of data recorded when a patient seeks medical treatment.

A **medical record** is a collection of data recorded when a patient seeks medical treatment. Hospitals, surgical centers, clinics, physicians' offices, and other facilities providing health care services maintain patients' medical records. Medical records serve many purposes:

- They are required by licensing authorities and provide a format for tracking, documenting, and maintaining a patient's communication data, both inside and outside a health care facility.
- They provide documentation of a patient's continuing health care, from birth to death.
- They provide a foundation for managing a patient's health care.
- They serve as legal documents in lawsuits.
- They provide clinical data for education, research, statistical tracking, and assessing the quality of health care.

Entries

As a legal document, a patient's medical record may be subpoenaed (via subpoena *duces tecum*) as evidence in court. When they are conscientiously compiled, medical records can prevail over a patient's recollection of events during a trial. When there is no entry in the record to the effect that something was done, there is a presumption that it was not done, and when there is an entry that something was done, the presumption is that it was done. Therefore, what is omitted from the record may be as important to the outcome of a lawsuit as what is included.

Records may be kept on paper, microfilm, or computer tapes or disks. For legal protection as well as continuity of care, the following information must be recorded in a patient's record:

- Contact and identifying information: the patient's full name, Social Security number, date of birth, and full address. If applicable, include e-mail address, home and work telephone numbers, marital status, and name and address of employer.

- Insurance information: name of policy member and relationship to patient, details such as certificate and group numbers, telephone numbers, copy of insurance card, Medicaid or Medicare numbers if applicable, and secondary insurance.

- Driver's license information, state, and number.

- Person responsible for payment and billing address.

- Emergency contact information.

- The patient's health history.

- The dates and times of the patient's arrival for appointments.

- A complete description of the patient's symptoms and reason for making an appointment.

- The examination performed by the physician.

- The physician's assessment, diagnosis, recommendations, treatment prescribed, progress notes, and instructions given to the patient, plus a notation of all new prescriptions the physician writes for the patient and of refills the physician authorizes.

- X-rays and all other test results.

- A notation for each time the patient telephoned the medical facility or was telephoned by the facility, listing date, reason for the call, and resolution.

- A notation of copies made of the medical record, including date copied and the person to whom the copy was sent.

- Documentation of informed consent, when necessary.

- Name of the guardian or legal representative to be contacted if the patient is unable to give informed consent.

- Other documentation, such as complete written descriptions; photographs; samples of body fluids, foreign objects, and clothing; and so on. All items should be carefully labeled and preserved.

- Condition of the patient at the time of termination of treatment, when applicable, and reasons for termination, including documentation if the physician-patient contract was terminated before completion of treatment.

Five Cs (Figure 6-1) can be used to describe the necessary attributes of entries to patients' medical records. These entries must be

1. Concise.
2. Complete (and objective).
3. Clear (and legibly written).
4. Correct.
5. Chronologically ordered.

Medical records should never include inappropriate personal judgments or observations or attempts at humor.

Photographs, Videotaping, and Other Methods of Patient Imaging

In today's health care environment, it has become increasingly common to record patients' images through the use of photography, videotaping, digital imaging, and other visual recordings. For example, surgeons may photograph, videotape, or otherwise record procedures used during an operation for purposes of education or review. Cosmetic surgeons and physicians who treat accident victims may want to document visually the patient's condition "before" and "after" the incident. Such images then become part of the patient's medical record, subject to the same requirement for written release as the rest of the record. (See the section in this chapter entitled "Release of Information," on page 154.)

Photographing or otherwise recording a patient's image without proper consent may be interpreted in a court of law as invasion of privacy. Invasion of privacy charges are most often upheld in court if the patient's image was used for commercial purposes, but such claims have also been upheld under public disclosure of embarrassing private facts. For example, "before" and "after" photographs published by a cosmetic surgeon may cause embarrassment to the patient if he or she did not give consent for the photographs to be published.

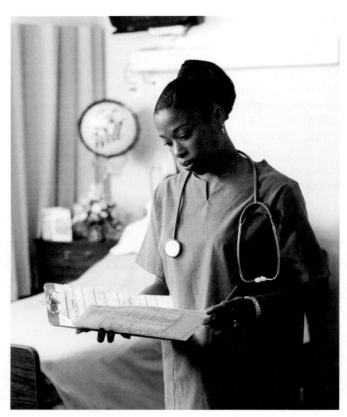

FIGURE 6-1 Always remember the five Cs of charting when recording patient information.

If a health care facility routinely photographs patients to document care, a special consent form should be signed stating that

- The patient understands that photographs, videotapes, and digital or other images may be taken to document care.

- The patient understands that ownership rights to the images will be retained by the health care facility, but that he or she will be allowed to view them or to obtain copies.

- The images will be securely stored and kept for the time period prescribed by law or outlined in the health care facility's policy.

- Images of the patient will not be released and/or used outside the health care facility without written authorization from the patient or his or her legal representative.

If the images will be used for teaching or publicity, a separate consent form should be used.

Corrections

Errors made when making an entry in a medical record or errors discovered later can be corrected, but corrections must be made in a specific manner, so that if the medical records are ever used in a medical malpractice lawsuit,

1. Define *medical record*.

   _____

   _____

2. List five purposes served by a patient's medical record.

   _____

   _____

   _____

   _____

   _____

3. As the person responsible for charting in a medical office, would you record a patient's statement that she often feels "woozy" and thinks she has "dropsy"? Why or why not?

   _____

   _____

4. If a reconstructive surgeon wants to publish "before" and "after" photographs of patients in a brochure left in the waiting room for distribution to prospective patients, what must she do?

   _____

   _____

5. If a patient makes critical remarks to you, a medical assistant, about your physician/employer, would you record the remarks in the patient's medical record? Why or why not?

   _____

   _____

it will not appear that they were falsified. Follow these guidelines when correcting errors in a client's medical record:

- Draw a line through the error so that it is still legible. Do not black out the information or use correction fluid to cover it up.
- Write or type in the correct information above or below the original line or in the margin. If necessary, you may attach another sheet of paper or another document with the correction on it. In this case, note in the record "See attached document A" to indicate where the corrected information can be found.
- Note near the correction why it was made (for example, "error, wrong date," or "error, interrupted by a phone call"). You can place this note in the margin or, again, add an attachment. Do not make a change in the record without noting the reason for it.
- Enter the date and time, and initial the correction.
- If possible, ask another staff member or the physician to witness and initial the correction to the record when you make it.

Ownership

Patients' medical records are considered the property of the owners of the facility where they were created. For example, a physician in private practice owns his or her records; records in a clinic are the property of the clinic. Hospital records are the property of the admitting hospital. The facility where the medical records were created owns the documents, but *the patient owns the information they contain.* Upon signing a release, patients may usually obtain access to or copies of their medical records, depending upon state law. However, under the **doctrine of professional discretion,** courts have held that in some cases, patients treated for mental or emotional conditions may be harmed by seeing their own records. Under HIPAA, patients who ask to see and/or copy their medical records must be accommodated, with a few exceptions. HIPAA is discussed in detail in Chapter 7, "Privacy Law and HIPAA." If patients need clarification, records may be reviewed in the presence of a trusted health care professional, but this is not a requirement for allowing patients to see their records.

When a physician in private practice examines a patient for a job-related physical, scheduled and paid for by the patient's employer or prospective employer, those records are still the physician's property, but the employer is entitled to a copy of the record that is pertinent to the job-related exam. Medical records should never be kept in an employer's general personnel files. The patient must obtain permission from the employer to release information contained in the records.

Under HIPAA, patients are entitled to access any health care information a physician generates about them, with a few exceptions, which are discussed in Chapter 7.

Retention and Storage

As a protection in the event of litigation, records should be kept until the applicable statute of limitations period has elapsed, which generally ranges from two to seven years. In some cases, this involves keeping the medical records for minor patients for a specified length of time after they reach legal age. Some states have enacted statutes for the retention of medical records. However, most physicians retain records indefinitely, since, in addition to their value as documentation in medical professional liability suits and for tax purposes, the patient's medical history may be vital in determining future treatment.

Confidentiality

Since medical office personnel have a duty to protect the privacy of the patient, medical records should not be released to a third party without written permission, signed by the patient or the patient's legal representative. Only the information requested should be released.

Requests for release of records may ask for records concerning a specific date or time span. Records may also be requested for a specific diagnosis, symptom, or body system, or for results of certain diagnostic tests. Medical records personnel should not send unsolicited records. They should carefully review the signed release form to ensure that the correct records are sent.

When medical records are requested for use in a lawsuit, a signed consent for the release of the records must be obtained from the patient, unless a court subpoenas the records. In this case, the patient should be notified in writing that the records have been subpoenaed and released.

doctrine of professional discretion A principle under which a physician can exercise judgment as to whether to show patients who are being treated for mental or emotional conditions their records. Disclosure depends on whether, in the physician's judgment, such patients would be harmed by viewing the records.

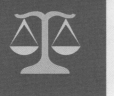

Court Case

Loss of Medical Records

A plaintiff brought a medical malpractice suit against a hospital in Massachusetts. During discovery, the plaintiff learned that the hospital had lost his medical records. An appeals court entered a default judgment in favor of the plaintiff as sanction for the hospital's loss of plaintiff's medical records, and the state supreme court upheld the lower court's decision. The supreme court stated that the missing records, which the defendant conceded were irreparably lost, contained the only documentation of the critical time period during which the alleged malpractice event occurred, making a determination based on the evidence impossible.

Note: Results of this decision were not published. It is likely that the hospital settled with the plaintiff out of court.

Keene v. Brigham & Women's Hosp., Inc. 439 Mass. 223 (2003).

HEALTH INFORMATION TECHNOLOGY (HIT)

When Hurricane Katrina, a Category 5 storm, hit the Louisiana and Mississippi coasts on August 29, 2005, the widespread destruction that resulted included countless numbers of paper medical records. Many of the survivors gathered in the Superdome couldn't remember the names of lost prescriptions, or when they had last been immunized against tetanus and other diseases. Katrina victims who reported to physicians had virtually no medical records, and reconstruction would take time.

Health information technology—electronic medical records—could prevent such huge medical record losses in the future, but as of September 2005, surveys showed that only approximately 14 percent of group practices and 13 percent of hospitals had converted to electronic medical records. One year later, after Katrina, that figure had not increased significantly, according to articles in *Information Week, PC World,* and other publications.

According to the U.S. Department of Health and Human Services, **health information technology (HIT)** is "the application of information processing involving both computer hardware and software that deals with the storage, retrieval, sharing, and use of health care information, data, and knowledge for communication and decision-making." The broad category *health information technology* also includes telemedicine and use of the Internet for health information purposes. A central component of HIT is the patient's medical file, and as electronic medical records become more widely adopted, confidentiality and privacy concerns must be addressed.

As of 2004, President George W. Bush had set a 10-year goal for the broad adoption of electronic health records in the United States.

Government-initiated steps toward broad adoption of electronic health information include the following:

1. **The Health Insurance Portability and Accountability Act (HIPAA).** Passed in 1996 and implemented in stages through 2005, HIPAA addresses privacy of health information and mandates certain

health information technology (HIT) The application of information processing, involving both computer hardware and software, that deals with the storage, retrieval, sharing, and use of health care information, data, and knowledge for communication and decision making.

procedures and standards for the electronic transmission and storage of health care information. (See HIPAA details in Chapter 7, "Privacy Law and HIPAA.")

2. **Executive Orders.** In April 2004, President George W. Bush signed an executive order establishing the position of National Coordinator for Health Information Technology. The coordinator was charged with the development, maintenance, and oversight of a plan for nationwide adoption of health information technology.

   In August 2006, a second executive order stated that all federal agencies would utilize, where available, health information technology systems and products meeting certain "recognized" standards. These HIT systems and products "shall be used for implementing, acquiring, or upgrading health information technology systems used for the direct exchange of health information between agencies and with nonfederal entities." The order further stipulated that federal agencies shall require in contracts or agreements with health care providers, health plans, or health insurance issuers that, where available, health information technology systems and products meeting recognized standards shall be used.

3. **Adoption of the Health Information Standards Developed by Health and Human Services (HHS).** As part of this effort, HHS has negotiated and licensed a comprehensive medical vocabulary and made it available to everyone in the United States at no cost. The results of these projects include standards for the following types of information:

   ▌ Transmitting X-Rays over the Internet: Today, a patient's chest X-ray can be sent electronically from a hospital or laboratory and read by the patient's doctor in his office.

   ▌ Electronic Laboratory Results: Laboratory results can be sent electronically to the physician for immediate analysis, diagnosis, and treatment, and could be automatically entered into the patient's electronic health record if one existed. For example, a doctor could retrieve this information for a hospitalized patient from his office, assuring a prompt response and eliminating errors and duplicative testing due to lost laboratory reports.

   ▌ Electronic Prescriptions: Patients will save time because prescriptions can be sent electronically to their pharmacists. By eliminating illegible handwritten prescriptions, and because the technology automatically checks for possible allergies and harmful interactions with other drugs, standardized electronic prescriptions help to avoid serious medical errors. The technology also can generate automatic approval from a health insurer.

4. **Use of the Federal Government to Foster the Adoption of Health Information Technology.** As one of the largest buyers of health care—in Medicare, Medicaid, the Community Health Centers program, the Federal Health Benefits program, veterans' medical care, and programs in the Department of Defense—the federal government can create incentives and opportunities for health care providers to use electronic records.

The federal government maintains that the broad use of health information technology will improve individual patient care by

▌ Improving health care quality.

▌ Preventing medical errors.

- Reducing health care costs.
- Increasing administrative efficiency.
- Decreasing paperwork.
- Expanding access to affordable care.

The above benefits can be seen in the following examples:

- When arriving at a physician's office, new patients do not have to enter their personal information, allergies, medications, or medical history, since these facts are already available.
- A parent, who previously may have had to carry a large folder containing the child's medical records and X-rays by hand when seeing a new physician, can now keep the most important medical history on a keychain, or simply authorize the new physician to retrieve the information electronically from previous health care providers.
- Arriving at an emergency room, an elderly patient with a chronic illness and memory difficulties can authorize her physicians to access her medical information from a recent hospitalization at another hospital—thus avoiding a potentially fatal drug interaction between the planned treatment and the patient's current medications.

Public health benefits will include

- Early detection of infectious outbreaks around the country. For example, three patients experience unusual sudden-onset fever and cough that would not individually be reported. They show up at separate emergency rooms, and through access to electronic health information, the trend is instantly reported to public health officials, who alert authorities of a possible disease outbreak or bioterror attack.
- Improved tracking of chronic disease management.
- Evaluation of health care based on comparisons of price and quality.

While the goal of widespread adoption of electronic health records by 2014 seems beneficial, many physicians and hospitals have not been eager to digitalize written records, because the process is expensive and often fraught with information technology headaches, such as susceptibility to hackers who would steal private information, software that doesn't always perform as expected, and other threats to confidentiality when medical records are maintained and transported electronically.

Technological Threats to Confidentiality

Increasingly, as the federal government mandates and encourages health information technology, modern health care facilities rely on technology for creating, maintaining, and transporting patients' medical information. The implementation of HIPAA imposes penalties for breaches of confidentiality regarding medical records that identify patients by name. The following guidelines can help ensure that confidentiality is not breached when employees use photocopiers, fax machines, computers, and printers to reproduce and send medical records.

Photocopiers

- Do not leave confidential papers anywhere on the copier where others can read the information.
- Do not discard copies in a shared trash container; shred them.

- If a paper jam occurs, be sure to remove from the machine the copy or partial copy that caused the jam.

Fax Machines

- Always verify the telephone number of the receiving location before faxing confidential material.
- Never fax confidential material to an unauthorized person.
- Do not fax confidential material if others in the room can observe the material.
- Do not leave confidential material unattended on a fax machine.
- Do not discard fax copies in a shared trash container; shred them.
- Use a fax cover sheet that states, "Confidential: To addressee only. Please return if received in error."

Computers

- Locate the monitor in an area where others cannot see the screen.
- Do not leave a monitor unattended while confidential material is displayed on the screen.
- Because it is difficult to ensure the privacy of e-mail messages, sending confidential patient information via e-mail is not recommended.

Printers

- Do not print confidential material on a printer shared by other departments or in an area where others can read the material.
- Do not leave a printer unattended while printing confidential material.
- Before leaving the printing area, check to be sure all computer disks containing confidential material and all printed material have been collected.
- Be certain that the print job is sent to the right printer location.
- Do not discard printouts in a shared trash container; shred them.

Release of Information

Medical information about a patient is often released for the following purposes:

Insurance Claims. The medical office supplies specific requested information, but does not usually send the patient's entire medical record. An authorization to release information, signed by the patient, is required before records may be released, but most health care providers incorporate the release into the patient registration form so that information can be provided in a timely manner.

Transfer to Another Physician. The physician may photocopy and send all records, or may send a summary. The patient must sign an authorization to release records.

Use in a Court of Law. When a subpoena *duces tecum* is issued for certain records (the subpoena commands a witness to appear in court and to bring certain medical records), the patient's written consent to release the records is waived.

The following classic court case illustrates that physicians who produce patients' medical records for use in court, or those who testify in court as expert witnesses, are not liable for breach of confidentiality.

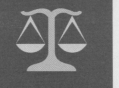

CLASSIC
Court Case

Not Guilty of Breach of Confidentiality

A physician cannot be sued for breach of confidentiality when required to produce a patient's medical records for use in court testimony.

A patient (Cruz) sued a physician (Agelides) for breach of fiduciary duty. (**Fiduciary duty** is a physician's duty to his or her patient, based upon trust and confidence.) In a previous malpractice action brought by Cruz against another physician, Agelides had given a sworn pretrial affidavit and video deposition in favor of the defending physician. The court held that Agelides was immune from any civil liability action as a result of his testimony as a witness in the previous trial.

Cruz v. Agelides, 574 So.2d 278 (Fla. App. 3 Dist., 1991).

fiduciary duty A physician's obligation to his or her patient, based on trust and confidence.

CHECK YOUR PROGRESS

6. Define *fiduciary duty.*

_____

_____

7. Who owns a patient's medical records?

_____

_____

8. Define *doctrine of professional discretion.*

_____

_____

9. You are charting after a patient's office visit and you are interrupted by a telephone call. The interruption causes you to incorrectly record results of the patient's blood tests. When you discover your mistake, can you correct it? If so, how?

_____

_____

10. You are photocopying a patient's medical record and an employee from the clinic's accounting department is reading over your shoulder while he waits to use the copier. What should you do?

_____

_____

The following court case is complicated, but it illustrates how breach of confidentiality may be charged, as well as negligence and defamation, when personal records are released to others. In this case, the court

Breach of Confidentiality Charged

As a result of a criminal complaint filed by his girlfriend for battery and disorderly conduct, a student in a physician assistant program was dismissed from the program. After his dismissal from the PA program, the plaintiff entered into a diversion agreement on the criminal charges, requiring him to participate in a men's abuse program at a family center. The former PA student signed a release allowing the family center coordinator to provide information concerning his progress to the District Attorney's Office.

The family center coordinator spoke with the student's girlfriend, learning that he took amphetamines daily; hit her at least 15 days in one month; called her names; forbade her to wear a seat belt in the car; and threatened to kill her. The coordinator then sent a letter to the District Attorney, quoting the girlfriend's statements and recommending that the former PA student spend more time in family center counseling programs.

The student then filed suit against the family center and the coordinator, alleging breach of confidentiality of health records, intentional infliction of emotional distress, professional negligence, and defamation.

A lower court granted summary judgment to the defendants for all claims. An appeals court upheld the summary judgment for claims of confidentiality of patient health care records and intentional infliction of emotional distress but reversed and remanded for further proceedings the defamation and professional negligence claims.

Note: The student's dismissal from the PA program was not at issue in this proceeding, but was upheld by a review committee at the school. The family center coordinator's letter was held not to be "patient health care records." The former PA student was, however, held to have defamation and professional negligence claims against the family center and its coordinator. No published results are available as to whether or not the former PA student pursued these claims in court.

Hart v. Kenneth Bennet and Family & Children's Center, Inc., 2003 WI App 231; 267 Wis. 2d 919, 672 N.W.2d 306; 2003 Wisc. Appl, LEXIS 984.

determined that the records in question were not "health care records" in the legal sense of the term.

Physicians receive subpoenas for patient medical records for a variety of reasons, including accidents involving patients, workers' compensation claims, and other non-medical-liability reasons. When this occurs, the medical office sends a photocopy of the patient's medical records to the attorney who issued the subpoena.

When a physician is sued for medical malpractice, however, responsibility to comply with a subpoena to produce specified medical records in court may fall to the medical office employee in charge of medical records. In that case, the person in charge of medical records should follow these guidelines:

▌ Check the subpoena to be sure the name and phone number of the issuing attorney and the court docket number of the case are listed.

▌ If a carbon copy of the subpoena is received, verify that it is the same as the original in every way.

▌ Verify that the patient named was a patient of the physician named.

▌ Verify the trial date and time as listed on the subpoena.

- Notify the physician that a subpoena was received, and then notify the physician's insurance company or attorney, if so directed.
- Check all subpoenaed records to be sure they are complete, but never alter them in any way.
- Document the number of pages in the record and itemize its contents. Make a photocopy of the original to be submitted, if permitted by state law and the court.
- Offer sworn testimony regarding the record, if so instructed by the court.

Confidentiality of Alcohol and Drug Abuse, Patient Records
A federal statute that protects patients with histories of substance abuse regarding the release of information about treatment.

Some state laws specifically address the release of confidential medical information, especially as it pertains to treatment for mental or emotional health problems, HIV testing, and substance abuse. In addition, the federal statute **Confidentiality of Alcohol and Drug Abuse, Patient Records** protects patients with histories of substance abuse regarding the release of information about treatment. Under no circumstances should information of this type be released without specific, written permission from the patient to do so. The patient also has the right to rescind (cancel) consent to release information, in which case the information should not be released.

CHECK YOUR PROGRESS

11. Name three reasons a medical office might be requested to release a patient's medical records.

_____

_____

_____

12. In which of the three situations named in question 11 might a patient's written consent to release records be waived?

_____

_____

13. What is needed before the medical office can send a patient's medical record to the insurer?

_____

_____

14. If an insurance company submits a request for medical records pertaining to an enrolled patient's outpatient foot surgery and you are responsible for sending the records, should you send the patient's entire file just to be on the safe side? Why or why not?

_____

_____

15. As the person who reviews requests for patients' medical records, do you need to know the purpose for which the data will be used? Explain your answer.

_____

_____

The following rules for authorizations for the release of medical records can serve as a general guide for medical assistants, health information technicians, and other health care practitioners:

I Authorizations should be in writing.

I Authorizations should include the patient's name, address, and date of birth.

I The patient should sign authorizations, unless he or she is not a legal, competent adult. In that case, parents or guardians should sign authorizations.

I Only the information specifically requested should be released.

I The patient has the right to rescind a consent to release information, in which case information should not be released.

Requests for information coming into the medical office from insurance companies, physicians, or other sources should

I Be witnessed and dated and include the complete name, address, and signature of the party requesting the information, as well as that of the party asked to release the information.

I Include a specific description of the information that is needed. List the purpose for which the data will be used and the date upon which the consent expires.

CONSENT

consent Permission from a patient, either expressed or implied, for something to be done by another.

By giving **consent,** the patient gives permission, either expressed (orally or in writing) or impl1ied, for the physician to examine him or her, to perform tests that aid in diagnosis, and/or to treat for a medical condition. When the patient makes an appointment for an examination, that patient has given implied consent for the physician to perform the exam. Likewise, when he or she cooperates with various diagnostic testing procedures, implied consent for the tests has been given.

Informed Consent

For surgery and for some other procedures, such as a test for HIV, implied consent is not enough. In these cases, it is important to ask the patient to sign a consent form, thereby establishing informed consent (see Figure 6-2).

doctrine of informed consent The legal basis for informed consent, usually outlined in a state's medical practice acts.

The **doctrine of informed consent** is the legal basis for informed consent and is usually outlined in a state's medical practice acts. Informed consent implies that the patient understands

I Proposed modes of treatment.

I Why the treatment is necessary.

I Risks involved in the proposed treatment.

I Available alternative modes of treatment.

I Risks of alternative modes of treatment.

I Risks involved if treatment is refused.

Informed consent involves the patient's right to receive all information relative to his or her condition and then to make a decision regarding treatment based upon that knowledge. Documents establishing that the patient gave informed consent prove that the patient was not coerced into treatment.

INFORMED CONSENT for SURGERY and PROCEDURES

1. I hereby authorize staff physicians and resident staff at _____ to
   _____ *(Name of Hospital or Facility)*

   perform upon _____, such treatment,
   (Name of Patient)

   procedures and/or operations necessary to treat or diagnose the condition(s) which appear indicated.

2. The operation(s) or procedure(s) necessary to treat and/or diagnose my condition and the risks, benefits/alternatives

   and options associated with them have been explained to me by _____,
   (Name of Physician or Provider)

   and I understand the operation(s) or procedure(s) to be: _____

   _____

3. **Different Provider:** ☐ Not Applicable
   I understand and approve that a different provider other than the physician named above may actually perform the procedure.

4. **Operative Side:** ☐ Not Applicable   ☐ Left   ☐ Right

5. **Sedation & Local Anesthetics:** I authorize the administration of sedation and the use of local anesthetics, drugs and medicines as may be deemed appropriate. If they will be used, the risks and benefits/alternatives of sedation have been explained to me by the procedural physician.

6. **Blood and Blood Products:** ☐ Not Applicable
   I understand certain surgeries, procedures, or illnesses may result in loss of blood. I authorize the administration of blood and/or blood components during the procedure as well as during the course of my hospital stay. If blood will be used, the risks, benefits/alternatives have been explained to me by the physician.

   Patient Initials: _____

7. **No Blood Products:** ☐ Not Applicable
   I request that NO blood derivative be administered to me. I hereby release the hospital, its personnel, the attending physician and its agents from any responsibility whatsoever for unfavorable reactions or any untoward results due to my refusal to permit the use of blood or its derivatives. The possible risks and consequences of such refusal on my part have been fully explained and I fully understand such risks and consequences may occur as a result of my refusal.

   Signature of Patient/Responsible Person: _____   Relationship: _____

8. **Unforeseen Conditions:** It has been explained to me that during the course of the operation(s) or procedure(s) unforeseen conditions may be revealed that necessitate an extension of the original procedure(s) or different procedure(s) than those set forth above. I am aware that the practice of medicine is not an exact science and I acknowledge that no guarantees have been made to me concerning the results of this operation(s) or procedure(s).

9. **Photography:** I consent to the use of photography, closed circuit television recording and to use the photographs and other materials for study, educational and scientific purposes, in accordance with ordinary practices of the facility.

10. I consent to have my procedure/operation observed, for educational purposes, by individual(s) other than those assisting the physician during the procedure/operation.

Physician or Provider Signature	Patient's Signature *(If competent)*		Witness		Date	Time
Signature of Interpreter *(If applicable)*	Date	Time	Signature of Person Responsible/Relationship		Date	Time
Witness *(Telephone consent)*	Date	Time	Second Physician or Provider Signature for Emergencies for Incompetent Patient and No Family		Date	Time

Physician must initial faxed copy

FIGURE 6-2   A Sample Consent Form

Adults of sound mind are usually able to give informed consent. Those individuals who cannot give informed consent include the following:

Minors, Persons Under the Age of Majority. Exceptions include

▌ Emancipated minors—those who are living away from home and responsible for their own support. A minor becomes "emancipated" through a court hearing where evidence is presented that the minor

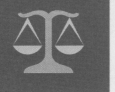
Medical Malpractice/Consent and Informed Consent

A woman who was 23 weeks pregnant went into labor and was admitted to a Texas hospital. An obstetrician and a neonatologist informed both parents that if the "baby were born alive and survived, she would suffer severe impairments." Based on that information, the parents orally requested that no heroic measures be performed on the baby after birth. The request was entered in the medical record, and the neonatologist was dismissed. However, the obstetrician later concluded that if the baby were born alive and weighed over 500 grams, the medical staff would be obligated by law and hospital policy to administer life-sustaining procedures, even if the baby's parents did not consent to such procedures. The obstetrician later stated that this caveat was explained to the parents. A second neonatologist who assisted in the delivery determined that the child was "viable" and "instituted resuscitative measures." The child survived birth but, as predicted, suffered severe physical and mental impairments.

The parents filed suit against the corporation that owned the hospital, alleging, among other claims, that the physicians had treated their newborn without their consent. A jury trial held the hospital corporation liable for the baby's injuries, and the court awarded the parents $29,400,000 in past and future medical expenses, $13,500,000 in punitive damages, and $17,503,066 in "prejudgment interest."

The hospital corporation appealed, claiming that no duty was owed to the plaintiffs and that the doctors and hospital personnel who resuscitated the baby were legally obligated to do so. The hospital corporation also alleged that the parents had no right to withhold life-sustaining medical treatment from their child.

The appellate court held that "as a general rule, parents have no right to refuse urgently-needed life-sustaining medical treatment to their non-terminally ill children." The court found that the physicians involved in resuscitating the newborn had acted reasonably and dismissed the vicarious liability action against the hospital corporation. Therefore, the parents received no award.

HCA, Inc. v. Miller, 36 S.W.3d 187 (2000).

should be emancipated, and a judge makes a determination that the minor has met certain criteria. The minor is then declared "emancipated" and can consent to his or her health care treatment just as any adult of sound mind determines his or her health care treatment.

- ▌ Married minors.
- ▌ Mature minors—those who, through the doctrine of mature minors, have been granted the right to seek birth control or care during pregnancy, treatment for reportable communicable diseases, or treatment for drug- or alcohol-related problems without first obtaining parental consent.

The rights of emancipated minors, married minors, and mature minors to consent to their own health care are discussed further in Chapter 10, "The Beginning of Life and Childhood."

The Mentally Incompetent. Individuals judged by the court to be insane, senile, mentally challenged, or under the influence of drugs or alcohol cannot give informed consent. In these cases, a competent person may be designated by the court to act as the patient's agent.

Those Who Speak Limited or No English. When a patient does not speak or understand English, an interpreter may be necessary in order to inform the patient and obtain his or her consent for treatment.

Other problems in obtaining informed consent may arise, in such situations as when foster children need medical attention or a spouse seeks

16. Who may give informed consent?

_____

_____

17. Who may not give informed consent?

_____

_____

18. Must consent to perform routine medical care, such as a physical examination, always be in writing? Explain your answer.

_____

_____

19. In which health care situations is implied consent not sufficient?

_____

_____

20. What consequences generally ensue if a legally competent adult is treated without consent and an adverse event occurs?

_____

_____

sterilization or an abortion. In each case, health care practitioners must determine who is legally able to give informed consent for treatment. When in doubt, seek legal advice.

Patient education is vital to the issue of informed consent. Stocking the medical office with brochures about various medical problems is not sufficient if the physician does not review the material with the patient. Patients who sue have successfully claimed lack of informed consent because they did not read the consent form they signed or did not read brochures handed to them. Health care personnel should be sure that patients understand all forms and all treatments/surgeries to be performed before signing.

The following U.S. Supreme Court decision illustrates the fact that before proceeding with treatment, health care practitioners must determine whether or not patients are competent to give informed consent.

Informed Consent and Abortion Law

In *Planned Parenthood v. Casey,* U.S. 833 (1992), the United States Supreme Court upheld a 24-hour waiting period, an informed consent requirement, a parental consent provision for minors, and a recordkeeping requirement for women seeking an abortion. At the same time, the Court struck down the spousal notice requirement of a Pennsylvania statute, in addition to other specific requirements. (Ten states, however, have unenforceable spousal consent or notice laws: Colorado, Florida, Illinois, Kentucky, Louisiana, North Dakota, Pennsylvania, Rhode Island, South Carolina, and Utah.)

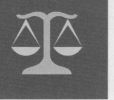

Patient Not Competent to Sign Forms

The U.S. Supreme Court overruled two lower federal courts, stating that a Florida mental patient had a cause of action. The patient claimed that he had been admitted to a state mental health treatment facility as a voluntary patient, based on forms he signed when he was heavily medicated, disoriented, and suffering from a psychotic disorder. He had been found wandering along a highway and appeared to be injured and disoriented. He was taken to a private mental health facility. While he was hallucinating, confused, and psychotic, he signed forms for admission.

The U.S. Supreme Court held that allegations that employees of the state hospital admitted him as a voluntary patient without taking steps to ascertain whether he was mentally competent to sign the admission forms stated a cause of action.

Zinermon v. Burch, 110 S.Ct. 975 (U.S. Sup. Ct., Feb. 27, 1990).

Casey and *Webster v. Reproductive Health Services* before it (1989), upheld *Roe v. Wade,* the 1973 Supreme Court decision that legalized abortion in the United States (see the following case), but allowed state regulation of abortion. A number of state legislatures took the cue and passed new abortion restrictions.

Among a long list of state-imposed abortion restrictions are laws that specify certain changes in informed consent. For example, some states require that a woman seeking an abortion be clearly informed of all alternatives to abortions and be told of all risks associated with such surgeries before she can give informed consent to the abortion. In addition, before a woman can consent to an abortion in many states, she must wait a certain length of time (usually 24 hours) before actually signing a consent form.

LANDMARK
Court Case

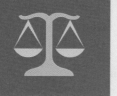

Case Legalizes Abortion

In 1970 a single woman in Texas became pregnant. She had difficulty finding work because of her pregnancy and feared the stigma of an illegitimate birth. Under the fictitious name "Jane Roe," the woman sued Henry Wade, the district attorney in Dallas County, Texas, claiming that she had limited rights to an abortion and sought an injunction against the Texas statute prohibiting abortion except to save a woman's life.

It took three years for the case to reach the United States Supreme Court, which struck down the Texas statute. The ruling came too late for Jane Roe to have the abortion she originally sought, of course, but it affected the rights of all women who would seek abortions from that time on. The Court held that the constitutional right to privacy includes a woman's decision to terminate a pregnancy during the first trimester (three months), but that states could impose restrictions and regulate abortions after that.

Roe v. Wade, 410 U.S. 113, 144 n.39 (1973).

TABLE 6-1 State Abortion Laws

Law	Description	States
General Abortion Bans	17 states have never repealed restrictive laws ruled unconstitutional by *Roe v. Wade* in 1973	AL, AZ, AR, CA, CO, DE, DC, MA, MI, MS, NH, MN, OK, TX, VT, WV, WI
*Partial-Birth Abortion Bans	24 states passed laws to prohibit partial-birth procedures during the second or third trimester, but such laws in approximately two-thirds of the 24 states have been temporarily or permanently enjoined by federal courts	AL, AK, AR, AZ, FL, GA, IL, IN, KS, LA, MS, MT, MI, NE, NJ, OH, RI, TN, SC, SD, TN, UT, VA, WI
Nonsurgical Abortions	Two states prohibit nonsurgical (also called chemical) abortions	RI, TN
Spousal Consent Required	A woman must either obtain spousal consent or notify her spouse in 10 states, but this law was rendered unenforceable by the 1992 Supreme Court decision in *Casey*	CO, FL, IL, KY, LA, ND, PA, RI, SC, UT
Detailed Informed Consent	Women must be thoroughly informed as to alternatives and risks in 30 states	AL, AK, CA, CT, DE, FL, ID, IN, KS, KY, LA, ME, MA, MI, MN, MS, MO, MT, NE, NV, ND, OH, PA, RI, SC, SD, TN, UT, VA, WI
Waiting Period	24 states have enacted a waiting period before a woman can consent to an abortion; in two of the 24 states—MA and MT—waiting period enforcement was permanently enjoined by court order, and the policy is not in effect	AL, AK, GA, ID, KS, KY, LA, , MI, MN, MS, NE, ND, OH, OK, PA, SC, SD, TX, UT, VA, WV, WI
Conscience Exceptions	46 states permit certain medical personnel and health facilities to refuse to participate in abortion on the basis of conscience or religious conviction	AK, AZ, AR, CA, CO, CT, DE, FL, GA, HI, ID, IL, IN, IA, KS, KY, LA, ME, MD, MA, MI, MN, MO, MT, NE, NV, NJ, NM, NY, NC, ND, OH, OK, OR, PA, RI, SC, SD, TN, TX, UT, VA, WA, WV, WI, WY

*Partial-birth abortion is a lay term. The medical term for the procedure is dilation and extraction (D&X). *Merriam-Webster's Medical Dictionary* defines partial-birth abortion as "an abortion in the second or third trimester of pregnancy in which the death of the fetus is induced after it has passed partway through the birth canal."

Since abortion law is constantly changing, health care practitioners must stay informed about current abortion laws in their respective states. Table 6-1 provides a quick look at a few of the abortion laws in various states, current as of August 1, 2008:

HIV and Informed Consent

State public health law varies for human immunodeficiency virus (HIV) testing, but, generally, health care practitioners must consider the following factors:

Can a minor (aged less than 18 in some states, 21 in others) consent to his or her own HIV test? Informed consent law for minors vary, but this determination may sometimes be made without regard to age, depending upon the minor's situation:

- Infants and young children do not have the capacity to consent, because they do not yet have the ability to make informed decisions. The person legally designated to make health care decisions for the child has the right to decide whether the child should be tested for HIV.
- Married minors, emancipated minors, and minor parents may have the right to give consent for HIV testing, depending on state law.

Can an HIV-infected minor consent to his or her own treatment? Generally, parental or guardian consent is required for a physician to treat a minor for HIV/AIDS, including treatment in school-based clinics. Married, emancipated, and mature minors can usually consent to their own care.

When Consent Is Unnecessary

In emergency situations, when the patient is in immediate danger, the physician is not expected to obtain consent before proceeding with treatment.

All 50 states have passed **Good Samaritan acts.** This protects physicians and, in some states, other health care practitioners and laypersons from charges of negligence or abandonment if they stop to help the victim of an accident or other emergency (Figure 6-3), provided they

- Give such care in good faith.
- Act within the scope of their training and knowledge.
- Use due care under the circumstances.
- Do not bill for their services. (If a physician treats a patient as a "Good Samaritan" and later bills the patient for services, he or she may be held as having established a physician-patient relationship and may not have the immunity from civil damages that a Good Samaritan law would otherwise provide.)

Good Samaritan acts State laws protecting physicians and sometimes other health care practitioners and laypersons from charges of negligence or abandonment if they stop to help the victim of an accident or other emergency.

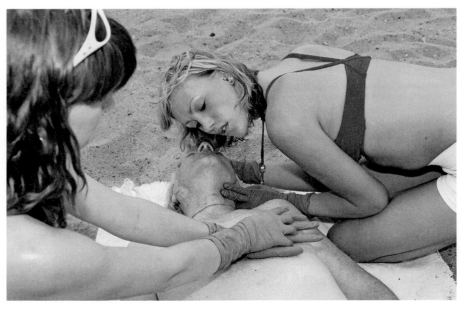

FIGURE 6-3 Good Samaritan laws protect health care practitioners who help patients in an emergency.

Court Case

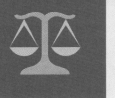

Good Samaritan Act

A woman's obstetrician induced her labor and left the delivery area. Another doctor who was not on call responded to a hospital page that a delivery was in progress without a doctor present. The baby was born paralyzed, and the mother sued the attending physician. The trial court granted the doctor's summary judgment motion, which alleged that he acted under the state's Good Samaritan act and was therefore immune from prosecution. The mother appealed, and the appeals court reversed the trial court's decision, deciding in favor of the mother.

The doctor appealed to the state supreme court, and the court held that the doctor was exempt from liability under the Good Samaritan act because he acted in good faith and without willful or wanton negligence in an emergency and because he did not and "would never have charged" the patient for his services. The supreme court remanded the case to the court of appeals for further proceedings consistent with the supreme court's opinion.

Note: Final disposition of the case was not published. The mother might have dropped the action after the supreme court's decision, or a hearing might have been scheduled for a date still in the future.

McIntyre v. Ramirez and Bocanegra, 109 S.W.3d 741; 2003 Tex. LEXIS 89; 46 (Tex. Sup. J. 854, June 26, 2003).

Ethics Issues

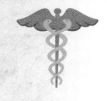

Medical Records and Informed Consent

A basic tenet of medical law and ethics is that patients have the right of self-determination. That right, however, can be effectively exercised only if patients have enough information to make an intelligent, informed choice about medical treatment. Health care practitioners do not have the right to withhold information, because full disclosure might prompt the patient to forgo needed therapy.

Dr. Carmen Paradis, a bioethicist with the Cleveland Clinic, says the following to health care practitioners regarding informed consent:

"Make information relevant to how the patient thinks. For example, '3 percent' may mean nothing to a patient, where '3 out of 100' will. You may also want to say, '97 out of 100 will not have this problem.'

"Benefits must be weighed against risks for the patient. How risky is the treatment under consideration? Is the benefit marginal? In addition, make the information available over time, so the patient is not overwhelmed with information all at once. And in addition to verbal explanations use alternative methods of giving information, such as videos, CDs, written material, and so on."

Medical providers at the Cleveland Clinic are fortunate, in that the clinic has an international center practitioners can call on for translations of medical documents into languages other than English, and for translators who can relate to a patient's native culture and language.

ETHICS ISSUE 1: A nurse working in a physician's office is helping the physician explain a medical diagnosis and proposed treatment plan to a middle-aged woman who is a recent immigrant from Thailand. The woman speaks no English, and her daughter is attempting to translate the conversation. The woman has metastasized lung cancer, and her prognosis is not good. The nurse notices a pronounced hesitation in the daughter's translation of this news to her mother, and she suspects the daughter has not relayed the information correctly, because the patient seems undisturbed by the news.

DISCUSSION QUESTIONS

1. As the nurse helping the physician in this scenario, what would you do?

_____

_____

2. Assume that the nurse and the physician must obtain informed consent from the patient in the above scenario. Should they rely solely on the daughter's ability to translate? Explain your answer.

_____

_____

ETHICS ISSUE 2: You are an LPN in a reproductive services clinic, and a pregnant patient is suffering a medical condition wherein the pregnancy threatens her life. Her physician suggests that she undergo an abortion.

DISCUSSION QUESTIONS

1. Will your personal values allow you to assist with the procedure? Explain your answer.

_____

_____

2. If your answer to question number 3 is no, what are your alternatives?

_____

_____

ETHICS ISSUE 3: You have observed an LPN with whom you work in a hospital attempting to erase an entry she has made in a patient's medical record. She asks you not to tell that you saw her attempting to erase the entry.

DISCUSSION QUESTION

1. What will you do next?

_____

_____

ETHICS ISSUE 4: You have faxed a patient's medical record to another physician's office and discover you have used the wrong fax number.

DISCUSSION QUESTION

1. What will you do next?

_____

_____

Go to www.mhhe.com/judson5e to practice your case review skills. Then read on for more information.

6 REVIEW

Applying Knowledge

Answer the following questions in the spaces provided.

1. Assume you are in charge of recording medical information in a patient's record after the patient has seen his or her physician. What seven items will you be sure to record?

_____

_____

_____

_____

_____

_____

_____

2. What are the five Cs for correctly entering information into a medical record?

_____

_____

_____

_____

_____

_____

3. After an entry in the medical record has been written or keyed and an error is discovered, what procedure should be followed to correct the error?

_____

_____

_____

_____

_____

4. Dr. Wellness works as an employee of Anytown Medical Clinic. Who owns the records of his patients?

_____

5. Dr. Wellness also sees patients at Anytown General Hospital, where he maintains records of hospital stays, procedures, and emergency room visits. To whom do these records belong?

_____

Jan B. sees Dr. Wellness on occasion for routine illnesses and physicals. She will soon be moving, and wishes to transfer these records to her new physician, Dr. Good.

6. Does Jan have the right to obtain copies of her own medical records?

_____

7. Who has ownership of the records before Jan moves?

_____

8. Who has ownership of the records after Jan moves?

_____

9. What procedure should be followed for the records to be transferred to Jan's new physician?

_____

_____

_____

10. What is the statute of limitations in your state for filing a medical malpractice suit?

_____

_____

11. Assume you are in charge of releasing medical information to a third party. What items will you note for the record?

_____

_____

_____

12. The copier malfunctions while you are photocopying a patient's medical records and prints too many copies of several pages. What will you do with the extra copies?

_____

_____

_____

13. You must fax part of a patient's medical record to a consulting physician in another city. What precautions will you follow?

_____

_____

_____

14. Give two examples of persons who would need an agent to give informed consent for them.

_____

_____

15. Assume you are in charge of explaining proposed medical treatment to a patient in order for him to give informed consent for the treatment. What six items will you need to explain?

_____

_____

_____

_____

16. State and federal laws protect patients with a medical history of drug or alcohol abuse, treatment for mental or emotional problems, or HIV/AIDS from release of confidential information about this history. What does the law generally require?

_____

_____

_____

_____

17. Medical records are often subpoenaed in court because a patient's medical record is what kind of document?

_____

18. In a court of law, which testimony will prevail, a patient's recollection of events or the written documentation in a medical record? Explain your answer.

_____

_____

19. May physicians, nurses, and other health care practitioners write any comment they choose in a patient's medical record? Why or why not?

_____

_____

20. What advantages does the federal government foresee for use of electronic health information in the area of public health?

_____

_____

Match the following statements with the correct terms by writing the appropriate letter in the space provided.

_____ 21. Addresses the electronic storage and transmission of health information.

_____ 22. Protects patients from being coerced into treatment.

_____ 23. Protects health care providers from lawsuits when providing care at an accident or emergency.

_____ 24. Provides for a continuum of medical care for patients.

_____ 25. Allows physicians to decide whether or not to show medical records to those patients treated for mental or emotional disorders.

_____ 26. A federal statute that protects the confidentiality of medical records of patients with histories of substance abuse.

a. Good Samaritan act

b. HIPAA

c. Uniform Anatomical Gift Act

d. Doctrine of informed consent

e. Confidentiality of Alcohol and Drug Abuse, Patient Records

f. Doctrine of professional discretion

g. Medical record

Case Study

Use your critical-thinking skills to answer the questions that follow each of the case studies.
A 10-year-old girl suffered from a rare malignancy in her brain and around her spinal cord. She had surgery, and most of the tumor mass was removed, but residual tumor remained in the brain and around the spinal cord. The girl's doctors informed her parents that chemotherapy and radiation were possible treatment options but could cause serious problems such as sepsis, a permanent loss of IQ and stature, and even death. The parents wished to proceed with the therapy.

While their child was undergoing aggressive chemotherapy and radiation, the parents did independent research and read of several drugs being administered for cancer in other states that were unapproved by the Federal Drug Administration (FDA) and were illegal in their home state but were touted by physicians using them as "miracle cures." The couple sued their child's physician for failure to disclose alternative treatments, thus depriving them of informed consent.

A court awarded summary judgment to the physician.

27. In your opinion, does the court's decision seem warranted? Why or why not?

_____

_____

_____

28. Did the physician involved follow the law? Did he act ethically? Explain your answer.

_____

_____

_____

29. Under the doctrine of informed consent, should a physician be responsible for informing patients of all treatment options, even if some of the treatments are illegal or not yet proven effective? Explain your answer.

_____

_____

_____

When Ruth applied for health insurance, she listed a colonoscopy examination as part of her medical history. The insurance company asked for more information. Ruth requested, in writing, that the clinic where she had been examined send only the colonoscopy records to her insurance company. In addition to the requested information on her colonoscopy, the clinic sent all of Ruth's medical records for the past five years, which included the diagnoses of fibrocystic breast disease and obesity. As a result, the insurance company issued Ruth a policy, but attached riders stipulating that it would not pay for any illnesses arising from the fibrocystic breast disease or obesity.

Ruth complained to the clinic administrator, explaining that she had requested that only those records concerning her colonoscopy be forwarded to the insurance company. The administrator apologized and assured Ruth that the clinic's policy concerning release of medical records would be reviewed. He also told Ruth that should she ever incur medical expenses for those conditions excepted in her insurance policy, she should contact him.

30. Did the clinic err in sending all of Ruth's medical records to the insurance company? Why or why not?

_____

_____

31. In your opinion, did Ruth have a legal cause for action against the clinic? Explain.

_____

_____

32. What would you do, in the clinic administrator's place, to rectify the situation and make sure that similar problems did not arise in the future?

_____

_____

A patient asked her dermatologist for the name of an internist. She visited the recommended internist several times and then learned that, without informing her, he had sent the dermatologist two detailed reports on her condition and family medical history. Since her gastrointestinal condition had nothing to do with her dermatological complaint, she believed the internist had sent the records to show his appreciation for the referral. She told the internist that she felt her privacy had been violated.

33. Do you agree with the patient? Why or why not?

_____

_____

Internet Activities

Complete the activities and answer the questions that follow.

34. Search online for "health information technology occupations." What occupations are listed under HIT? List three advantages to pursuing an education in HIT. If your primary interest is in patient care, would a career in HIT interest you? Explain your answer.

_____

_____

_____

_____

35. Visit the Web site for the American Medical Informatics Association (AMIA) at www.amia.org/inside/code/. Locate the association's Code of Ethics and briefly describe the AMIA's stance on maintaining confidentiality of electronic records.

_____

_____

_____

_____

CHAPTER 7

Privacy Law and HIPAA

Learning Outcomes

After studying this chapter, you should be able to:

1. Discuss federal privacy laws that pertain to health care.

2. Discuss the four standards of HIPAA.

3. Determine which covered entities must comply with HIPAA provisions.

4. Summarize the provisions of the Privacy Rule and how they apply to your profession.

5. Recognize and dispel some of the more prevalent myths concerning HIPAA.

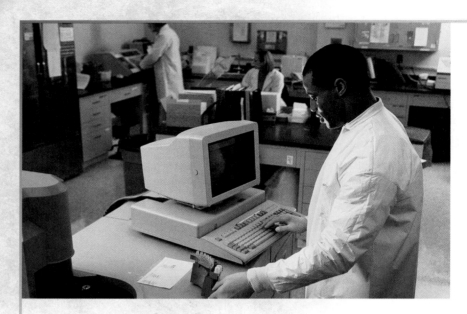

Key Terms

code set

covered entities

covered transaction

de-identify

designated record set

electronic data
    interchange (EDI)

electronic transmission

encryption

firewalls

Health Insurance Portability and
    Accountability Act (HIPAA)

limited data set

minimum necessary

Notice of Privacy Practices (NPP)

permission

privacy

protected health information (PHI)

rule

security

standard

state preemption

transaction

treatment, payment, and health
    care operations (TPO)

verification

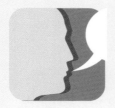

Voice of Experience

HIPAA and Privacy Officer Discusses Compliance

Tom is the Health Insurance Portability and Accountability Act (HIPAA) Compliance Coordinator and Privacy and Information Security Officer for a midwestern regional hospital. Tom emphasizes that health care facilities have always been concerned with information privacy and patient confidentiality, but says that with the enactment of HIPAA, "the force of the law is behind privacy."

Tom has a degree in computer information systems and has added national training sessions for HIPAA privacy and security to his résumé. Different providers will comply with HIPAA in different ways, Tom says. Early in the compliance process, Tom trained 4,500 hospital employees. He trains all new hires, students, and volunteers in HIPAA compliance and conducts continuing departmental training as necessary. The initial training is all instructor led, but update sessions are a combination of instructor-led and computer-based self-study.

The most frequently asked question from hospital staff members, Tom says, is "Can I talk to this person?" Before releasing information, Tom advises staff members to "refer to your policies or, if in doubt, check with compliance. There are few restrictions on sharing health care information with other health care providers, but we have to understand who is a 'health care provider.' For example, some assisted care facilities may not provide health care, and we can't always release information to them."

Since implementation of HIPAA, many situations require clarification before information can be released. For instance, can the person working at the hospital information desk tell a caller from the police department if a certain person is a patient in the hospital? "It depends," Tom answers. "If the police call and say a suspect fell out of a window during a robbery and may have broken his arm, and they ask if we have anyone like that who was recently in the emergency room, we can give them names and addresses, but we can't release information about medical treatment administered. Victims of a crime or witnesses to a crime are treated differently. The hospital cannot release any information regarding a victim unless the release is required by law (as it is for gunshot wounds) or the victim authorizes us to make the release."

The privacy portion of HIPAA means protecting the protected health information (PHI) that the facility has collected, "no matter what form or medium it is in, including paper, electronic, and verbal forms," Tom tells hospital staff. "HIPAA security is an entirely different matter. Security relates to information technology and electronic security. It does not address things like conversations or paper charts. We have had to develop policies and goals that meet HIPAA security standards. . . . Appropriate security involves items like unique passwords, antivirus protection and firewalls at Internet service provider (ISP) levels ."

One of the more difficult issues to address from the security perspective is the fact that the hospital employs telecommuters. Says Tom, "They must meet the minimum standard for working from home. For example, they must have operating system updates sufficient for protection of information." This can be difficult to enforce if telecommuters are using their personal computers as opposed to hospital-provided equipment.

"Encryption [scrambling] of information is provided for in HIPAA," Tom adds. "We encrypt patient lists sent to outside contractors, such as the survey company and billing service we use. We are moving toward more encryption."

"Total HIPAA compliance is our goal," Tom states. "It's ongoing and never completely accomplished because 100 percent security is unachievable."

So far, Tom sums up, HIPAA enforcement, handled by the Office of Civil Rights, has not resulted in major penalties for health care facilities. "They are taking a 'helping hand' approach to resolving issues as opposed to a strict enforcement action."

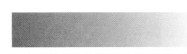

PRIVACY AND THE UNITED STATES CONSTITUTION

privacy Freedom from unauthorized intrusion.

Contrary to popular belief, the term **privacy** (freedom from unauthorized intrusion) does not appear in the U.S. Constitution or the Bill of Rights. However, the U.S. Supreme Court, the court responsible for determining constitutional issues, has ruled in favor of privacy interests (and occasionally against them), deriving the right to privacy from the First, Third, Fourth, Fifth, Ninth, and Fourteenth Amendments to the Constitution. The U.S. Supreme Court first declared that a constitutional right to privacy was implied in the following case *Griswold v. Connecticut.*

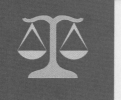

The Right to Privacy Decided

In November 1961, the executive director and the medical director of a Planned Parenthood clinic in Connecticut were charged with violating a state statute prohibiting the dispensing of contraceptive devices to a married couple. The defendants were convicted and fined $100 each. The U.S. Supreme Court heard the case in March 1965 and issued a written opinion on June 7, 1965. William O. Douglas, writing the majority opinion for the Court, held that the Connecticut statute was an unconstitutional violation of the right of privacy. Douglas noted that many rights are not expressly mentioned in the Constitution, but the Court has nevertheless found that persons possess such a right. In reviewing the many rights that Americans possess, Douglas noted the existence of "penumbras" or "zone(s) of privacy created by several fundamental constitutional guarantees."

As a result of the Supreme Court's decision in *Griswold v. Connecticut*, patients possess certain rights which affect the delivery of medical services and health care. For example, persons have the right to refuse medical treatment, and courts now recognize a person's right to die.

Griswold v. Connecticut, 381 US 479, 85 S. Ct 1978, 14 L. Ed2d 510 (1965).

The following amendments to the United States Constitution have particular implications in science, medicine, and the delivery of health care:

First Amendment: "Congress shall make no law respecting an establishment of religion, or prohibiting the free exercise thereof; or abridging the freedom of speech, or of the press; or the right of the people peaceably to assemble, and to petition the Government for a redress of grievances."

The First Amendment guarantees that information relevant to science and medicine can freely flow throughout the international marketplace of ideas. Furthermore, as a result of the Establishment and Freedom of Religion clauses, the government *cannot* fund or show preference for any religion (or discriminate against any religion), and religious tests are prohibited for anyone seeking a public office. Similarly, persons testifying in court or serving on juries cannot be required to take a religious oath or swear to a belief in any god.

Third Amendment: "No Soldier shall, in time of peace be quartered in any house, without the consent of the Owner, nor in time of war, but in a manner to be prescribed by law." This amendment has certain implications for privacy, but the U.S. Supreme Court has never had to decide a Third Amendment case.

Fourth Amendment: "The right of the people to be secure in their persons, houses, papers, and effects, against unreasonable searches and seizures, shall not be violated, and no Warrants shall issue, but upon probable cause, supported by Oath or affirmation, and particularly describing the place to be searched, and the persons or things to be seized."

The Fourth Amendment protects persons from unreasonable searches. As a result, patient records are private, and the government must in most cases have a search warrant to obtain such records. Rules of evidence also govern the use of information obtained as a result of the doctor-patient relationship. Because of state licensing laws for medical offices, however, such offices are subject to administrative oversight by licensing agencies.

Fifth Amendment: "No person shall be held to answer for a capital, or otherwise infamous crime, unless on a presentment or indictment of a Grand Jury, except in cases arising in the land or naval forces, or in the Militia, when in actual service in time of War or public danger; nor shall any person be subject for the same offence to be twice put in jeopardy of life or limb; nor shall be compelled in any criminal case to be a witness against himself, nor be deprived of life, liberty, or property, without due process of law; nor shall private property be taken for public use, without just compensation."

The Miranda warning ("You have the right to remain silent. . . ."), so often heard recited on television crime shows, was derived from this amendment. The Fifth Amendment applies solely to criminal arrests and prosecutions. Since medical malpractice cases are argued in civil court, however, health care practitioners may be required to answer questions or submit documents to attorneys during the course of such a case.

Ninth Amendment: "The enumeration in the Constitution, of certain rights, shall not be construed to deny or disparage others retained by the people." That is, if a certain right is not explicitly mentioned in the Constitution, that does not mean it doesn't exist. This amendment has not been used to uphold a specific right. Some constitutional scholars believe, however, that rights such as the right to health care or housing are implicit in the Ninth Amendment.

Fourteenth Amendment, Section 1: "All persons born or naturalized in the United States, and subject to the jurisdiction thereof, are citizens of the United States and of the State wherein they reside. No State shall make or enforce any law which shall abridge the privileges or immunities of citizens of the United States; nor shall any State deprive any person of life, liberty, or property, without due process of law; nor deny to any person within its jurisdiction the equal protection of the laws."

All states must provide rights for citizens that are at least equal to those in the U.S. Constitution, and under the philosophy called federalism, states may grant citizens additional rights not specifically granted in the U.S. Constitution.

The court case on page 176 is an example of a privacy action that the United States Supreme Court decided in 2003.

FEDERAL PRIVACY LAWS

Concern about privacy has led to the enactment of federal and state laws governing the collection, storage, transmission, and disclosure of personal data. Common points in most of these laws include the following:

1. Information collected and stored about individuals should be limited to what is necessary to carry out the functions of the business or government agency collecting the information.

2. Once it is collected, access to personal information should be limited to those employees who must use the information in performing their jobs.

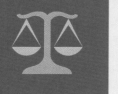
Privacy Loses to Security

Under the Alaska Sex Offender Registration Act of 1994, any sex offender or child kidnapper incarcerated in the state must register with the Department of Corrections within 30 days before his release, providing his name, address, and other information. The person must register with local law enforcement authorities within a working day of his conviction, if he remains free, or if he enters the state after being released from incarceration in another state. If he was convicted of an aggravated (made worse by more serious circumstances, such as deadly force, violence, or the commission of another crime) sex offense or of two or more sex offenses, he must register for life and verify the information quarterly. If he was convicted of a single, nonaggravated sex crime, the offender must provide annual verification of the specified information for 15 years.

The offender's information is forwarded to the Alaska Department of Public Safety, which maintains a central registry of sex offenders. Some of the data, such as fingerprints, anticipated change of address, and whether the offender has had medical treatment after his conviction, are kept confidential. However, the following information is published on the Internet: the offender's name, aliases, address, photograph, physical description, driver's license number, motor vehicle identification numbers, place of employment, date of birth, crime, date and place of conviction, length and conditions of sentence, and a statement as to whether the offender is in compliance with the Act's update requirements or cannot be located. Both the Act's registration and notification requirements are retroactive (apply to those convicted before the Act was passed).

Two sex offenders convicted of aggravated sex offenses were released from an Alaska prison and completed rehabilitative programs for sex offenders. They were convicted before the Act's passage, and sought in court to have the Act declared void in their cases, both because they believed the Act violated privacy and because they believed it should not be retroactive.

A District Court granted the petitioners summary judgment. The state appealed, and the Ninth Circuit Court reversed the District Court's decision, holding that because the Alaska Sex Offender Registration Act is nonpunitive, its retroactive application is upheld. The appeals court also held that the public safety issue was more important than the petitioners' privacy. The petitioners appealed, and the case reached the United States Supreme Court, which upheld the Ninth Circuit Court's decision. The petitioners must register as required under the Alaska Act.

Smith v. Doe, 123 S.Ct. 1140, 71 USLW 4182 (2003).

3. Personal information cannot be released outside the organization collecting it unless authorization is obtained from the subject.

4. When information is collected about a person, that person should know that the information is being collected and should have the opportunity to check the information for accuracy.

Table 7-1 is a summary of the major U.S. government laws concerning privacy.

As you can see from Table 7-1, most federal privacy laws have dealt with financial and credit information or the theft or illegal disclosure of electronic information. All states have laws governing the confidentiality of medical records, but laws vary greatly from state to state. The HIPAA of 1996 was the first *federal* legislation to deal thoroughly and explicitly with the privacy of medical records. To ensure compliance, HIPAA provides for civil and criminal sanctions for violators of the law.

TABLE 7-1 Major Federal Privacy Laws

Date Enacted	Law	Purpose
1970	Fair Credit Reporting Act	Prohibits credit reporting agencies from releasing credit information to unauthorized people, and allows consumers to review their own credit records.
1974	Family and Privacy Act Educational Rights	Gives students and parents access to school records and limits disclosure of records to unauthorized parties.
1974	Privacy Act	Forbids federal agencies from allowing information to be used for a reason other than that for which it was collected.
1978	Right to Financial Privacy Act	Strictly outlines procedures federal agencies must follow when looking at customer records in banks.
1984	Computer Fraud and Abuse Act	Forbids unauthorized access of federal government computers.
1984	Cable Communications Policy Act	Regulates disclosure of cable television subscriber records.
1986	Electronic Communications Privacy Act (ECPA)	Provides privacy protection for new forms of electronic communications, such as voice mail, e-mail, and cellular telephone.
1988	Video Privacy Protection Act	Forbids retailers from releasing or selling video rental records without customer consent or a court order.
1991	Telephone Consumer Protection Act	Restricts activities of telemarketers.
1992	Cable Act	Extends the privacy provisions of the Cable Communications Policy Act of 1984 to include cellular and other wireless services.
1994	Computer Abuse Amendments Act	Amends the 1984 act to forbid transmission of harmful computer code such as viruses.
1996	National Information Infrastructure Protection Act	Penalizes theft of information across state lines, threats against networks, and computer system trespassing.
1996	Health Insurance Portability and Accountability Act (HIPAA)	Guarantees that workers who change jobs can obtain health insurance. Increases efficiency and effectiveness of the U.S. health care system by electronic exchange of administrative and financial data. Improves security and privacy of patient-identifying information. Decreases U.S. health care system transaction costs.
1997	No Electronic Theft (NET) Act	Closed a loophole in the law that let people give away copyrighted material (such as software) on the Internet without legal repercussions.

(continued)

TABLE 7-1 *continued*

Date Enacted	Law	Purpose
1998	Digital Millennium Copyright Act (DMCA)	Makes it illegal to bypass antipiracy measures in commercial software, and outlaws the sale of devices that copy software illegally.
1999	Gramm-Leach Bliley Act	Requires all financial institutions and insurance companies to clearly disclose their privacy policies regarding the sharing of nonpublic personal information with affiliates and third parties.
2001	Provide Appropriate Tools Required to Intercept and Obstruct Terrorism (PATRIOT) Act	Gives law enforcement broad leeway in monitoring people's activities, including Internet use, e-mail, and library habits.
First enacted in early 1970s, revised in 2002	Code of Federal Regulations (CFR), 42 (Public Health), Part 2	Provides for the confidentiality of medical records of patients treated for drug and alcohol dependency.
2003	Do Not Call Implementation Act	Allows individuals to opt out of receiving calls from telemarketers by placing phone numbers on a national registry.

CHECK YOUR PROGRESS

1. Name four common points in most federal and state privacy laws.

_____

_____

2. The first federal law to deal thoroughly and explicitly with the privacy of medical records is

_____

_____

HEALTH INSURANCE PORTABILITY AND ACCOUNTABILITY ACT (HIPAA)

Circumstances that led to the 1996 passage of federal **Health Insurance Portability and Accountability Act (HIPAA)** legislation include the following:

▌ Health care has become a complicated business. Health care employees are faced with a quagmire of complex billing codes, a multitude of software programs in use for storing medical records and for processing billing and payment, and more time spent on administrative chores (and less on patient issues).

▌ Managed care adds yet another level to the many administrative duties necessary to administer patient care; personnel include case reviewers, claims and coding experts, billing personnel, committees to review every

Health Insurance Portability and Accountability Act (HIPAA) A federal law passed in 1996 to protect privacy and other health care rights for patients. The act helps workers keep continuous health insurance coverage for themselves and their dependents when they change jobs, and protects confidential medical information from unauthorized disclosure and/or use. It was also intended to help curb the rising cost of health care fraud and abuse.

facet of service, employees trained to handle patient complaints, and so on. Before HIPAA was passed, nurses had assumed many of the duties associated with health care services reporting and administration, and both physicians and nurses had less time to spend on patient care.

▌ Patients gather information from television ads and the Internet, often expecting their physicians to prescribe medications and treatments not appropriate for their medical problems. A side effect has been that medical malpractice and risk management issues threaten to put some physicians and health care facilities out of business, due to the high cost of medical malpractice insurance and the rising costs of staying in the health care business.

▌ Health care consumers were and are increasingly dismayed over the rising cost of medical care and health insurance, to the point that millions of Americans do not seek necessary medical care for treatment their insurance plans will not cover, are underinsured, or do not have health insurance.

In the mid-1990s when groups of health care professionals, consumers, and others confronted members of the U.S. Congress about solving these serious health care problems, Congress responded with passage of the Health Insurance Portability and Accountability Act of 1996, to be administered by the *U.S. Department of Health and Human Services (HHS)*. HHS has assigned enforcement activities for the Privacy Rule to the *U.S. Office for Civil Rights (OCR)*. A second agency within HHS, the *Centers for Medicare and Medicaid Services (CMS)*, has enforcement authority for other HIPAA Administrative Simplification Standards, including transactions, code sets, identifiers, and security.

HIPAA LANGUAGE

Covered Entities

covered entities Health care providers and clearinghouses that transmit HIPAA transactions electronically, and must comply with HIPAA standards and rules.

In HIPAA language, health plans, health care clearinghouses, and all health care providers that transmit HIPAA standard transactions electronically are called **covered entities.** Covered entities include

▌ Hospitals, including academic medical centers
▌ Nursing homes
▌ Hospices
▌ Pharmacies
▌ Physician practices
▌ Dental practices
▌ Chiropractors
▌ Podiatrists
▌ Osteopaths
▌ Physical therapists
▌ Alternative medicine practitioners (acupuncturists, massage therapists)
▌ Laboratories
▌ Health plans (payers)
▌ Health care clearinghouses

Covered entities are people, businesses, or agencies that must comply with the HIPAA Standards and Privacy Rule. HIPAA offers no exclusion from the covered entity determination for small practices. If a health care practice exchanges even one of the standard transactions via electronic means with any payer, that practice is a covered entity.

Table 7-2 can help health care practitioners and facilities determine if they are covered entities. For more complete information for determining covered entities, visit the home page for the Centers for Medicare and Medicaid Services at www.cms.hhs.gov/.

Covered Transactions

covered transactions Electronic exchanges of information between two covered-entity business partners using HIPAA-mandated transaction standards.

Electronic exchanges of information between two covered-entity business partners using HIPAA-mandated transaction standards (explained below) are called **covered transactions.** HIPAA Standard Transactions include, but are not limited to, the following:

- A physician submitting an electronic claim to a health plan.
- A physician sending a referral or authorization electronically to another physician, lab, or hospital.
- A physician sending patient-identifying information to a billing service or to another physician.
- Any health care provider that employs another entity, such as a clearinghouse or billing agency, to send claims to payers or health plans.

Table 7-2 provides some guidelines for determining whether a practice is a covered entity.

Note that a patient sending an e-mail message to a physician that contains patient-identifying information would not be a HIPAA standards-covered transaction, because patients are not covered entities.

Any physician, health care practitioner, or health care facility, regardless of size, that files even one electronic claim is a covered entity and must use HIPAA electronic transaction and code set standards.

Other Important HIPAA Terms

designated record set Records maintained by or for a HIPAA-covered entity.

A **designated record set** includes records maintained by or for a covered entity, including medical records and billing records about individuals; a health plan's enrollment, payment, 10 claims adjudication, and case or medical management record systems; and records used by or for the covered entity to make decisions about an individual.

Notice of Privacy Practices (NPP) A written document detailing a health care provider's privacy practices.

Notice of Privacy Practices (NPP) is a written document detailing a health care provider's privacy practices. Under HIPAA's Privacy Rule, every patient visiting his or her health care provider after April 14, 2003 must have received an NPP. The patient is asked to sign the form, and it is filed with the patient's medical records.

protected health information (PHI) Information that contains one or more patient identifiers.

de-identify To remove all information that identifies patients from health care transactions.

Protected health information (PHI) refers to information that contains one or more patient identifiers and can, therefore, be used to identify an individual. The Privacy Rule (see below) says that PHI must be protected whether it is written, spoken, or in electronic form. It is possible to **"de-identify"** health information, by removing the patient identifiers from it. Once patient identifiers are removed, the information is not considered PHI. Information that includes one or more of the following makes a patient's medical record identifiable:

- Name
- Zip code
- Date of birth

TABLE 7-2 How to Determine Covered Entities

Column A: Question	Column B: Answer to the Question, Is the practice described in Column A a covered entity?	
Do you furnish, bill, or receive payment for health care in the normal course of business?	No Not a covered entity	Yes Probably a covered entity
Does your practice conduct covered transactions?	No Not a covered entity	Yes Covered entity
Are any of the covered transactions conducted in electronic format?	No Not a covered entity	Yes Covered entity
Does the practice conduct all of the following transactions *on paper, by phone, or by fax* (from a dedicated fax machine, as opposed to faxing from a computer)? • Submitting claims or managed care encounter information • Checking claim status inquiry and response • Checking eligibility and receiving a response • Checking referral certifications and authorizations • Enrolling and disenrolling in a health plan • Receiving health care payments and remittance advice • Providing coordination of benefits	No Covered entity if even one transaction is conducted electronically	Yes Not a covered entity (no electronic transactions)
Is the practice a small provider with fewer than 10 full-time equivalent employees?	No, unless health information is transmitted electronically. In that case, the practice is a covered entity, regardless of size.	Yes, if health information is transmitted electronically. Covered entity, even though the practice has fewer than 10 full-time equivalent employees.

- Dates of treatment
- Telephone numbers
- Fax numbers
- E-mail addresses
- Social Security number
- Medical record numbers
- Health plan beneficiary numbers
- Birth certificate and driver's license
- Vehicle identification number and license plate number
- Web site address
- Fngerprints and voiceprints
- Photos

state preemption If a state's privacy laws are stricter than HIPAA privacy standards, the state laws take precedence.

treatment, payment, and health care operations (TPO) A HIPAA term for qualified providers, disclosure of PHI to obtain reimbursement, and activities and transactions among entities. *Treatment* means that a health care provider can provide care; *payment* means that a provider can disclose PHI to be reimbursed; *health care operations* refers to HIPAA-approved activities and transactions.

State preemption means that if a state's privacy laws are stricter than HIPAA privacy standards and/or guarantee more patients' rights, the state laws will take precedence.

Treatment, payment, and health care operations (TPO) is another important term. Within HIPAA, *treatment* means that a health care provider can provide care. *Payment* means that a provider can disclose PHI to obtain reimbursement for health care. *Health care operations* refers to a number of activities and transactions within and among entities, including conducting quality assessments, reviewing the competence or qualifications of health care practitioners, and managing the business.

Business associates are not covered entities, but covered entities must have contracts or agreements with business associates that conduct certain activities on behalf of those covered entities. Contracts must specify that the business associate will safeguard protected health information according to HIPAA requirements. The agreement should include recourse provisions for the covered entity if the business associate accidentally or intentionally releases patient-identifying information entrusted to it.

Business associates of covered entities include, but are not limited to, services engaged in

accounting	dictation and transcription
accreditation	legal consultation
benefit management	practice management
billing	processing or administration
claims processing	quality assurance
consulting	repricing
data aggregation	utilization review
data analysis	

CHECK YOUR PROGRESS

3. Distinguish between *covered entities* and *covered transactions*.

_____

_____

4. Give two examples of a covered entity.

_____

_____

5. Give two examples of covered transactions.

_____

_____

6. Define *state preemption*.

_____

_____

HIPAA STANDARDS

standard A general requirement under HIPAA.

rule A document that includes the HIPAA standards or requirements.

HIPAA contains four sets of standards, with rules that health care facilities must implement within a designated time frame. Under HIPAA, a **standard** is a general requirement; a **rule** is a document that includes the standards. Each rule begins with a Notice of Proposed Rule-Making (NPRM) that HHS presents for public comment and suggested revisions. HHS publishes the final rule in the *Federal Register*. Health care providers then have 24 months to comply with the rule. The four HIPAA standards are presented in Table 7-3.

TABLE 7-3 HIPAA Standards and Timelines

Standard Name	Purpose	Deadline for Implementation	Comments
1. Transactions and Code Sets	Primary goal is Administrative Simplification. Provides for uniformity and simplification of billing and coding for health care services, and requires the use of standard formats and data content for transmitting files electronically.	10/16/2002 10/16/2003 4/16/2003	Implementation time could be extended to the latest date, but by 4/16/2003 health care providers had to have started testing transactions. HHS established contingency plans that extended past the deadline to ease the transition from nonstandard to standard transactions.
2. Privacy Rule	Protecting the privacy of patient-identifying information in any form or medium. Gives certain rights to patients, as explained below.	4/14/2003	HHS continues to release guidance to clarify the Privacy Rule. The Rule allows for an update only once yearly.
3. Security Rule	Provides for the security of electronic Protected Health Information (ePHI). It does this by requiring general and specific protections for data stored and transmitted electronically. Some of the security measures listed include use of firewalls, antivirus software, encryption, password protection, and other measures. (Terms defined below.)	4/21/2005	Security safeguards required by the Privacy Rule must be in place by 4/14/2003, even though the date for compliance with the Security Rule is 2005.
4. National Identifier Standards	To provide uniform national identifiers for the movement of electronic transactions. The 4 national identifiers are provider, health plan, employer, and individual	7/30/2004	As of May 2008, Standard 4 is fully implemented.

*See the government Web site for Medicare and Medicaid Services at www.cms.hhs.gov/ for any updates to Standard 4 and other information about HIPAA.

transaction Transmission of information between two parties for financial or administrative activities.

code set Under HIPAA, terms that provide for uniformity and simplification of health care billing and record keeping.

A **transaction** refers to the transmission of information between two parties to carry out financial or administrative activities. A **code set** is "any set of codes used to encode data elements, such as tables of terms, medical concepts, medical diagnostic codes, or medical procedure codes. A code set includes the codes and the descriptors of the codes." HIPAA provisions say that codes must now be uniform throughout the country, to make filling out insurance claim forms and billing for services much easier than before.

Before HIPAA, medical facilities filing and collecting on claims used different formats; this often held up payment while codes were explained and further information was submitted. (By the mid-1990s, there were over 400 different software formats for coding and billing in medical facilities.) Now, through HIPAA, the law says that all health care providers must ensure that they can send and receive information using standard data formats and data content. Health care providers, not software vendors, are responsible for compliance.

Code Sets

Under HIPAA, all local code sets are eliminated. Code sets now fall into four categories:

1. Coding systems for diseases, impairments, or other health problems.
2. Causes of injuries, diseases, impairments, or other health problems.
3. Actions taken to prevent, diagnose, treat, or manage diseases, injuries, and impairments.
4. Substances, equipment, supplies, or other items used to perform these actions.

Health care practitioners required to use HIPAA code sets will need to consult HIPAA compliance officers in their facilities or areas for reference to HIPAA publications on coding.

Transaction Requirements

The HIPAA Transaction Standard was finalized on August 17, 2000, giving covered entities until October 16, 2003, to comply. Extensions were possible (see Table 7-3), but covered entities that applied for the extensions were required to begin testing of electronic transactions and code set standards by April 16, 2003. The act also specified that physicians with 10 or more full-time equivalent employees were required to file electronically for Medicare reimbursement, unless "no method [was] available" to file electronically, and in that case, such covered entities could file on paper.

electronic transmission The sending of information from one network-connected computer to another.

electronic data interchange (EDI) The use of uniform electronic network protocols to transfer business information between organizations via computer networks.

Complying with HIPAA Transaction Standards means that covered entities must use the HIPAA-defined standards when using *electronic data interchange (EDI)* for electronic transmissions. **Electronic transmission** refers to the sending of information from one network-connected computer to another. **Electronic data interchange (EDI)** is the use of uniform electronic network protocols (formats) to transfer business information between organizations. Banking, financial, and retail businesses first began using electronic data interchange to transmit information in the mid-1960s, and it has been the transmission method of choice for businesses since the mid-1990s.

Under HIPAA, if a health care provider conducts one of the following general types of covered transactions electronically, that provider must use the HIPAA standards:

1. Claims or encounter information.
2. Eligibility requests.
3. Referrals and authorizations.
4. Claim status inquiries.

Health plans and clearinghouses must be able to receive the above transactions and must also be able to conduct four additional transactions electronically:

1. Premium payment.
2. Claim payment and remittance advice.
3. Enrollment and disenrollment.
4. Coordination of benefits.

Since converting electronic transmissions to HIPAA standards is highly technical, health care practitioners and facilities need to rely on information technology (IT) staff or outside IT experts to be sure they are in compliance.

Advantages to using standard EDI protocols to transmit PHI electronically include these:

- EDI protocols ensure that protected information travels between linked computers as intended, because everyone is using a common language.
- EDI protocols are compatible with firewall and encryption features that help ensure confidentiality of PHI.

There are many advantages for health care providers and consumers in using uniform transaction formats and code sets to transmit health information:

- Uniform coding ensures consistency in the language used to identify diseases.
- Uniform coding helps HHS track disease trends for public health purposes.
- Uniform coding speeds communication between payers and health care providers and speeds the payment process.
- Uniform coding ensures that covered entities can communicate without confusion and long delays.
- Uniform coding helps track how drugs are used and evaluate quality of health care.
- Once codes are learned, employees responsible for coding will find their jobs easier.

STANDARD 2. PRIVACY RULE

As the electronic age progresses, individuals have become increasingly concerned about the privacy of their medical records. However, patient fears are not the underlying reason for the HIPAA Privacy Rule. Because Congress recognized that electronic transmission of health information is the rule in today's computerized society, legislators paid particular attention to ensuring that confidentiality of medical records would not be violated through electronic transmission or storage.

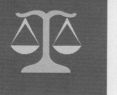
U.S. Attorney General Denied Medical Records

In 2000, the U.S. Supreme Court found the Nebraska version of a partial birth abortion ban unconstitutional, on grounds that this type of abortion may, in certain circumstances, be the safest means by which a medically necessary abortion can be performed, and the Nebraska law lacked such a safety clause. (The law defines "partial birth abortion" as a method of abortion in which a second- or third-trimester fetus partially exits the womb and is then destroyed.)

When the U.S. Supreme Court has ruled, the matter is usually settled, but in response to the Court's Nebraska decision, Congress passed the federal Partial Birth Abortion Ban Act in 2003. Congress claimed it had made new factual findings that "partial-birth abortion is never necessary to preserve the health of a woman. . . ."

Immediately after President George W. Bush signed the act, a group of abortion providers challenged it in court. A federal district judge in New York City granted the group an injunction to stop enforcement of the law. In March 2004, however, the matter was ordered to trial to see if the Supreme Court's view of the facts still prevailed.

To defend the federal partial birth abortion ban in court, United States Attorney General John Ashcroft sought the medical records of 45 patients at a Chicago hospital. He needed the records to dispute expert testimony for the plaintiffs' case, and he claimed that because he sought the records without patient-identifying information, he was not violating privacy laws.

However, on March 26, 2004, the United States District Court for the Northern District of Illinois disagreed. The court held that the Justice Department is not entitled to request patients' medical records, even with names and other identifying information removed.

In his opinion for the court, Judge Richard Posner explained that anonymity and privacy are not identical. Therefore, while the Justice Department would view the women's records without identifying information, the court still deemed their production a privacy violation.

While the court case settling the abortion providers' challenge to the federal Partial Birth Abortion Ban Act had not yet gone to court in June 2004, Ashcroft's petition to obtain medical records was denied. (In 2007, the Supreme Court issued a decision upholding the nationwide ban on partial birth abortion enacted by Congress in 2003.)

Northwestern Memorial Hospital v. Ashcroft (Appeal from the United States District Court, for the Northern District of Illinois, Eastern Division, No. 04 C 55, Argued March 23, 2004, Decided March 26, 2004).

permission A reason under HIPAA for disclosing patient information.

Health care providers and plans can use and disclose patient information (PHI), HIPAA legislators said, but they must identify a **permission**—a reason for each use and disclosure.

To *use* PHI means that you use patients' protected health information within the facility where you work in the normal course of conducting health care business. To *disclose* PHI means that patients' protected health information is sent outside of the office for legitimate business or health care reasons.

PERMISSIONS

Using and disclosing PHI must fall within the following 11 HIPAA-defined permissions:

1. Required disclosures

    HIPAA *requires* just two types of PHI disclosures. The first is that you disclose PHI to representatives from HHS that want to see your books,

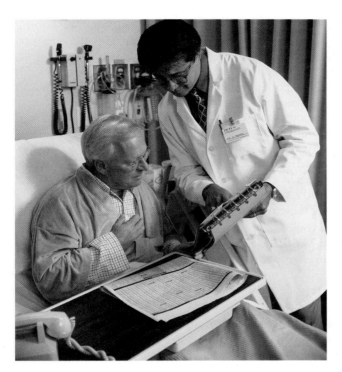

FIGURE 7-1 HIPAA requires that information be disclosed to a patient who asks to see his or her medical records.

records, accounts, and other documents. You must permit HHS representatives to see the documents they request, but you should ask HHS representatives to show identification, and you should record the reason for the requested disclosure to HHS. The second type of PHI disclosure that HIPAA *requires* is to individual patients upon request. (See number 2 below, "Disclosures to patients.")

Written authorization to disclose PHI to HHS representatives is not required.

2. Disclosures to patients

The second disclosure HIPAA *requires* is that PHI be disclosed to any patient who asks to see his or her own medical records (Figure 7-1). (Unless the health care provider believes that access will do harm to the patient.) This includes talking to the patient about his or her diagnosis, treatment, and medical condition, as well as allowing the patient to review his or her entire medical record. There are exceptions, however. Patients do not have the right to access

▌ Psychotherapy notes (see below for a definition of *psychotherapy notes*).

▌ Records that are being compiled for a civil, criminal, or administrative action.

▌ Records that are exempt from the Clinical Laboratory Improvement Act of 1988 (CLIA). CLIA requires clinical labs to disclose test results or reports only to authorized persons—usually to the person who ordered the test.

If you deny access to PHI to a patient, a review process may be instituted to determine whether or not you acted reasonably. However, under HIPAA, a patient cannot challenge a decision to deny access to his or her PHI if

▌ Any of the above restrictions exist.
▌ The patient is a prison inmate.
▌ The PHI was obtained through clinical research that includes treatment. This applies only during the research and only if limitation of access is agreed to in advance.
▌ The PHI is a government record.
▌ The PHI was obtained under a promise of confidentiality.

Decisions to deny access to a patient's PHI may be reviewed when challenged if

▌ The patient will be harmed if access is withheld.
▌ Someone else is mentioned in the record and that person will be harmed if access is withheld.
▌ The person making the request is the patient's personal representative, and you believe the patient or someone else may be harmed if the personal representative is allowed access.

Written authorization to disclose PHI to patients (as when a patient asks to see his or her medical record) is recommended, and you should ask to see identification for individuals requesting disclosure.

3. Use or disclosure for treatment, payment, or health care operations (TPO)

Health care practitioners need to use PHI within the medical office, hospital, or other health care facility for coordinating care, consulting with another practitioner about the patient's condition, prescribing medications, ordering lab tests, scheduling surgery, or for other reasons necessary to conduct health care treatment or business.

PHI may also be disclosed within a facility for the purpose of obtaining information about a patient's insurance coverage, inquiring about copayments, billing, claims management, and so on.

Health care operations—those activities the provider participates in that relate to business functions—may also require disclosure of PHI. These activities include quality assessments, case management, care coordination, contacting providers and patients with alternative treatment information, certification, accreditation, licensing or credentialing, medical reviews, legal service, auditing for fraud and abuse and for other purposes, and so on.

PHI disclosures for these purposes do not require written authorization.

4. Others' treatment, payment, operations

If other covered entities contact you or your employer for access to PHI, such as insurance plans, attorneys, medical survey representatives, and pharmaceutical companies, you must have the patient's written authorization to release PHI.

5. Personal representatives (friends, family)

Use professional judgment to determine if a family member, friend, or personal representative is participating in the care of a patient. For example, you saw the patient invite another person into the exam room, or you heard the patient ask that individual to pick up his or her prescription. You may share information with these individuals, in proportion to their involvement in the care of the patient. You should verify with the patient, if possible, before sharing information. If the patient objects, honor his or her wishes.

If a person claims to have the legal right to make medical decisions for a patient, including the right to review medical records, ask to see the legal document, and verify the representative's identity. A signature authorizing disclosure is recommended. If the patient is able, you can also verify with the patient.

6. Disaster relief organizations

Unless the patient objects, health care providers may disclose PHI to persons performing disaster relief notification activities. If the situation involves TPO, no authorization is needed.

7. Incidental disclosures

In December 2002, HHS released guidelines for clarifying when incidental disclosures of PHI are permitted without authorization from patients. For example, permitted disclosures include

- Nursing care center staff members can speak about patients' care if they take reasonable precautions to prevent unauthorized individuals, such as visitors in the area, from overhearing.
- Nurses and other health care practitioners can talk to patients on the phone or discuss patients' medical treatment with other providers on the phone if they are reasonably sure that others cannot overhear.
- Health care practitioners can discuss lab results with patients and other health care practitioners in a joint treatment area if they take reasonable precautions to ensure that others cannot overhear.
- Health care practitioners can leave messages on answering machines or with family members, but information should be limited to the amount necessary for the purpose of the call. (For detailed messages, it may be prudent to simply ask the patient to return a call.)
- You can ask patients to sign in, and you can call patients by name in waiting rooms, but a sign-in sheet must not ask for the reason for the visit.

- You can announce patients by name in a waiting room or use a public address system to ask patients to come to a certain area.
- You can use an X-ray light board at a nursing station if it is not visible to unauthorized individuals in the area.
- You can place patient charts outside exam rooms if you use reasonable precautions to protect patient identity: face the chart toward the wall or place the chart inside a cover while it is in place.

8. Public purpose

   Health care practitioners and facilities may be asked to disclose PHI "for the public good." If a state law does not prohibit releasing specific PHI, HIPAA allows this type of disclosure without patient authorization. Such disclosures include

   - When disclosure is required by law. You should limit the PHI disclosed to the requirements of the law. Verify identification of representatives asking for PHI.
   - Public health authority. Public health representatives are authorized by law to collect information to prevent or control disease, injury, birth, death, and for other public health investigations.
   - Child abuse or neglect. You may release this information to public health authorities that are authorized to receive reports of child abuse or neglect.
   - Victims of abuse, neglect, or domestic violence. If a health care practitioner has reason to believe a patient is a victim of abuse, neglect, or domestic violence, he or she may disclose PHI if
     - The disclosure is required by law.
     - The individual agrees to disclosure.
     - The disclosure is necessary to prevent serious harm, or the individual is physically or mentally unable to consent to disclosure. If PHI is disclosed in this situation, health care practitioners must notify the patient that they made the disclosure.
   - Food and Drug Administration (FDA). Health care practitioners may disclose PHI to the FDA for safety, quality, or effectiveness such as reporting adverse events, product defects, product recalls, or monitoring patient response to a drug.
   - Communicable diseases. If authorized by law to notify persons who may have been exposed to a communicable disease or are at risk of spreading a disease, health care practitioners may disclose PHI.
   - Employee workplace medical surveillance. Health care practitioners may disclose PHI to a patient's employer under certain conditions. Consult the privacy officer for those conditions.
   - Health oversight activities. These activities include audits, investigations, inspections, licensure, and disciplinary actions. You cannot disclose PHI about the person who is the subject of an investigation.
   - Judicial and administrative proceedings. HIPAA adds special criteria that must be included in most subpoenas. Court orders generally have no additional criteria added by HIPAA. Consult your privacy official or your legal department if you receive a subpoena or court order to release PHI.
   - Law enforcement. There are eight circumstances that apply concerning the disclosure of PHI to law enforcement officials:
     - Required by law, such as gunshot wounds, child abuse or neglect, or domestic violence.
     - Warrant or process.
     - Government agency request.

- Identifying a suspect or material witness.
- Victims of a crime.
- Suspicious death.
- Crime on the premises.
- Medical emergency.

Consult your privacy official or legal department if law enforcement representatives ask for PHI.

- **Coroners and funeral directors.** You may disclose PHI to a coroner or medical examiner to identify a deceased person and to funeral directors to help them carry out their duties.
- **Organ, eye, or tissue donation.** You can disclose PHI to appropriate agencies to facilitate organ and tissue donations.
- **Research.** Consult your privacy officer for special conditions that apply.
- **Avert a serious and imminent threat to health or safety.** You can disclose PHI if you believe a serious and imminent threat to health or safety exists.
- **Special government functions.** Special circumstances apply to individuals in the military, veterans, and prison inmates. Consult your privacy officer to determine the appropriate response.
- **Workers' compensation.** You can disclose PHI to comply with state workers' compensation laws.

9. Authorization

   A valid patient authorization allows you to disclose PHI. Use or disclose PHI as limited by the authorization. When in doubt, check with the privacy officer, and always document use or disclosure and those instances when access to PHI is denied.

10. De-identification

   You can disclose certain types of patient information when identifying information has been removed, because once the identifiers have been removed, the data is no longer considered protected by the HIPAA regulation. Check with your privacy officer for circumstances that require de-identification.

11. Limited data set

   A **limited data set** is protected health information from which certain specified, direct identifiers of individuals and their relatives, household members, and employers have been removed. A limited data set may be used and disclosed for research, health care operations, and public health purposes, provided the recipient enters into an agreement promising specified safeguards for the protected health information within the limited data set.

limited data set Protected health information from which certain patient identifiers have been removed.

SPECIAL REQUIREMENTS FOR DISCLOSING PROTECTED HEALTH INFORMATION

As discussed above, each use and disclosure of PHI must fall within one of the 11 permissions. However, before using or disclosing PHI you must also review any special restrictions that were agreed to and requirements

7. Briefly summarize the four HIPAA standards.

_____

_____

8. Which of the four standards is most concerned with confidentiality of medical records?

_____

_____

9. What are the two required disclosures of health care information that HIPAA mandates?

_____

_____

10. What information must be included in health care facility privacy notices?

_____

_____

verification The requirement under HIPAA that a patient's identity be verified before protected health information is released.

minimum necessary Term referring to the limited amount of patient information that may be disclosed, depending on circumstances.

for disclosing information for certain purposes, such as marketing or fundraising. These special requirements follow.

1. **Verification**

   Ask any person who requests access to PHI to show identification if the request is made in person. If a person asks over the telephone for you to fax PHI and you don't know that person, use common sense. If a patient is making the request, ask for information that you can verify by checking the medical record. If an outside company representative, such as an insurance employee, is making the request, say that you will return the call, and call the insurance office's business telephone number (not a number the caller gave you) to verify that the employee works there. Once you have verified that a patient has made the request, or that the request is legitimate, call the receiving office to say that you are faxing PHI. Fax only the information the patient has requested from the medical record. After you send the fax, request confirmation that it was received. Note the request in the patient's record.

2. **Minimum Necessary**

   This refers to the limited amount of patient data that may be disclosed as required by circumstances. For example, within a medical office a receptionist may only need to know that a patient's insurance information is up to date. An insurance clerk may only need to know a patient's insurance coverage. A billing clerk may only need to know the patient's copay and related contact information. The insurance company only need to access those portions of the medical record that concern the reason for a patient's visit. (The company does not need the entire medical record, for instance, to pay for a child's immunization visit.)

   When responding to requests to provide PHI, remember to provide only the information the patient has requested and to provide only the information necessary for workplace duties to be fulfilled. Everyone requesting information does not need to see a patient's entire medical record. If a patient has requested, in writing, that certain individuals not be allowed access to his or her PHI, you must honor the request. Therefore, before disclosing PHI, check the patient's record for special requirements. Always use the "minimum necessary" standard when disclosing PHI.

3. Marketing

Pharmaceutical and survey companies and other organizations may request patient information in order to target marketing efforts toward certain patient groups or to communicate general health information. These disclosures are generally not allowed without a patient authorization.

Communications such as mammogram reminder mailings, newsletters about childhood vaccinations, or news about health fairs and classes are not considered marketing and may be conducted without a patient authorization, although if a patient requests that you stop such communications, you should honor the request. If you have the patient's authorization to send additional marketing materials, you may do so. These authorizations are commonly granted at the time of treatment, but you may not make treatment dependent upon the patient's signing the authorization. Consult your privacy officer before using patient lists for nontreatment, payment, or health care operations communications.

4. Psychotherapy Notes

HIPAA defines *psychotherapy notes* as those notes that are

1. Recorded by a health care provider who is a mental health professional documenting or analyzing the contents of conversation during a private counseling session or a group, joint, or family counseling session.

2. Maintained separately from the medical record.

Protected psychotherapy notes do *not* include

a. Medication prescription and monitoring.
b. Counseling session start and stop times.
c. The modalities and frequencies of treatment furnished.
d. Results of clinical tests.
e. Any summary of diagnosis, functional status, the treatment plan, symptoms, prognosis, and progress to date.

Health care providers may *not* use or disclose psychotherapy notes for any purpose, including most treatment, payment, or health care operations, without written authorization from the patient. Exceptions include

▌ The person who originated the notes wants to review them.
▌ Counseling training programs want to use PHI to help trainees improve their skills.
▌ Using the notes as a defense in a legal action or other proceedings brought by the patient.
▌ The Secretary of HHS wants to see them.
▌ Use or disclosure is required by law.
▌ A health care practitioner needs to report a serious threat to health or safety, under specific conditions.

Consult your privacy officer for guidance if you are asked to disclose psychotherapy notes.

5. Policies and Procedures Consistent with Notice of Privacy Practices

HIPAA requires health care providers to have in place written policies and procedures on how to handle privacy. These internal policies and procedures must be consistent with the written privacy notification provided to every patient. If you work in a dentist's office, for example, and you will send appointment reminders to patients, the practice's privacy notification must state that the reminders will be sent. HIPAA compliance officers and privacy officers can provide advice on how to implement consistent privacy policies and notifications.

6. State Laws

All HIPAA compliance policies and procedures must be consistent with both state and federal laws. If state and federal laws conflict, you must follow either the law that offers the greater privacy protection or that which offers more patient rights. If a state law is more stringent or offers more patient rights than federal laws, the state law must be followed. Conversely, if HIPAA conflicts with state laws, and HIPAA is more limiting or grants more patient rights, follow the HIPAA regulations. Consult HIPAA compliance officers, privacy officers, and attorneys to develop consent forms compatible with laws in your state.

The following court case was adjudicated after HIPAA was passed in 1996, but before it was fully implemented by health care practitioners nationwide.

Court Case

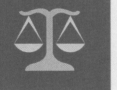

EMT Liable for Violating Patient's Privacy

An EMT employed by a volunteer fire department provided emergency treatment to a female patient for a possible drug overdose. The unresponsive patient was transported to a hospital. The EMT returned home and later spoke to a friend, telling her that she had assisted in taking a specific patient to the hospital emergency room for treatment for a possible drug overdose.

Prior to the emergency, the EMT had never met the patient. However, about two weeks prior to the incident, the EMT had heard about the patient and her medical problems at a social event. The woman who spoke about the patient was apparently a friend, and it was this person that the EMT telephoned, after the patient's overdose.

The patient sued the EMT and her insurance company, alleging that she had defamed her and violated her privacy by publicizing information concerning her medical condition and making untrue statements indicating that she had attempted suicide. The patient claimed that she had been and was continuing to undergo medical care due to illness, and that the apparent overdose she suffered was a "reaction to medication."

The insurance company claimed the EMT's actions were within the scope of her employment. The EMT argued that she had not acted recklessly or unreasonably in contacting the patient's friend regarding her care.

The EMT offered to settle for $5,000, but the plaintiff refused, and the matter went to a jury trial. The jury found that the EMT had violated the plaintiff's right of privacy, as alleged. The jury also awarded the plaintiff/patient $37,909.86 in compensatory damages and attorney fees.

The EMT and her insurance company appealed. An appeals court upheld the judgment of the lower court.

Pachowitz v. Ledoux, 2003 WL 21221823 (Wis.App., May 28, 2003).

PATIENT RIGHTS

HIPAA has also put in writing six important patient rights that must be explained in health care provider privacy notifications, and health care providers may not ask patients to waive their rights. These rights are found in Table 7-4.

STANDARD 3. SECURITY RULE

security The use of policies and procedures to protect electronic information from unauthorized access.

Privacy refers to those policies and procedures health care providers and their business associates put in place to ensure confidentiality of electronic, written, and oral protected health information. **Security** refers to those policies and procedures health care providers and their business associates use to protect electronically transmitted and stored PHI from unauthorized

TABLE 7-4 Patients' Rights Under the HIPAA Privacy Rule

Patient Right	Comments	Documentation Required	Documentation Recommended
Access to medical records and the right to copy them	Access to records is guaranteed under HIPAA, but there are some limitations, as mentioned above.	No	Yes
Request for amendment to designated record set	A patient has the right to request amendments to his or her PHI or other personal information. Unless a provider has grounds to deny the request, amendments must be made.	Yes	
Request for an accounting of disclosures of PHI	You are required to account for certain disclosures. Check with your privacy officer for a list. You have up to 60 days to provide the disclosure list.	Yes. Always keep a record of the appropriate disclosures, and make a copy of the disclosure report for the patient's file.	
Request to be contacted at an alternate location	Patients can request to have you contact them at places other than work or home. You can deny the request if you cannot reasonably comply.	Yes. Obtain a request from the patient in writing. Note in the patient's electronic medical record and in a paper communication for staff members who do not have access to the patient's electronic medical record. Document reasons for denying the request if it is denied.	
Requests for further restrictions on who has access to PHI	A patient can request that certain persons or entities do not have access to his or her medical record. You may deny the request if you cannot reasonably comply.	Yes. Ask the patient to complete an opt-out form that is then filed with electronic and paper records. Document reasons for denying the request if it is denied.	
Right to file a complaint	Enforcement of the Privacy Rule is complaint-driven. Patients should be encouraged to work first with the provider. Retaliation is prohibited.	Yes. Refer the complaint to the Privacy Officer. Document the complaint in a privacy complaint log. Evaluate the complaint and determine how best to solve it.	

access. The Security Rule was finalized on February 20, 2003. The compliance date for covered entities was listed as April 20, 2005. For small health plans, the compliance date was April 20, 2006.

Maintaining security of electronic data is complex, and specific technical knowledge and experience is required to implement the requirements of this rule. The Security Rule is flexible, allowing small health care providers to use different security procedures than larger providers. All health care providers must conduct security risk assessment surveys to determine their specific vulnerabilities, and to determine the appropriate responses. Security aspects that must be considered include

▌ Has a security officer for the practice been appointed?

▌ Are passwords that allow access to electronic information protected?

▌ Risk assessment should include evaluating how each person protects the password.

▌ Passwords should not be posted for all to see.

▌ Passwords should not be unnecessarily divulged to others.

▌ Are appropriate security measures, such as firewalls, encryption, and anti-virus software in place, and are they checked and updated regularly?

For example, some covered entities and their business associates use private networks that are not subject to traffic and security problems common with Internet use. Telecommunications networks that transmit electronic data from business to business are often direct links between senders and receivers, called *value-added networks (VANs)*. VANs operate over dedicated, secure communication lines leased from the telephone company especially for this purpose.

firewalls Hardware, software, or both designed to prevent unauthorized persons from accessing electronic information.

encryption The scrambling or encoding of information before sending it electronically.

Other entities and associates use the Internet, but they use **firewalls** (hardware or software designed to keep out unauthorized users) and encryption software to keep information private. **Encryption** software translates information into a code that can be decoded by the recipient but cannot be read by unauthorized viewers.

▌ Are security measures "reasonable and appropriate" for the health care practice and are they periodically reviewed?

▌ Have security breaches occurred in the past? If so, what caused the breaches, and have causes been remedied?

▌ Are security measures in place for business associates that have access to PHI?

▌ Have staff members been trained in maintaining security of electronic information?

▌ Are internal sanctions in place for security breaches, and have staff members been informed of such sanctions?

As stated earlier, the implementation of the HIPAA Security Rule can be a technically daunting task. It is best to involve the appropriate technical person or department as early as possible in the process, to ensure that the appropriate security level has been achieved and documented.

STANDARD 4. NATIONAL IDENTIFIER STANDARDS

The purpose of the National Identifier Standards is to provide unique identifiers (addresses) for electronic transmissions. Just as Web sites you visit on the Internet have unique "addresses," called uniform resource locators (URLs), this standard gives certain health care-related entities identifying numerical or alphanumerical addresses. The standard was fully implemented as of May 2008.

These identifiers are kept in a central databank and include unique "addresses" for employers, providers, and health plans.

FREQUENTLY ASKED QUESTIONS ABOUT HIPAA

For fear of government prosecution, HIPAA compliance overkill has been a problem in some cases. Myths and misinterpretations often must be dispelled as health care providers implement HIPAA standards and rules. For example, it is not true in all cases that health care providers cannot issue the names of hospital patients and patient condition updates to family members. Nor is it true that health care providers cannot correspond about a patient's care, or that police 911 dispatchers cannot give EMTs a patient's name. Here are a few frequently asked questions about HIPAA provisions that can help dispel myths.

Q: May one physician's office send a patient's medical records to another physician's office without the patient's consent?

A: Yes.

Q: Does the HIPAA Privacy Rule prohibit or discourage doctor-patient e-mails?

A: Health care practitioners can continue to correspond with patients via e-mail, but appropriate electronic safeguards must be in place.

Q: May a patient be listed in a hospital's directory without the patient's consent, and may the directory be shared with the public?

A: The HIPAA Privacy Rule allows hospitals to continue providing directory information to the public, unless the patient has specifically chosen not to be included. Hospital directories can include the patient's name, location in the facility (such as hospital floor and room number), and condition in general terms. The information can also be disclosed to callers who ask for the patient by name, but the patient must be informed in advance of this use and disclosure and must have the opportunity to opt out.

Q: May clergy members learn whether members of their congregation or religious affiliation are hospitalized?

A: Hospitals may continue disclosing directory information to members of the clergy, unless the patient has objected to such disclosure.

Q: Is a hospital allowed to share patient information with the patient's family without the patient's express consent?

A: HIPAA provides that a health care provider may "disclose to a family member, other relative, or a close personal friend of the individual, or any other person identified by the individual," medical information directly relevant to such person's involvement with the patient's care or payment related to the patient's care.

Q: May a patient's family member pick up prescriptions for the patient?

A: The Privacy Rule allows family members or others to "pick up filled prescriptions, medical supplies, X-rays, or other similar forms of protected health information."

Q: Does the Privacy Rule mandate many new disclosures of PHI?

A: HIPAA *requires* just two disclosures of PHI: One to HHS representatives who ask to review provider information, and the second to patients who ask to review their own medical records. Disclosure is permitted, but not mandated, in other situations, as discussed above.

Q: Is the HIPAA Privacy Rule prohibitively expensive to implement?

A: A 2002 White House report estimated the costs of implementing privacy over 10 years at about $18 billion. Savings incurred through implementation were estimated at about $29.9 billion over 10 years. However, some sources disagree with these figures, estimating it could cost around $43 billion over 10 years for health care providers to comply with HIPAA.

Q: Can patients sue health care providers who do not comply with the HIPAA Privacy Rule?

A: The HIPAA Privacy Rule does not give patients the express right to sue. Instead, the person must file a written complaint with the Secretary of Health and Human Services through the Office for Civil Rights. The HHS Secretary then decides whether or not to investigate the complaint. Patients may have other legal standings to sue, under state privacy laws.

Q: Are there legal penalties for health care providers who violate the HIPAA Privacy Rule?

A: HHS may impose civil penalties ranging from $100 to $25,000 per offense. The U.S. Department of Justice may enforce criminal sanctions ranging from $50,000 to $250,000 for each offense, with corresponding prison terms.

Q: If a patient refuses to sign an acknowledgment stating that he or she received the health care provider's Notice of Privacy Practices, must the health care provider refuse to provide services?

A: The Privacy Rule gives the patient a "right to notice" of privacy practices for protecting identifying health information. It requires that providers make a "good faith effort" to have patients acknowledge receipt of the notice, but the law does not give health care practitioners the right to refuse treatment to people who do not sign the acknowledgment.

Q: May the media still access public information from hospitals about accident or crime victims?

A: HIPAA lets hospitals continue to make public certain patient directory information, as specified above in the question about hospital directories. If the patient specifically opts out of having such information made public, then the hospital must respect his or her wishes.

Q: If I need emergency assistance from the police or fire department, is the 911 dispatcher prohibited from giving my name to rescue units or EMTs?

A: No. Names and addresses should be given to rescue or EMT staff for help in locating patients and treating their medical problems as quickly as possible.

Q: As a patient, how can I protect the privacy of my health care information?

A: Privacy experts recommend that you

▌ Read notices of privacy practices carefully to become aware of the uses and disclosures of your information that may be made.

- Tell your health care provider your confidentiality concerns.
- Ask how large health care organizations share your information.
- Read authorization forms carefully before you sign; edit them to limit the sharing of information if you wish. Initial and date your revisions.
- Register your objection to disclosures you consider inappropriate. You can file a complaint with the provider, plan, or Department of Health and Human Services.
- Request a copy of your medical record, and review it carefully to be sure the information is correct. You can request amendments or corrections.
- Be cautious when visiting Web sites. If you participate in surveys or health screenings on medical information Web sites, look for and read privacy policies. Don't participate if you don't know how the information will be used and who will have access to it.
- Request a copy of your file from the Medical Information Bureau (MIB). MIB is an organization of insurance companies. MIB compiles reports on individuals with serious medical conditions or other factors that could affect longevity, such as participating in dangerous sports. If MIB has a file on someone, that person has a right to see and correct misinformation in the file. To obtain a copy of your file, if one exists, contact MIB Inc., P. O. Box 105, Essex Station, Boston MA 02112; (866) 692-6901; www.mib.com.
- Educate yourself about medical privacy issues.

Providers' HIPAA compliance and privacy officers are best qualified to answer specific questions about HIPAA and medical privacy. Other sources include the following Web sites and publications.

Web Sites

www.hhs.gov/ocr/hipaa

www.hhs.gov/ocr/privacysummary.pdf

www.hhs.gov/news/facts/privacy.html

www.healthprivacy.org

www.ama-assn.org/ama/pub/category/4234.html (Or at www.ama-assn.org, do a search for HIPAA to reach the current page.)

Publications

Kevin Beaver and Rebecca Herold, *Practical Guide to HIPAA Privacy and Security Compliance* (CRC Press, 2003).

Carolyn P. Hartley, MLA, CHP, and Edward D. Jones III, *HIPAA Plain & Simple: A Compliance Guide for Health Care Professionals* (AMA Press, 2004).

Carolyn Hartley, David C. Kibbe, Jan Root, and Michael Hubbard, *Field Guide to HIPAA Implementation,* revised edition (AMA Press, 2003).

Uday Ali Pabrai, *Getting Started With HIPAA* (Premier Press, 2003).

Ethics Issues

Privacy Law and HIPAA

Laurinda Beebe Harman, PhD, RHIA, Associate Professor and Chair, Department of Health Information Management (HIM), at Temple University in Philadelphia, is editor of a 2006 text for health care students and practitioners, titled *Ethical Challenges in the Management of Health Information,* 2nd edition.

"There are many ethical issues that health care providers and HIM practitioners face," says Harman, "including those related to coding, quality review, research, public health, managed care, clinical care, the electronic health record, adoption, genetic and behavioral health." Health care practitioners also face many ethical issues in the special roles they assume, Harman continues, "including management, entrepreneurship, advocacy, and working with vendors. The legal system is a necessary but often insufficient resource when facing these issues."

For example, although HIPAA spells out specific requirements for privacy and confidentiality of medical records, like any law it cannot anticipate or address every possible situation. "It is within these voids that ethics must prevail and guide our decisions. . . .

"There must be a constant balancing between protecting privacy and releasing information, in accordance with federal privacy legislation, to authorized users so that business functions that support health care can be accomplished."[1]

Furthermore, "Several important criteria should be used when evaluating requests for the release of information, including the 'need-to-know' (minimum necessary) criterion."

ETHICS ISSUE 1: HIPAA has made it illegal, under threat of penalty, for health care practitioners to disclose confidential health information about patients to unauthorized sources.

DISCUSSION QUESTIONS

1. Sharon, a second-year nursing student, is completing a surgical rotation in a community hospital. At the breakfast table, Sharon's husband asks her to find out what is wrong with one of his employees, who has been hospitalized for several days. He is interested in knowing when the man may be able to return to work. Is it ethical for Sharon to give her husband this information? Explain your answer.

_____

_____

2. What should health care practitioners do when family members or friends ask them for information about others that they have discovered in the course of their employment?

_____

_____

ETHICS ISSUE 2: HIPAA requires health care providers to issue privacy notices to patients.

DISCUSSION QUESTION

1. You are the medical office employee responsible for giving patients your employer's privacy notice. Even though you have explained why an elderly patient has been given the privacy notice, he complains about yet another "health care form" and refuses to read it. How will you respond?

_____

_____

[1]Laurinda B. Harman, "Privacy and Confidentiality," in *Ethical Challenges in the Management of Health Information,* 2nd ed., by Laurie A. Rinehart-Thompson and Laurinda B. Harman (Sudbury, MA: Jones & Bartlett, 2006), Chapter 3.

ETHICS ISSUE 3: Some sources distinguish between *privacy* in health care and *confidentiality*. According to Harman, privacy refers to the right of an individual to be let alone and to the fact that patients must authorize release of information. Confidentiality refers to limiting disclosure to authorized persons and ensuring protection of records documenting communication between providers and patients.

DISCUSSION QUESTIONS

1. Why are privacy and confidentiality so important to patients and to health care practitioners?

_____

_____

2. With the implementation of HIPAA, the extensive federal law mandating certain privacy and security precautions, is privacy for protected health information now guaranteed? Explain your answer.

_____

_____

3. The health care practitioners listed below have followed the letter of HIPAA law. Have they also acted ethically? Explain why or why not.

A patient asks to see her medical records and a medical office records assistant complies, but slams the records down in front of the patient and mutters about being "too busy" for this service.

_____

_____

A physician does not refuse to see a patient who declares that he will not complete his notification preference form, but his abrupt manner discourages the patient from continuing to see the physician.

_____

_____

A patient asks for a list of disclosures his physician has made of his health information within the past six years, and he is politely asked to submit his request in writing.

_____

_____

The person responsible for faxing a patient's protected health information from one physician's office to another sends the information to the wrong fax number.

_____

_____

 Go to www.mhhe.com/judson5e to practice your case review skills. Then read on for more information.

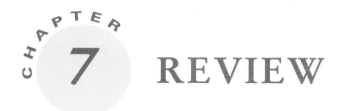

REVIEW

Applying Knowledge

Answer the following questions in the spaces provided.

1. HIPAA stands for _____ .

2. The department of the federal government responsible for supervising HIPAA compliance and implementation is _____ .

3. Patient complaints about privacy must be directed to which government agency?

_____

4. Which federal government agency deals with compliance and implementation of the National Identifier Standard?

_____

5. What is the determining factor in deciding whether or not health care providers are considered *covered entities* under HIPAA?

_____

_____

6. What is an *electronic transmission,* and how and why does HIPAA address it?

_____

_____

7. What is the primary objective of Administrative Simplification?

_____

_____

8. Which of the four HIPAA Standards addresses Administrative Simplification?

_____

_____

9. A document that informs patients on how a health care provider intends to use and disclose patient information and also informs patients of their rights is called

_____

_____

10. Protected health information (PHI) refers to

_____

_____

11. If a state law and HIPAA's federal law disagree, which law should you follow?

_____

12. The primary reason for the Security Rule is

_____

Circle the correct answer for each of the following multiple-choice questions.

13. A *business associate* is
    a. A person, group, or organization outside the medical practice that has a HIPAA-approved reason to see protected health information.
    b. A health care practitioner's financial advisor.
    c. Anyone who sells products related to health care.
    d. None of the above

14. You could unintentionally expose content on your personal computer or your employer's system network by
    a. Shopping on the Internet while you are at work.
    b. Downloading games from the Internet.
    c. Sending and receiving unsecured e-mails to and from friends.
    d. All of the above

15. If a patient complains that his privacy was breached, what should you ask that he do?
    a. Call a lawyer.
    b. Speak to your privacy officer to try to handle the complaint in the office.
    c. Immediately file a complaint with the Office for Civil Rights.
    d. Discuss the problem with someone else in the office.

16. Which of the following are the privacy officer's responsibilities?
    a. Researching the Privacy Rule.
    b. Helping to develop the Notice of Privacy Practices.
    c. Training staff on privacy policies and procedures.
    d. All of the above

17. Which of the following is *not* covered by HIPAA's Security Rule?
    a. The content of all documents pertaining to patient privacy.
    b. Maintaining electronic security for networked computers.
    c. Using HIPAA standards for electronic transmission of protected health information.
    d. None of the above

18. Which of the following is *not* considered marketing under HIPAA provisions?
    a. A pharmaceutical company wants to send special mailings to a provider's diabetic patients to announce a new blood sugar testing device.
    b. A reminder to female patients when their mammograms should be scheduled.
    c. Cholesterol screening results sent to patients through the mail.
    d. None of the above.

19. Which of the following is *not* a violation of HIPAA's Privacy Rule?
    a. You call across a crowded waiting room to tell a patient he has forgotten his prescription for dilantin, a drug used to control seizures.
    b. You are a medical assistant for a physician's private practice, and you tell a friend, who is a bank teller, that a mutual friend has seen your employer and is pregnant.
    c. A telephone caller identifies himself as an insurance plan representative and requests PHI. You do not know the caller, but you comply.
    d. All of the above are violations of HIPAA's Privacy Rule.

20. An unauthorized person (a computer hacker) manages to access the computers in the hospital where you work and downloads information. Who is the most likely person to handle the disaster?
    a. The privacy officer.
    b. The hospital administrator.
    c. The security officer.
    d. The medical records supervisor.

21. Which of the following is true under HIPAA?
    a. HIPAA language states unequivocally that patients have no standing to sue under the law.
    b. Patients must submit complaints to the Secretary of Health and Human Services through the Office of Civil Rights.
    c. Only a court of law can hear patient complaints.
    d. None of the above

22. HIPPA's Privacy Rule protects PHI
    a. Only in electronic form.
    b. Only in written form.
    c. Only in spoken form.
    d. In all of the above forms.

23. Circle the letter for the statement that is *not* true of HIPAA:
    a. HIPAA requires that health care practitioners change a medical record if a patient complains.
    b. If a patients asks to see his or her medical record, the request must be honored.
    c. Health care practitioners must supply patients who ask with a list of those who have received copies of the patient's medical record.
    d. Under HIPAA, any health care facility that transmits protected health information electronically is a covered entity.

Match each description that follows with the correct answer by writing the appropriate letter in the space provided.

_____ 24. The HIPAA-mandated standard for electronic transmissions.

_____ 25. A valid reason to disclose protected health information.

_____ 26. This person evaluates, manages, and reports on the security of a health provider's electronic data.

_____ 27. Networks closed to the Internet that are provided by the telephone company.

_____ 28. Covered entities.

_____ 29. Covered transactions.

_____ 30. Refers to providing only as much patient information as needed for a request or to conduct health care business.

_____ 31. One of two types of PHI access mandated by HIPAA.

_____ 32. One of a patient's six rights mandated by HIPAA.

_____ 33. To remove patient-identifying information from PHI.

a. File a complaint

b. value-added networks

c. physicians and pharmacists

d. minimum necessary

e. de-identify

f. billing patients and filing insurance claims

g. HIPAA representatives ask to see PHI

h. security officer

i. privacy officer

j. permission

k. electronic data interchange (EDI)

Case Study

Use your critical-thinking skills to answer the questions that follow each of the case studies.

Mona frequently travels for her job, and even when she is in town, she's usually reached most easily on her mobile phone. She has three teenagers at home and doesn't want them to pick up her health care messages. She also wants her medical bills sent to her work address.

34. What should Mona's health care provider do to accommodate her requests?

_____

_____

Lewis received a basketball scholarship to attend college, and he signed a form giving the university health service permission to access his health care records. Lewis now wants to know what is included in his health care records.

35. What should Lewis's health care provider do?

_____

Shirley, an EMT, is off duty and is driving her private vehicle on the interstate in a snowstorm. The car ahead of Shirley hits an icy patch and skids off the road, overturning as it hits the ditch. Shirley stops to help and dials 911 on her mobile phone. The lone woman in the wrecked car has scratches and bruises and an obviously broken arm. While Shirley is helping the woman, a news van stops and a television reporter films the wreck for the evening news. The injured driver refuses to answer questions, so the reporter turns to Shirley, who knows the injured driver's name.

36. May Shirley tell the television reporter the injured woman's name without violating federal law? Why or why not?

_____

37. Rescue services arrive while the television reporter is there. Can the ambulance attendants, who are also EMTs, tell the television reporter the apparent extent of the woman's injuries? Why or why not?

_____

You are a nurse and a teenaged patient's mother tells you she wants access to her daughter's medical records.

38. What will you do?

_____

_____

Internet Activities

Complete the activities and answer the questions that follow.

39. In 2007, medical records of two celebrities—George Clooney and Paris Hilton—were leaked to the press by health care employees who had access to the records. Visit the Web site at http://inside.duke.edu/article.php?IssueID=38&ParentID=1384. Read the article and answer the following questions:

What is the correct answer to the ethical question posed at the beginning of the article? Why is this the correct answer?

_____

_____

Take the HIPAA quiz at the above-listed Web site, under "Get Hip on HIPAA," and report your answers below or in class.

_____

_____

_____

40. Visit www.hhs.gov/faq/. Access "Frequent Questions," select number 2, and choose a category. Prepare a list of 10 questions you would most like to have answered. List the answers to the questions you have chosen.

_____

_____

_____

_____

_____

_____

_____

_____

PART

3

Professional, Social, and Interpersonal Health Care Issues

Physicians' Public Duties and Responsibilities

Learning Outcomes

After studying this chapter, you should be able to:

1. List at least four vital events for which statistics are collected by the government.

2. Discuss the procedures for filing birth and death certificates.

3. Explain the purpose of public health statutes.

4. Cite examples of reportable diseases and injuries, and explain how they are reported.

5. Discuss federal drug regulations, including the Controlled Substances Act.

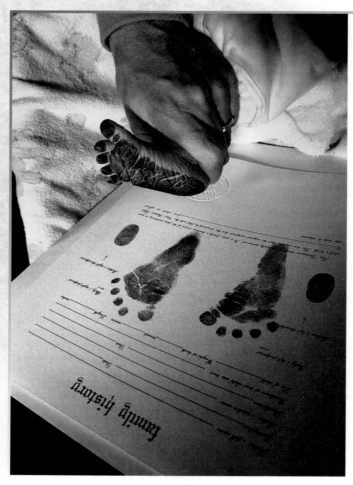

Key Terms

administer

Amendments to the Older Americans Act

autopsy

Child Abuse Prevention and Treatment Act

Controlled Substances Act

coroner

dispense

Drug Enforcement Administration (DEA)

Food and Drug Administration (FDA)

forensics

medical examiner

National Childhood Vaccine Injury Act

National Vaccine Injury Compensation Program (VICP)

prescribe

Unborn Victims of Violence Act

vital statistics

Voice of Experience
Community Health Nurse Practices Diplomacy

Mary, RN, BSN, is a community health nurse working for a county health department in a rural area of a northwestern state. She says that tact, understanding, and diplomacy are necessary when contacting individuals who may have been exposed to a sexually transmitted disease (STD).

"When a patient sees a physician who diagnoses an STD, the physician discusses test results with the patient, then reports the case to the health department. If the patient lives in the area we serve, then we visit that person and try to determine recent sexual partners. We emphasize that information will be kept confidential and hope that the person will feel a sense of responsibility so that their sexual partners can see a physician. Most do, but some are reluctant for one reason or another.

"We then contact all the named sexual partners of the person diagnosed with an STD and encourage them to see a physician or visit a clinic for examination, even if they have no symptoms," Mary continues. "Of course, we also ask them for names of their sexual partners, so they can also be contacted. Unfortunately, lists can be long, and some individuals may not even recall everyone with whom they have been intimate. It's a difficult task, because it's embarrassing and upsetting for everyone involved, but it's also necessary, to see that people who have been exposed [to STDs] get treatment."

[Note that contact procedures differ from state to state. In some states, for instance, "community disease specialists," who may or may not be nurses or other health care practitioners, contact individuals named as sexual partners by those diagnosed with STDs.]

VITAL STATISTICS

vital statistics Numbers collected for the population of live births, deaths, fetal deaths, marriages, divorces, induced terminations of pregnancy, and any change in civil status that occurs during an individual's lifetime.

In order to assess population trends and needs, state and federal governments collect **vital statistics.** Vital events for which statistics are collected include live births, deaths, fetal deaths, marriages, divorces, induced terminations of pregnancy, and any change in civil status that occurs during an individual's lifetime. Health care practitioners help in gathering this information and in filling out forms for filing with the appropriate state and federal agencies.

The information provided through the reporting of vital statistics is useful to educational institutions, governmental agencies, research scientists, private industry, and many other organizations and individuals. For example, the recording of vital statistics allows for tracking population composition and growth, measuring educational standards, and monitoring communicable diseases and other community and environmental health problems. Health care practitioners play an important role in collecting and recording valuable health data required by law; therefore, it is important that they know the correct methods and procedures for reporting public health information.

Birth and death certificates are permanent legal records, and a copy of a person's birth certificate is required to obtain certain government documents, such as a passport, driver's license, voter registration card, or Social Security card. Guidelines for completing the forms are as follows:

- Type or legibly print all entries. In some states, only black ink may be used.
- Leave no entries blank. Each state has specific requirements for recording information.
- Avoid corrections and erasures.
- Where requested, provide signatures. Do not use rubber stamps or initials in place of signatures.

- File only originals with state registrars.
- Verify the spelling of names.
- Avoid abbreviations, except those recommended in instructions for specific items.
- Refer any problems to the appropriate state officials.

Births

All live births must be reported to the state registrar. Figure 8-1 illustrates a sample birth certificate. In some states, separate birth and death certificates must be filed for stillbirths, while in others there are special forms for stillbirths that include both birth and death information. Generally, birth and death certificates are not required for fetal deaths in which the fetus has not passed the twentieth week of gestation.

Hospitals file birth certificates for babies born to mothers who have been admitted as patients. The attending physician must verify all medical information. For nonhospital births, the person in attendance is responsible for filing the birth certificate.

Deaths

After a person is pronounced dead, the attending physician must complete the medical portion of the certificate of death, which generally includes the following information:

- Disease, injury, and/or complication that caused the death and how long the decedent was treated for this condition before death occurred.
- Date and time of death.
- Place of death.
- If decedent was female, presence or absence of pregnancy.
- Whether or not an autopsy was performed. An **autopsy** is a postmortem examination to determine the cause of death or to obtain physiological evidence, as in the case of a suspicious death.

In most states it is against the law for an attending physician to sign a death certificate if the death was

- Possibly due to criminal causes.
- Not attended by a physician within a specified length of time before death.
- Due to causes undetermined by the physician.
- Violent or otherwise suspicious.

If any of these situations exist, the coroner or medical examiner (see below) must sign the death certificate. If a death occurs under suspicious circumstances, permission from next of kin is *not* needed for an autopsy to be performed. If the death did not occur under suspicious circumstances, however, consent from next of kin or a legally responsible party must be obtained for an autopsy to be performed.

When death has occurred under normal circumstances, after authorization has been obtained from the next of kin or from a legally responsible party, the body can be removed to a funeral home. In many states, the death certificate must be signed within 24 to 72 hours. The *mortician* or *undertaker* (person trained to attend to the dead) files the death certificate with the state. (See Figure 8-2 for a sample death certificate.)

autopsy A postmortem examination to determine the cause of death or to obtain physiological evidence, as in the case of a suspicious death.

Ohio Department of Health
VITAL STATISTICS
CERTIFICATE OF LIVE BIRTH
TYPE OR PRINT IN PERMANENT *BLACK* INK

Reg. Dist. No. _____
Primary Reg. Dist. No. _____
Registrar's No. _____

Birth No. 134 —

VOID

CHILD

1. CHILD - NAME First Middle Last | 2. SEX | 3a. DATE OF BIRTH (Month, Day, Year) | 3b. TIME OF BIRTH M

4a. FACILITY NAME - (If not institution, give street and number) | 4b. CITY, VILLAGE OR LOCATION OF BIRTH | 4c. COUNTY OF BIRTH

5. PLACE OF BIRTH
☐ Hospital ☐ Freestanding Birthing Center ☐ Clinic/Doctor's Office ☐ Residence ☐ Other (Specify) _____

6. REGISTRAR'S SIGNATURE | 7. DATE FILED BY REGISTRAR (Month, Day, Year)

ATTENDANT

8a. I certify that the above named child was born alive at the place and time and on the date stated above. SIGNATURE | 8b. DATE SIGNED | 8c. ATTENDANT ☐ M.D. ☐ D.O. ☐ C.N.M. ☐ OTHER MIDWIFE ☐ OTHER (Specify)

8d. ATTENDANT - NAME (Type or Print) | 8e. MAILING ADDRESS (Street or R.F.D. No., City or Village, State, Zip)

MOTHER

9a. MOTHER'S NAME (First, Middle, Last) | 9b. MAIDEN NAME | 10a. DATE OF BIRTH (Month, Day, Year) | 10b. AGE

11. BIRTHPLACE (State or Foreign Country) | 12a. RESIDENCE - STATE | 12. COUNTY | 12c. CITY, TOWN, OR LOCATION

12d. STREET AND NUMBER | 12e. INSIDE CITY LIMITS? ☐ Yes ☐ No | 13. MOTHER'S MAILING ADDRESS (If same as residence, enter zip code only)

FATHER

14. FATHER'S NAME (First, Middle, Last) | 15a. DATE OF BIRTH (Month, Day, Year) | 15b. AGE | 16. BIRTHPLACE (State or Foreign Country)

INFORMANT

17. I certify that the personal information provided on this certificate is correct to the best of my knowledge and belief. (ENTER INFORMANT'S NAME OR WHEN REQUIRED BY LAW, PARENTS' SIGNATURES.)

INFORMATION FOR MEDICAL AND HEALTH USE ONLY

MOTHER
FATHER

18. OF HISPANIC ORIGIN? (Specify No or Yes - if yes, specify Cuban, Mexican, Puerto Rican, etc.)
18a. ☐ NO ☐ YES Specify:
18b. ☐ NO ☐ YES Specify:

19. RACE American Indian, Black, White, etc. (Specify below)
19a.
19b.

20. EDUCATION (Specify only highest grade completed) Elementary/Secondary (0-12) College (1-4 or 5+)
20a.
20b.

21. OCCUPATION AND BUSINESS/INDUSTRY (Worked during last year) Occupation | Business/Industry
21a. | 21b.
21c. | 21d.

22. PREGNANCY HISTORY (Complete each section)

23. MOTHER MARRIED? (At birth, conception, or any time between) (Yes or No)

24. DATE LAST NORMAL MENSES BEGAN (Month, Day, Year)

LIVE BIRTHS (Do not include this child)
OTHER TERMINATIONS (Spontaneous and induced at any time after conception)

25. TOTAL PRENATAL VISITS (If none, so state)

22a. NOW LIVING NUMBER ☐ NONE | 22b. NOW DEAD NUMBER ☐ NONE | 22d. NUMBER ☐ NONE

25. MONTH OF PREGNANCY PRENATAL CARE BEGAN First, Second, Third, etc. (Specify) | 26b. CITY | 26c. COUNTY

27. BIRTH WEIGHT IN GRAMS | 28. CLINICAL ESTIMATE OF GESTATION (Weeks)

22c. DATE OF LAST BIRTH (Month, Year) | 22e. DATE OF LAST OTHER TERMINATION (Month, Year) | 29a. PLURALITY - Single, Twin, Triplet, etc. (Specify) | 29b. IF NOT SINGLE BIRTH - Born First, Second, Third, etc. (Specify)

30. APGAR SCORE | 31a. MOTHER TRANSFERRED PRIOR TO DELIVERY? ☐ No ☐ Yes If yes, enter name of facility and city transferred FROM
30a. 1 MINUTE | 30b. 5 MINUTES | 31b. FACILITY NAME | 31c. CITY

31d. INFANT TRANSFERRED? ☐ No ☐ Yes If yes, enter name of facility and city transferred TO.
31e. FACILITY NAME | 31f. CITY

MULTIPLE BIRTHS Enter State File Number for Male(s) LIVE BIRTH(S) FETAL DEATH(S)

32a. MEDICAL RISK FACTORS FOR THIS PREGNANCY (Check all that apply)
Anemia (Hct. < 30/Hgb. < 10) ... 01 ☐
Cardiac disease ... 02 ☐
Acute or chronic lung disease ... 03 ☐
Diabetes ... 04 ☐
Genital herpes ... 05 ☐
Hydramnios/Oligohydramnios ... 06 ☐
Hemoglobinopathy ... 07 ☐
Hypertension, chronic ... 08 ☐
Hypertension, pregnancy-associated ... 09 ☐
Eclampsia ... 10 ☐
Incompetent cervix ... 11 ☐
Previous infant 4000 + grams ... 12 ☐
Previous preterm or small-for-gestational-age infant ... 13 ☐
Renal disease ... 14 ☐
Rh sensitization ... 15 ☐
Uterine bleeding ... 16 ☐
None ... 00 ☐
Other (Specify) ... 17 ☐

32b. OTHER RISK FACTORS FOR THIS PREGNANCY (Complete all items)
Tobacco use during pregnancy ... Yes ☐ No ☐
Average number cigarettes per day _____
Alcohol use during pregnancy ... Yes ☐ No ☐
Average number drinks per week _____
Weight gained during pregnancy _____ lbs.
Pre-Pregnancy weight _____ lbs.

33. OBSTETRIC PROCEDURES (Check all that apply)
Amniocentesis ... 01 ☐
Electronic fetal monitoring ... 02 ☐
Induction of labor ... 03 ☐
Stimulation of labor ... 04 ☐
Tocolysis ... 05 ☐
Ultrasound ... 06 ☐
None ... 00 ☐
Other (Specify) ... 07 ☐

34. COMPLICATIONS OF LABOR AND/OR DELIVERY (Check all that apply)
Febrile (>100° F. or 38° C.) ... 01 ☐
Meconium, moderate/heavy ... 02 ☐
Premature rupture of membrane (>12 hours) ... 03 ☐
Abruptio placenta ... 04 ☐
Placenta previa ... 05 ☐
Other excessive bleeding ... 06 ☐
Seizures during labor ... 07 ☐
Precipitous labor (<3 hours) ... 08 ☐
Prolonged labor (>20 hours) ... 09 ☐
Dysfunctional labor ... 10 ☐
Breech/Malpresentation ... 11 ☐
Cephalopelvic disproportion ... 12 ☐
Cord prolapse ... 13 ☐
Anesthetic complications ... 14 ☐
Fetal distress ... 15 ☐
None ... 00 ☐
Other (Specify) ... 16 ☐

35. METHOD OF DELIVERY (Check all that apply)
Vaginal ... 01 ☐
Vaginal birth after previous C-section ... 02 ☐
Primary C-section ... 03 ☐
Repeat C-section ... 04 ☐
Forceps ... 05 ☐
Vacuum ... 06 ☐

36. ABNORMAL CONDITIONS OF THE NEWBORN (Check all that apply)
Anemia (Hct. < 39/Hgb. < 13) ... 01 ☐
Birth injury ... 02 ☐
Fetal alcohol syndrome ... 03 ☐
Hyaline membrane disease/RDS ... 04 ☐
Meconium aspiration syndrome ... 05 ☐
Assisted ventilation < 30 min ... 06 ☐
Assisted ventilation ≥ 30 min ... 07 ☐
Seizures ... 08 ☐
None ... 00 ☐
Other (Specify) ... 09 ☐

37. CONGENITAL ANOMALIES OF CHILD (Check all that apply)
Anencephalus ... 01 ☐
Spina bifida/Meningocele ... 02 ☐
Hydrocephalus ... 03 ☐
Microcephalus ... 04 ☐
Other central nervous system anomalies (Specify) ... 05 ☐
Heart malformations ... 06 ☐
Other circulatory / respiratory anomalies (Specify) ... 07 ☐
Rectal atresia / stenosis ... 08 ☐
Tracheo-esophageal fistula / Esophageal atresia ... 09 ☐
Omphalocele / Gastroschisis ... 10 ☐
Other gastrointestinal anomalies (Specify) ... 11 ☐
Malformed genitalia ... 12 ☐
Renal agenesis ... 13 ☐
Other urogenital anomalies (Specify) ... 14 ☐
Cleft lip / palate ... 15 ☐
Polydactyly / Syndactyly / Adactyly ... 16 ☐
Club foot ... 17 ☐
Diaphragmatic hernia ... 18 ☐
Other musculoskeletal / integumental anomalies (Specify) ... 19 ☐
Down's syndrome ... 20 ☐
Other chromosomal anomalies (Specify) ... 21 ☐
None ... 00 ☐
Other (Specify) ... 22 ☐

37a. PARENT(S) REQUEST ISSUANCE OF A SOCIAL SECURITY NUMBER FOR THIS CHILD ☐

38. NAME OF PROPHYLACTIC USED IN EYES OF CHILD | 39. DATE OF APPROVED TEST FOR SYPHILIS, IF NONE, STATE REASON | 40. DATE OF APPROVED TEST FOR GONORRHEA, IF NONE, STATE REASON

HEA 2703 5112.06 (REV. 7/92)

FIGURE 8-1 A Sample Birth Certificate

Ohio Department of Health
VITAL STATISTICS
CERTIFICATE OF DEATH

DO NOT WRITE IN MARGIN RESERVED FOR ODH DATA CODING

Reg. Dist. No. _____

Primary Reg. Dist. No. _____

State File No. _____

Registrar's No. _____

a. ____
b. ____
c. ____
d. ____
e. ____

DECEDENT

1. DECEDENT'S NAME *(First, Middle, LAST)*		2. SEX	3. DATE OF DEATH *(Month, Day, Year)*

4. SOCIAL SECURITY NUMBER	5a. AGE - Last Birthday *(Years)*	5b. UNDER 1 YEAR		5c. UNDER 1 DAY		6. DATE OF BIRTH *(Month, Day, Year)*	7. BIRTHPLACE *(City and State or Foreign Country)*
		Months	Days	Hours	Minutes		

8. WAS DECEDENT EVER IN U.S. ARMED FORCES? ☐ Yes ☐ No	9a. PLACE OF DEATH *(Check only one)*

HOSPITAL: ☐ Inpatient ☐ ER/Outpatient ☐ DOA   OTHER ☐ Nursing Home ☐ Residence ☐ Other *(Specify)*

9b. FACILITY NAME *(If not institution, give street and number)*	9c. CITY, VILLAGE, TWP., OR LOCATION OF DEATH	9d. COUNTY OF DEATH

IF DEATH OCCURRED IN INSTITUTION, GIVE RESIDENCE BEFORE ADMISSION →

10. MARITAL STATUS - Married, Never Married, Widowed, Divorced *(Specify)*	11. SURVIVING SPOUSE *(If wife give maiden name)*	12a. DECEDENTS USUAL OCCUPATION *(Give kind of work done during most of working life. Don't use retired.)*	12b. KIND OF BUSINESS/INDUSTRY

13a. RESIDENCE - STATE	13b. COUNTY	13c. CITY, TOWN, TWP., OR LOCATION	13d. STREET AND NUMBER

13e. INSIDE CITY LIMITS? *(Yes or No)*	13f. ZIP CODE	14. WAS DECEDENT OF HISPANIC ORIGIN? *(Specify No or Yes - If yes, specify Cuban, Mexican, Puerto Rican, etc.)* ☐ No ☐ Yes Specify:	15. RACE - American Indian, Black, White, etc. *(Specify)*	16. DECEDENT'S EDUCATION *(Specify only highest grade completed)* Elementary/Secondary (0-12) College (1-4 or 5+)

PARENTS

17. FATHER'S NAME *(First, Middle, Last)*	18. MOTHER'S NAME *(First, Middle, Maiden Surname)*

INFORMANT

19a. INFORMANT'S NAME *(Type/Print)*	19b. MAILING ADDRESS *(Street and Number or Rural Route Number, City or Town, State, Zip Code)*

DISPOSITION

20a. METHOD OF DISPOSITION ☐ Burial ☐ Cremation ☐ Removal from State ☐ Donation ☐ Other *(Specify)*	20b. PLACE OF DISPOSITION *(Name of cemetery, crematory, or other place)*	20c. LOCATION - City or Town, State

20d. DATE OF DISPOSITION	21a. NAME OF EMBALMER	21b. LICENSE NUMBER

22a. SIGNATURE OF FUNERAL DIRECTOR OR OTHER PERSON ►	22b. LICENSE NUMBER *(of Licensee)*	23. NAME AND ADDRESS OF FACILITY

REGISTRAR

f. ____
g. ____
h. ____
i. ____

24. REGISTRAR'S SIGNATURE ►	25. DATE FILED *(Month, Day, Year)*

26a. SIGNATURE OF PERSON ISSUING PERMIT ►	26b. DIST. No.	27. DATE PERMIT ISSUED

CERTIFIER

28a. CERTIFIER *(Check only one)*	☐ CERTIFYING PHYSICIAN To the best of my knowledge, death occurred at the time, date, and place, and due to the cause(s) and manner as stated.
	☐ CORONER On the basis of examination and/or investigation, in my opinion, death occurred at the time, date, and place, and due to the cause(s) and manner as stated.

28b. TIME OF DEATH M	28c. DATE PRONOUNCED DEAD *(Month, Day, Year)*	28d. WAS CASE REFERRED TO CORONER? ☐ Yes ☐ No

j. ____
k. ____
l. ____
m. ____

28e. SIGNATURE AND TITLE OF CERTIFIER ►	28f. LICENSE NUMBER	28g. DATE SIGNED *(Month, Day, Year)*

29. NAME AND ADDRESS OF PERSON WHO COMPLETED CAUSE OF DEATH *(Type/Print)*

CAUSE OF DEATH

n. ____
o. ____
p. ____
q. ____
r. ____
s. ____
t. ____
u. ____

30. **PART I.** Enter the diseases, injuries, or complications that caused the death. Do not enter the mode of dying, such as cardiac or respiratory arrest, shock, or heart failure. List only one cause on each line. TYPE OR PRINT IN PERMANENT INK	Approximate Interval Between Onset and Death
IMMEDIATE CAUSE (Final disease or condition resulting in death) → a. _____ DUE TO (OR AS A CONSEQUENCE OF):	
Sequentially list conditions, if any, leading to immediate cause. Enter **UNDERLYING CAUSE** (Disease or injury that initiated events resulting in death) LAST b. _____ DUE TO (OR AS A CONSEQUENCE OF):	
c. _____ DUE TO (OR AS A CONSEQUENCE OF):	
d.	

SEE INSTRUCTIONS ON OTHER SIDE

PART II. Other *significant* *conditions* contributing to death but not resulting in the underlying cause given in Part I.	31a. WAS AN AUTOPSY PERFORMED? ☐ Yes ☐ No	31b. WERE AUTOPSY FINDINGS AVAILABLE PRIOR TO COMPLETION OF CAUSE OF DEATH? ☐ Yes ☐ No

32. MANNER OF DEATH ☐ Natural ☐ Pending Investigation ☐ Accident ☐ Suicide ☐ Could not be Determined ☐ Homicide	33a. DATE OF INJURY *(Month, Day, Year)*	33b. TIME OF INJURY M	33c. INJURY AT WORK? ☐ Yes ☐ No	33d. DESCRIBE HOW INJURY OCCURRED
	33e. PLACE OF INJURY - At home, farm, street, factory, office building, etc. *(Specify)*			33f. LOCATION *(Street and Number or Rural Route Number, City or Town, State)*

HEA 2717
5152.06 Rev. 2/89

FIGURE 8-2 A Sample Death Certificate

coroner A public official who investigates and holds inquests over those who die from unknown or violent causes; he or she may or may not be a physician, depending on state law.

medical examiner A physician who investigates suspicious or unexplained deaths.

forensics A division of medicine that incorporates law and medicine and involves medical issues or medical proof at trials having to do with malpractice, crimes, and accidents.

If the deceased has not been under a physician's care at the time of death, the appropriate county health officer—usually the coroner or medical examiner—is responsible for completing the death certificate. A **coroner** is a public official who investigates and holds inquests over those who die from unknown or violent causes. He or she may or may not be a physician, depending upon state law.

The purpose of a coroner's inquest is to gather evidence that may be used by the police in the investigation of a violent or suspicious death. It is not a trial, but it is a criminal proceeding, in the nature of a preliminary investigation.

Some states employ a medical examiner instead of a coroner. A **medical examiner** is a physician, frequently a pathologist, who investigates suspicious or unexplained deaths in a community. As a physician, the medical examiner can order and perform autopsies.

Forensic Medicine

Forensics is a division of medicine that incorporates law and medicine and involves medical issues or medical proof at trials having to do with malpractice, crimes, and accidents. Forensic scientists investigate crime scenes and present medical proof at trials and hearings. Crime scene investigators are specifically trained to determine cause of death or injury and to help identify a criminal, a victim, and others involved in crimes. Specialists in forensic medicine study such subjects as forensic pharmacology, doping control, postmortem toxicology, blood spatter interpretation, DNA (deoxyribonucleic acid) analytical techniques, and expert testimony procedures. They work for police departments and other criminal investigative bureaus, medical examiners' offices, universities, and other facilities and government agencies.

Court Case

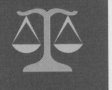

Autopsy Performed without Permission Leads to Lawsuit

A 47-year-old cleaning company supervisor passed out at work. He was taken to a hospital emergency room, but the attending physician was unable to revive him. The doctor issued a Notice of Death at 2:15 A.M., listing cardiac arrest as the cause of death. The deceased's relatives arrived at the hospital 30 minutes after the patient died and told hospital personnel of both their Muslim faith and their desire to take the body to a mosque. The relatives were told to return to the hospital at 8:00 A.M. and they did, but the hospital no longer had the body; at 7:00 A.M. it had been sent to the medical examiner's office. An autopsy was performed at 2:00 P.M. that same day. The relatives filed suit against the hospital and the patient's attending physician for inflicting emotional injuries, alleging that the autopsy was unauthorized.

The plaintiffs sought partial summary judgment on the issue of liability, and the court granted the motion because state law limited the right of a hospital and its physicians to perform an autopsy without the consent of a deceased patient's survivors.

Note: A final disposition of the case was not available, but since the defendants were found liable for performing an autopsy without consent, it is likely that the suit was settled out of court.

Lirjie Juseinoski, et al., v. New York Hospital Medical Center of Queens, et ano, Defendants, 2002 NY Slip Op 50441U; 2004 N.Y. Misc. LEXIS 631.

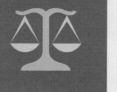

Did the Press Have the Right to Information Involving the Drug Testing of Olympic Athletes?

The crux of the following case was that parties engaged in litigation have a First Amendment right, under the United States Constitution, to disseminate information they obtain in discovery, unless a judge has issued a protective order against releasing such information. Also at issue was the fact that the filing of a document with a court gives rise to a presumptive right of public access.

In 2002, the former director of drug control administration for the United States Olympic Committee (USOC) sued the USOC for wrongful termination, in addition to certain contract claims. Discovery materials included athletes' drug testing results, since the plaintiff alleged that the USOC had asked him to violate rules for releasing the information and, when he refused, had fired him. The USOC filed a motion for a protective order, so that the press would not gain access to discovery materials related to drug testing in Olympic athletes.

The decision in this case was that the athletes who were tested did not have a reasonable expectation of privacy with respect to drug testing, or in the information they gave to the USOC for drug testing purposes, because they signed a form revealing medications they were taking—a precursor to drug testing. The form clearly stated that it was not confidential. Therefore, the court held, a protective order would not be issued.

Another factor in the court's decision not to issue a protective order was that the USOC is a public body, charged with obtaining the most competent amateur athletic representation possible for the United States and with encouraging and supporting research and dissemination of information in the areas of sports medicine and sports safety.

The result of the court's decision was that the press could publish the drug testing information filed as discovery information in the plaintiff's lawsuit against the USOC.

Note: The case is complicated, but it illustrates the fact that under First Amendment rights, in certain circumstances the press has access to health-related information that might otherwise be confidential, if such information is deemed to be within "public access."

Wade F. Exum, M.D. v. United States Olympic Committee, 209 F.R.D. 201; 2002 U.S. Dist. LEXIS 14716, May 23, 2002.

CHECK YOUR PROGRESS

1. Define *vital statistics.*

_____

_____

2. Define *autopsy.*

_____

_____

3. Define *coroner.*

_____

_____

4. Define *medical examiner.*

_____

_____

5. Define *forensics.*

_____

_____

6. Where are birth certificates and death certificates filed?

_____

_____

7. Birth certificates must be filed for _____.

Requirements vary with states for _____.

8. Name three circumstances in which an attending physician may not legally complete a death certificate.

_____

_____

_____

PUBLIC HEALTH STATUTES

In all states, to help guarantee the health and well-being of citizens, physicians or other health care practitioners must report births, deaths, certain communicable diseases, specific injuries, and child and drug abuse to the appropriate local, state, and federal authorities. Public health statutes vary with states concerning the reporting of fetal deaths and stillbirths, time limits for filing reports, and the manner in which information must be recorded. However, all provide for

▮ Guarding against unsanitary conditions in public facilities.

▮ Inspecting establishments where food and drink are processed and sold.

▮ Exterminating pests and vermin that can spread disease.

▮ Checking water quality.

▮ Setting up measures of control for certain diseases.

▮ Requiring physicians, school nurses, and other health care workers to file certain reports for the protection of citizens.

Communicable and Other Notifiable Diseases

Under each state's public health statutes, physicians, other health care practitioners, and anyone who has knowledge of a case must report to county or state health agencies the occurrence of certain diseases that, if left unchecked, could threaten the health and well-being of the population.

The list of reportable diseases is long and varies with the state. Requirements for reporting, such as time lapses and whether to report by telephone,

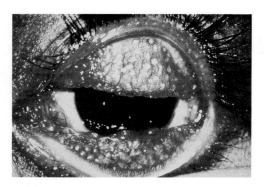

FIGURE 8-3 Primary ocular chlamydial infection of the eye. STDs are often systemic infections.

mail, or online, also vary, so medical office personnel should be familiar with the specific requirements for reporting communicable diseases in their county and state of employment. Requirements for reporting and forms for reporting by mail are available from county and state health departments, either by mail or, in most cases, online. Those communicable diseases most likely to have mandated reporting by state statutes are diphtheria, cholera, meningococcal meningitis, plague, smallpox, tuberculosis, anthrax, HIV and AIDS, brucellosis, infectious and serum hepatitis, leprosy, malaria, rubeola, poliomyelitis, psittacosis, rheumatic fever, rubella, typhoid fever, trichinosis, and tetanus. Other diseases that may have mandated reporting if a higher than normal incidence occurs are influenza and streptococcal and staphylococcal infections.

Certain sexually transmitted diseases (STDs), also called venereal diseases, must be reported whenever diagnosed. *Sexually transmitted disease* is a general term that refers to any disease transmitted through sexual contact. Many STDs are transmitted through genital contact, which may or may not include sexual intercourse. For example, practicing oral sex can transmit gonorrhea from the genitals of one partner to the mouth and throat region of the other. Reportable STDs differ with states but generally include gonorrhea, syphilis, chlamydia, lymphogranuloma venereum (Figure 8-3), chancroid, granuloma inguinale (genital warts), scabies, pubic lice, and trichomonas. Public health practitioners use reported cases to find and treat others who may have been infected through sexual contact with the named individual.

Most of the 50 states now have laws that require individuals infected with HIV to notify past and present sexual partners. The following case illustrates how Michigan's HIV notification law was tested in court.

Court Case

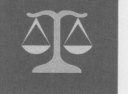

State Law Mandates Notification of Sexual Partners by HIV Carrier

Michigan passed a state law requiring individuals who know they are HIV-infected to notify their sexual partners before sexual activity. A defendant was convicted of having sexual contact as defined under the act without notifying her partner of her HIV status. She was sentenced from 2 years 8 months to 4 years in prison on each of three counts.

The defendant appealed, claiming that the statute is unconstitutionally broad because it applies to both consensual and nonconsensual sexual acts and because it does not require intent. The appeals court addressed the issue of intent by comparing killing someone with a car while driving drunk to the defendant's having sexual contact with someone without telling them of her HIV status. The comparison made was that the statute against driving while intoxicated does not require an intent to kill but recognizes that there is intent in the reckless action of driving drunk. The court found that the intent in the HIV notification statute is satisfied by the reckless action of having sexual contact without warning one's partner about exposure to HIV. The court held that the statute was constitutional and that punishment in this case was appropriate under the law.

People v. Jensen, 231 Mich.App. 439, 586 N.W.2d 748 (Mich.App., Aug 28, 1998). Appeal denied, *People v. Jensen,* 595 N.W.2d 850 (Mich. May 25, 1999).

Reporting requirements for communicable diseases are usually more stringent for patients who are employed in restaurants, cafeterias, day care centers, schools, health care facilities, and other places where contagion can be rampant.

Through extensive vaccination programs, many communicable diseases that decimated world populations in the past have largely been eradicated. In the United States, for example, smallpox has virtually disappeared, and very few cases of poliomyelitis, typhoid fever, diphtheria, or measles are reported annually.

In some states, certain noncommunicable diseases must also be reported, to allow public health officials to track causes and/or treatment or to otherwise protect the public's health and safety. These diseases include cancer (to determine environmental causes); congenital metabolic disorders in newborns, such as phenylketonuria, congenital hypothyroidism, and galactosemia (to allow for prompt treatment); epilepsy and some other diseases that cause lapse of consciousness (to determine eligibility to drive a vehicle); and pesticide poisoning.

The National Childhood Vaccine Injury Act of 1986

Parents usually begin programs of vaccination against certain communicable diseases for their children when they are infants. When children reach school age, most states ask for proof of vaccination for children entering the public school system for the first time. Since a small percentage of vaccinated children suffer adverse effects from the vaccine administered, parents or guardians are informed of risks associated with each vaccine and must sign consent forms allowing health care practitioners to **administer** the vaccine (see Figure 8-4).

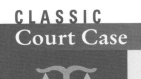
administer To instill a drug into the body of a patient.

CLASSIC
Court Case

Case Establishes Right of State to Quarantine

A California man was diagnosed with pulmonary tuberculosis, a reportable, communicable disease. A state health officer served the man with a quarantine order, and he was admitted to a hospital. The patient deserted the hospital one month later, but he still had tuberculosis. The man was subsequently arrested, tried, and convicted of violating the Health and Safety Code of California. He was sentenced to 180 days in jail, but the sentence was suspended and he was placed on a 3-year probation. The health officer again served the man with an order of isolation, and he was returned to the hospital, this time to the security section. The county public health officer then served the man with successive orders of isolation for periods of six months each.

The man asked for a writ of habeas corpus, claiming that the Health and Safety Code of California was unconstitutional, and, therefore, the health officer had no legal authority to issue consecutive certificates of quarantine and isolation.

The court held that it is the "duty of the state to protect the public from the danger of tuberculosis"; therefore, the Health and Safety Code of California was not unconstitutional. The court also held that, "The health officer may make an isolation or quarantine order whenever he shall determine in a particular case that quarantine or isolation is necessary for the protection of the public health." The petition for a writ of habeas corpus was denied.

In re Halko, 246 Cal. App. 2d 553, 54 Cal. Rptr. 661 (Cal. App. Dist. 2, Nov. 18, 1966).

Patient Name _____

Address _____

Birth Date _____

Patient's Name _____

Phone Number _____ Physician _____

Clinic Name/Address

Health care providers, health care facilities, federal or state agencies, welfare agencies, schools, or family day care facilities may have access to this information. Immunization records remain confidential, and any person who fails to protect the confidentiality of this information is guilty of a Class 1 misdemeanor.

REFUSAL TO RELEASE INFORMATION: I have read or had explained to me the immunization information system. I understand the benefits of allowing my child's immunization record to be shared with other primary care providers and public health officials. However, I choose NOT to have my child's immunization record shared with other providers.

Signature (parent or legal guardian if minor): _____ Date: _____

Reviewed with parent by (initials): _____ Date: _____

Vaccine	Date Given	Vaccine Mfg.	Vaccine Lot No.	Site Given	*Initials	Parent/Guardian Sig.@
DT DTP DTaP 1						
DT DTP DTaP 2						
DT DTP DTaP 3						
DT DTP DTaP 4						
DT DTP DTaP 5						
MMR 1						
MMR 2						
*Hep B-P 1						
Hep B-P 2						
Hep B-P 3						
*Hep B-H 1						
Hep B-H 2						
Hep B-H 3						
OPV EIPV 1						
OPV EIPV 2						
OPV EIPV 3						
OPV EIPV 4						
OPV EIPV 5						

*Initials: Initials indicate VIS were provided & vaccine administered.

Signature of Vaccine Administrator

_____

@ I have been provided a copy of, and have read or have had explained to me, information about the diseases and the vaccines listed above. I have had a chance to ask questions that were answered to my satisfaction. I believe I understand the benefits and risks of the vaccines cited and ask that the vaccine(s) listed above be given to me or the person named above (for whom I am authorized to make this request).

FIGURE 8-4 Sample Vaccination Consent Form

The **National Childhood Vaccine Injury Act** of 1986 created the **National Vaccine Injury Compensation Program (VICP)**. The VICP is a no-fault system designed to compensate those individuals, or families of individuals, who have been injured by childhood vaccines. The program serves as an alternative to suing vaccine manufacturers and providers. Vaccines covered by the original act include diphtheria, tetanus, pertussis, measles, mumps, rubella, and polio. Vaccines added to the program from 1997 to 1999 include hepatitis B, haemophilus influenza type b, varicella, rotavirus, and pneumococcal conjugate vaccines. A rule was published in 1997 which provides for the automatic addition of future vaccines recommended by the Centers for Disease Control and Prevention (CDC) for routine administration to children. Following is a complete list of vaccinations recommended by the American Academy of Pediatrics, the American Academy of Family Practice, and the Advisory Committee on Immunization Practices of the United States Centers for Disease Control and Prevention (CDC):

- Hepatitis B (HepB or HBV): Four doses as follows: the first soon after birth; the second at one month of age; the third at 4 months of age; and the fourth at 6 to 18 months of age.
- Diphtheria, Tetanus (lockjaw), and Pertussis (whooping cough) (DTP): Five doses administered at 2, 4, and 6 months; at 15 to 18 months; and at 4 to 6 years. Tetanus/Diphtheria booster at age 11. Tetanus booster at 10-year intervals thereafter.
- Haemophilus influenza type b (Hib): Administered at age 4 months and again at 2 years.
- Inactivated Polio: Four doses: at 2 months, at 4 months, at between 6 and 18 months, and at 4 to 6 years.
- Measles, mumps (Figure 8-5), and rubella (MMR): Two doses, one administered at 12 to 15 months and the second at 4 to 6 years.
- Varicella (chickenpox): Administered during any doctor's visit at or after 12 to 18 months of age.
- Pneumococcal conjugate vaccine (PCV7): To protect against pneumonia, blood infections, and meningitis (a serious infection of the lining of the brain or spinal cord) caused by the pneumococcus bacterium. Four doses: at 2, 4, and 6 months of age, and at 12 to 15 months. Another form of the vaccine is given to children aged 2 years and over whose immune systems are vulnerable.
- Hepatitis A: Administered to children and adolescents in selected states and regions and to certain high-risk groups.
- Influenza: Administered annually to children aged 6 to 23 months who have certain risk factors, such as asthma, heart disease, sickle cell disease, human immunodeficiency virus (HIV), and diabetes.

In 2006, the FDA licensed a vaccine for the prevention of infection with the human papilloma virus (HPV), administered via three injections over six months. Certain types of the virus can cause genital warts and other STDs in both sexes and cancer of the cervix in women. Because of the risk of cervical cancer, vaccination is recommended for females ages 9 to 26 years of age. For optimum protection, the vaccine should be given to girls before they become sexually active.

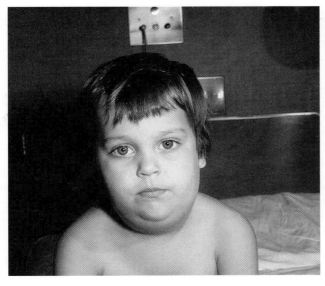

FIGURE 8-5 Swollen parotid glands in a child with mumps.

Vaccination as a Bioethics Issue

Whether or not to have their children vaccinated has become a dilemma for some parents. Since we seldom see diseases such as polio any more, and some parents have never seen measles, we may tend to fear harmful effects caused by vaccines, rather than the disease itself. For example, several years ago, a British physician, Andrew Wakefield, noticed that 6 of the 12 children he was treating for a bowel disease also had autism (a brain disorder that appears early in childhood and affects communication, imaginative play, and social interaction). All 12 children Wakefield was treating had received the measles, mumps and rubella (MMR) vaccine. Although the group he observed was small and Wakefield did not conduct a formal study, he published his speculation about a relationship between the MMR vaccine and autism in the British medical journal *The Lancet*. The media disseminated the idea of a relationship between autism and childhood vaccinations, possibly caused by a mercury preservative used in vaccines, and many parents became fearful that vaccinations could cause autism.

Later studies, including an often-cited study by Brent Taylor and colleagues at the Department of Community Child Health, University College, London, UK (published in the June 12, 1999, issue of *The Lancet*), have concluded that there is no relationship between the MMR vaccine and autism. The Centers for Disease Control and Prevention continue to maintain that there is no relationship, and the American Academy of Pediatrics continues to recommend the MMR vaccine for young children, but some parents remain fearful of vaccinations, even though the use of mercury as a vaccine preservative has been largely discontinued.

Children may be declared exempt from vaccination programs on medical grounds, such as HIV infection, organ transplants, or allergies to eggs used to prepare vaccines. Furthermore, since vaccination laws vary with states, in some states it is relatively easy for parents to opt out of vaccinating their children on nonmedical grounds. The downside of vaccination exemption is that children who are not vaccinated, or whose vaccinations are not up to date, are vulnerable to contracting serious infectious diseases that they can then pass on to others. The vaccination issue then becomes a public health concern.

The National Childhood Vaccine Injury Act initiated programs to educate the public about vaccine benefits and risks. The act requires physicians and other health care providers administering vaccines to report adverse events following vaccination and to keep permanent records on vaccines administered and health problems occurring after vaccination. Vaccine administrators are required to document in the patient's permanent medical record:

- The date the vaccine was administered.
- The vaccine manufacturer.
- The vaccine lot number.
- The name, address, and title of the health care provider who administered the vaccine.

The Vaccine Adverse Events Reporting System (VAERS), operated by the Food and Drug Administration and the Centers for Disease Control and Prevention, should be notified of any adverse event by the filing of a VAERS reporting form. Health care providers must report the following events:

- Any event listed in the Vaccine Injury Table, available at the Health Resources and Services Administration Web site and from the Health Resources and Services Administration Bureau of Health Professions, 5600 Fishers Lane, Rockville, Maryland 20857.

- Any contraindicating event listed in the manufacturer's package insert.

Reportable Injuries

In all states, physicians must immediately report to law enforcement officials medical treatment of patients whose injuries resulted from certain acts of violence, such as assault, rape, or domestic violence, so that authorities can investigate the incident. (In most states, spousal abuse is reportable only if the patient says his or her injuries are due to spousal abuse.) Reportable acts of domestic violence include child abuse, spousal abuse, and elder abuse.

Child Abuse

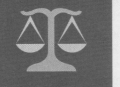

Child Abuse Prevention and Treatment Act A federal law passed in 1974 requiring physicians to report cases of child abuse and to try to prevent future cases.

To help prevent violence against children, in 1974 Congress passed the **Child Abuse Prevention and Treatment Act,** mandating the reporting of cases of child abuse. All states have enacted legislation making child abuse a crime and requiring that teachers, physicians, and other licensed health care practitioners report child abuse and neglect. The report must immediately be made to the proper authorities—either in person or by telephone—and a written report is generally required within a specified time frame, such as 72 hours. Any individual reporting suspected child abuse is granted absolute immunity from criminal and civil liability resulting from the reported incident. Depending upon state law, failure to report suspected cases of child abuse may be a misdemeanor.

Spousal Abuse

Unlike cases of child abuse, most state laws do not specifically require a physician to report spousal abuse, unless a spouse states that his or her injuries were the result of spousal abuse. Legal remedies available to battered spouses vary from state to state, but all states have laws protecting victims of domestic abuse. Advocacy programs can explain legal options to

---

Court Case

Court Says Military Must Get Consent for Anthrax Vaccinations

After the terrorist attacks on the World Trade Center towers and the Pentagon on September 11, 2001, and the anthrax scare immediately thereafter, when eight people died from anthrax distributed anonymously through the mail, Americans' fears of chemical and biological attacks increased. As preparations were underway to attack Iraq, military enrollees and some civilian employees of the military were ordered to undergo vaccinations against anthrax. Because the vaccine in use at that time was considered experimental, and because many people feared side effects of the vaccine, some active duty personnel, other National Guardsmen, and some civilian contract employees of the Department of Defense (DoD) filed suit against Donald Rumsfeld, Secretary of Defense; Tommy Thompson, Secretary of Health and Human Services; and Mark McClellan, Commissioner of the Food and Drug Administration. Plaintiffs alleged that the vaccine was experimental and unlicensed for use and that the Anthrax Vaccine Immunization Program violated federal law and an executive order. They asked the court to issue a preliminary injunction to stop the DoD from inoculating them without their informed consent.

The court granted the plaintiffs' motion for a preliminary injunction, holding that the vaccine was an "investigational" drug and unapproved for use against inhalation anthrax. The court decision read, "In the absence of a presidential waiver, defendants are enjoined from inoculating service members without their consent." After this decision, members of the military and others could be vaccinated against anthrax only with their informed consent.

John Doe #1 et al., Plaintiffs v. Donald H. Rumsfeld, et al. Defendants, F. Supp.2d, 2003 West Law 22994225, decided by United States District Court for the District of Columbia, December 22, 2003.

victims and can help them cope with the legal system. Courts may issue protective, or restraining, orders, or they may issue injunctions that direct the batterer to stop abusing the victim. In some states, police may be required to arrest batterers under certain conditions. Depending on laws within the jurisdiction and the type of offense committed, a batterer may be criminally prosecuted for assault, battery, harassment, intimidation, rape, or attempted murder.

Elder Abuse

Amendments to the Older Americans Act A 1987 federal act that defines elder abuse, neglect, and exploitation, but does not deal with enforcement.

The Older Americans Act was signed into law by President Lyndon B. Johnson in 1965. The act created the Administration on Aging and outlined 10 objectives aimed at preserving the rights and dignity of older citizens. The 1987 **Amendments to the Older Americans Act** defines elder abuse, neglect, and exploitation, but does not deal with enforcement. The year 2000 *Amendments to the Older Americans Act* includes a 5-year reauthorization for funding, maintains the original 10 objectives, and adds the National Family Caregiver Support Program for addressing the needs of caregivers to the elderly.

All 50 states and the District of Columbia have enacted legislation instituting reporting systems to identify domestic and institutional elder abuse, neglect, and exploitation. In most states, reporting suspected elder abuse is mandatory for certain professionals, including physicians. (If not mandated by state law, reporting may be voluntary.) Physical, sexual, and financial abuses of the elderly are considered crimes in all states. Some forms of emotional abuse and types of neglect may be considered crimes in some states.

In addition to laws regarding child, spousal, and elder abuse, some states have passed laws protecting vulnerable adults, such as mentally ill and mentally challenged individuals. Some states also have statutes dealing with the prevention of fetal abuse stemming from sniffing paint and other chemicals, taking drugs, or drinking alcohol while pregnant.

The Unborn Victims of Violence Act

Unborn Victims of Violence Act Also called Laci and Conner's Act, a 2004 federal law that provides for the prosecution of anyone who causes injury to or the death of a fetus in utero.

In April 2004, Congress passed and President George W. Bush signed into law the **Unborn Victims of Violence Act,** also called "Laci and Conner's Act," after the December 24, 2002 murder of Laci Peterson, a pregnant woman, and her nine-month-old fetus, Conner. The act provides for the prosecution of anyone who causes injury to or the death of a fetus in utero. It also states that "the punishment for that separate offense is the same as the punishment provided under Federal law for that conduct had that injury or death occurred to the unborn child's mother." Before this federal law was passed, in most states a person accused of injuring or killing a pregnant woman was tried for offenses against the mother, but not for injuring or killing her fetus as a separate individual.

Identifying Abuse

Health care practitioners should be alert for signs of physical abuse, for purposes both of mandatory reporting and of possible intervention on behalf of the victim. It is imperative, however, that medical personnel not jump to conclusions and make unsubstantiated abuse reports.

Physical signs of abuse may include but are not limited to these:

▌ Unexplained fractures.

▌ Repeated injuries, especially those in unusual places or those shaped like objects such as electrical cords, hairbrushes, belt buckles, and so forth.

- Burns with unusual shapes (such as a circle, that may have been caused by a cigarette, or the mark of an object such as an iron).
- Friction burns apparently caused by a rope or cord.
- Bite marks.
- Signs of malnutrition or dehydration, such as extreme weight loss, dry skin, or red-rimmed, sunken eyes.
- Torn or bloody underwear.
- Pain or bruising in the genital area.
- Unexplained venereal disease or other genital infections.

Behavioral signs of abuse may include the following:

- Illogical or unreasonable explanations for injuries.
- Frequently changing physicians and/or missing medical appointments.
- Attempts to hide injuries with heavy makeup or sunglasses.
- Frequent anxiety, depression, or loss of emotional control.
- Changes in appetite; problems at school or on the job.

Observation of individuals who accompany the patient may also identify a potential abuser. One might suspect abuse, for example, if, in the presence of additional evidence, an alleged victim of abuse is accompanied by someone who smells of alcohol, exhibits pensive or obsessive behavior, seems unusually or inappropriately emotional, or shows aggressive or otherwise suspicious body language toward the patient.

When a health care practitioner suspects abuse, care and tact must be used in eliciting information from patients. Direct, open-ended questions such as, "Has someone harmed you?" may encourage a patient to relate what has caused his or her injuries.

Health care practitioners should emphasize to the patient that information offered will be kept confidential, as required by physician-patient confidentiality, except in those cases in which the law mandates reporting abuse. Reporting requirements for abuse should be explained during the patient's first visit. Some sources recommend having patients sign a statement indicating that they understand the reporting requirements and agree with them.

Forcing the issue to encourage an adult to leave a batterer is not always the immediate answer. Similarly, providing hotline numbers, information on safe houses, or handouts about abuse may not be helpful if the batterer is waiting in the reception area for the patient or may later find the material and be further enraged. Instead, many medical facilities have bulletins posted in restrooms, telling patients where to call for help. If tear strips with the telephone number are provided, a victim can tear off the small, easily concealed strip for future reference.

Drug Regulations

The federal government has jurisdiction over the manufacture and distribution of drugs in the United States. The **Food and Drug Administration (FDA),** an agency within the Department of Health and Human Services, tests and approves drugs before releasing them for public use. This agency also oversees drug quality and standardization.

Both federal and state governments regulate the sale and use of certain drugs. At the federal level, the **Drug Enforcement Administration (DEA),** a branch of the Department of Justice, regulates the sale and use of drugs

Food and Drug Administration (FDA) A federal agency within the Department of Health and Human Services that oversees drug quality and standardization and must approve drugs before they are released for public use.

Drug Enforcement Agency (DEA) A branch of the U.S. Department of Justice that regulates the sale and use of drugs.

Controlled Substances Act
The federal law giving authority to the Drug Enforcement Agency to regulate the sale and use of drugs.

prescribe To issue a medical prescription for a patient.

dispense To deliver controlled substances in some type of bottle, box, or other container to a patient.

by the authority granted in the Comprehensive Drug Abuse Prevention and Control Act of 1970, commonly called the **Controlled Substances Act.**

General regulations mandated by the Controlled Substances Act require physicians who purchase, **prescribe, dispense,** administer, or in any way handle controlled drugs to follow these procedures:

- Register with the Drug Enforcement Administration through a division office. (A list of division offices is available online at the DEA Web site.) The physician will receive a registration number that must appear on all prescriptions for controlled substances and must be renewed periodically for a specified fee. Each DEA number is issued for a specific physician in a specific location. That location is the only one at which the physician may store controlled substances, including salespeople's samples. If a physician practices in more than one state, he or she needs a DEA number for each state. The physician must notify the appropriate state authorities and the DEA whenever he or she moves from a registered location.

- Keep records concerning the administering or dispensing of a controlled drug on file for two years. Such records must include the patient's full name and address, the reason for use of the drug, the date of the order, the name of the drug, the dosage form and quantity of the drug, and whether the drug was administered or dispensed.

- Note on a patient's chart when controlled substances are administered or dispensed.

- Make a written inventory of drug supplies every two years, and keep such records an additional two years.

- Keep drugs in a locked cabinet or safe, and report any thefts immediately to the nearest DEA office and the local police.

The Controlled Substances Act

The Controlled Substances Act is a federal law that regulates drugs under five schedules, based upon their potential for abuse and their medical usefulness. If a drug has no potential for abuse, it is not listed as controlled. The five schedules for controlled substances are as follows.

CHECK YOUR PROGRESS

9. What two federal agencies control the manufacture and standardization of drugs and their sale and use?

_____

_____

Use these three terms correctly in the sentences that follow: prescribe, dispense, administer.

10. Dr. Wellness will _____ the drug to his patient, Mrs. Doe, when he starts an intravenous injection.

11. Under the law, medical assistants may not _____ drugs for patients but may _____ or _____ them under a physician's direct order.

12. When a pharmacist fills a patient's prescription, he or she then _____ the drug to the patient.

Schedule I: Potential for abuse is high and there is no currently accepted medical use of the drug or substance in the United States. Schedule I substances have been used strictly for research. Potential for abuse is determined by the following criteria:

1. There is evidence that individuals are taking the drug or other substance in amounts sufficient to create a hazard to their health or to the safety of other individuals or to the community; or
2. There is significant diversion of the drug or other substance from legitimate drug channels; or
3. Individuals are taking the drug or other substance on their own initiative rather than on the basis of medical advice from a practitioner licensed by law to administer such drugs; or
4. The drug is a new drug so related in its action to a drug or other substance already listed as having a potential for abuse to make it likely that the drug will have the same potential for abuse as such drugs. Of course, evidence of actual abuse of a substance is indicative that a drug has a potential for abuse.

Examples of Schedule I drugs include heroin, lysergic acid diethylamide (LSD), marijuana, and methaqualone

Schedule II: Potential for abuse of these narcotic drugs is high, but there are currently accepted medical uses for the drug or substance in the United States, but often with severe restrictions. Severe psychological and physical dependence is possible. Examples of Schedule II drugs include morphine, phencyclidine (PCP), cocaine, methadone, and methamphetamine.

A subdivision of Schedule II, called IIn, refers to nonnarcotic drugs with a high potential for abuse. Examples of such drugs include Dexedrine®, Desoxyn®, Preludin®, Ritalin®, and pentobarbital.

Schedule III: The drug or other substance has less potential for abuse than the drugs or other substances in Schedules I and II, and has currently accepted medical uses in the United States.

Abuse of the drug or other substance may lead to moderate or low physical dependence or high psychological dependence. Examples of Schedule III substances include anabolic steroids, codeine and hydrocodone with aspirin or Tylenol®, and some barbiturates.

Schedule IIIn refers to nonnarcotic central nervous system depressants. These drugs include glutethhimide, methyprylong, and barbiturates not listed in other schedules, as well as anorectant agents (suppositories) not listed elsewhere.

Schedule IV: The drug or other substance has a low potential for abuse relative to the drugs or other substances in Schedule III, and has currently accepted medical uses in the United States.

Abuse of the drug may lead to limited physical dependence or psychological dependence Examples of Schedule IV drugs include Darvon®, Talwin®, Equanil®, Valium®, and Xanax®.

Schedule V: The drug or other substance has a low potential for abuse relative to the drugs or other substances in Schedule IV, and has a currently accepted medical use in the United States.

Abuse of the drug or other substances may lead to limited physical dependence or psychological dependence relative to the drugs or other substances in Schedule IV. Cough medicines with codeine are examples of Schedule V drugs, as well as antitussive, antidiarrheal, and analgesic drugs.

Drugs included in Schedule II and IIn require a properly executed, manually signed prescription. No refills are permitted on these prescriptions.

All other scheduled drugs (Schedules III through V) may be prescribed on written or oral orders, and refills are generally permitted with certain limitations.

Whenever prescriptions are written for controlled substances, a copy should be filed with the patient's record. When a physician discontinues practice, he or she must return the registration certificate and any unused order forms (preferably marked "void") to the DEA. When it is necessary to dispose of controlled drugs, the physician or employee charged with disposal should contact the nearest field office of the DEA and the responsible state agency for disposal information.

State laws governing controlled substances may be as strict as or stricter than federal laws. Physicians may be required to register with the appropriate state agency as well as the DEA, and must follow all state and federal requirements in prescribing, dispensing, and administering controlled substances. Whenever state and federal regulations differ, the more stringent regulation must be followed. For example, if federal law requires that records be held for two years and state law specifies five years, the state law takes precedence.

Since violation of a law dealing with a state-controlled and/or federally controlled substance is a criminal offense and can result in fines, jail sentences, and loss of license to practice medicine, physicians, other health care practitioners, and medical office employees should be familiar with all state and federal narcotics laws.

The role of the medical assistant concerning compliance with DEA regulations is to remind the physician of license renewal dates, to keep accurate records for scheduled drugs, to maintain an accurate inventory and inventory records, and to ensure the security of scheduled drugs kept in the office. This is accomplished by

- Checking to be sure that all controlled substances are kept in a locked cabinet or safe.
- Reminding the physician to keep his or her "black bag" in a safe place.
- Keeping all prescription blanks, especially those used for narcotics, under lock and key.
- Ordering prescription blanks that are serially numbered or otherwise printed to help detect alterations and theft.
- Reporting to the physician any behavior by patients that would suggest an attempt to secure addictive drugs.
- Checking patients' records to verify all prescriptions that may be questioned by a pharmacist.

Ethics Issues

Physicians' Public Duties and Responsibilities

Two principles are often at odds when health care practitioners must deal with public health issues: the autonomy of each patient and beneficence. *Autonomy* refers to the individual's right to make his or her own decisions. *Beneficence* refers to the moral obligation to act in ways that promote the health and welfare of others. As stated in Harman's *Ethical Challenges in the Management of Health Information*, "Beneficence and the closely allied principle of nonmaleficence ['first do no harm'] are among the primary justifications supporting public policies that interfere with the autonomy of individuals."

ETHICS ISSUE 1: In 2007, Andrew Speaker, a personal injury attorney, flew via public transportation from Atlanta, Georgia, to Paris, to get married. He returned to the United States on a flight from Prague, Czech Republic, to Montreal, Canada, then crossed the border into the United States. Speaker was thought to have an extremely contagious and untreatable form of multidrug-resistant tuberculosis, diagnosed before he left the United States. Upon Speaker's return to the United States, the Centers for Disease Control used a provision of the Public Health Service Act to involuntarily hospitalize and isolate him. Speaker's diagnosis was later corrected: He had a treatable form of drug-resistant tuberculosis. At least nine individuals who were passengers on the flights Speaker took later filed civil suits against him for knowingly exposing them to the disease. Speaker was the first person to be quarantined by the CDC since 1963.

DISCUSSION QUESTIONS

1. In your opinion, did the CDC act within its ethical and legal authority in involuntarily quarantining Mr. Speaker? Explain your answer.

_____

_____

2. In your opinion, should Mr. Speaker's concern for others have superseded his plans to fly to Europe to get married? Explain your answer.

_____

_____

3. Thinking as a health care practitioner, in your opinion should Mr. Speaker's autonomy as a person have taken precedence over the CDC's desire to enforce public health law? Explain your answer.

_____

_____

ETHICS ISSUE 2: A minor is admitted to the hospital as a result of a sexual assault, which she says was perpetrated by an uncle who lives in the household. The minor's mother indicates that the uncle is under treatment for gonorrhea with a local physician. A caseworker with Children's Protective Services is called and she has asked the local physician named for permission to review the uncle's medical records.

DISCUSSION QUESTIONS

1. Should the caseworker be allowed to review the uncle's medical records? Why or why not?

_____

_____

2. Does the minor's best interest supersede the alleged offender's right to privacy? Explain your answer.

_____

_____

3. What values are involved in Ethical Issue 2?

_____

_____

4. What is the first duty of health care practitioners caring for the minor in Ethical Issue 2?

_____

_____

ETHICS ISSUE 3: Laws that require the reporting of cases of suspected abuse of children and elderly persons often create a dilemma for health care practitioners. The parties involved, both the suspected offenders and the victims, will often plead that the matter be kept confidential and not be disclosed or reported for investigation by public authorities.

DISCUSSION QUESTIONS

1. Assume you are a member of the health care team that has repeatedly treated a woman for injuries that appear to have been inflicted by another. How might you phrase an opening question in order to learn whether or not she is the victim of abuse?

_____

_____

2. If the woman protests that she is simply "accident prone," how might you phrase your response? Would you drop the matter at this point or continue to question the woman?

_____

_____

3. What could you do to protect the woman if she does not admit abuse, but you are reasonably sure that she is being abused?

_____

_____

 Go to www.mhhe.com/judson5e to practice your case review skills. Then read on for more information.

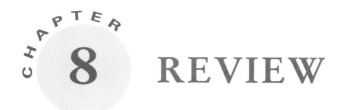

Applying Knowledge

Answer the following questions in the spaces provided.

1. Four vital statistics that the government collects are _____, _____
_____, _____, and _____.
Of these, the physician should be concerned with documenting _____ and
_____ .

2. List eight federal recommendations to be followed in completing birth and death certificates.

3. After a person is pronounced dead, the attending physician must complete the medical portion of the
death certificate. What information does this generally include?

_____

_____

_____

_____

4. Explain the difference between a coroner and a medical examiner.

_____

_____

_____

5. List four situations in which a death certificate must be completed by a medical examiner or coroner.

_____

_____

_____

_____

6. What is the purpose of a coroner's inquest?

_____

_____

_____

7. List five physical and five behavioral clues that may indicate that a patient has been a victim of abuse.

_____   _____

_____   _____

_____   _____

_____   _____

_____   _____

8. Give five examples of noncommunicable diseases for which reporting may be mandated in certain states.

_____

_____

_____

9. The _____ is responsible for testing and approving drugs for public use, while the _____ regulates the sale and use of drugs.

10. There are _____ schedules of controlled drugs. Schedule _____ drugs are the most addicting and have the most stringent controls. Schedule _____ drugs have the least potential for abuse of all the schedules for controlled substances.

11. Does your community have a coroner or a medical examiner? Is this an elective or an appointive office? Where will you find this information?

_____

_____

12. What are the reportable diseases mandated by law in your state? Where did you find this information?

_____

_____

_____

13. What regulations apply in your state to the reporting of HIV and AIDS cases? Is identity of the patient protected by law? Where did you find this information?

_____

_____

14. Are public health statutes in all states the same? Why or why not?

_____

_____

15. Who may legally file birth certificates for newborns?

_____

_____

16. Should a physician report to the state a greater than normal influenza outbreak in his or her community? Why or why not?

_____

_____

17. Which physicians must register with the federal Drug Enforcement Administration?

_____

_____

18. Referring to the drug schedules, name the category/categories of drugs for which prescriptions may not be renewed.

_____

19. If physicians may not prescribe Schedule I drugs for patients, what is the value of those drugs?

_____

20. Which federal agency tests and approves drugs before releasing them for public use and oversees drug quality and standardization?

_____

21. In the medical office, who is generally responsible for keeping accurate records concerning prescribing and dispensing drugs?

_____

Match each of the following descriptions with the correct term by writing the appropriate letter in the space provided.

_____ 22. Tests and approves drugs for public use.

_____ 23. Also known as the Comprehensive Drug Abuse Prevention and Control Act of 1970.

_____ 24. As a branch of the Department of Justice, regulates the sale and use of drugs.

_____ 25. Require reports of communicable diseases and certain injuries, as mandated by state laws.

_____ 26. Mandates reporting of child abuse.

_____ 27. Created a no-fault compensation program for citizens injured or killed by vaccines, as an alternative to suing vaccine manufacturers and providers.

_____ 28. The federal law that makes killing or injuring a fetus a crime separate from killing or injuring the pregnant mother.

a. Unborn Victims of Violence Act

b. Drug Enforcement Administration (DEA)

c. National Childhood Vaccine Injury Act of 1986

d. Food and Drug Administration (FDA)

e. Amendments to the Older Americans Act

f. Controlled Substances Act

g. Child Abuse Prevention and Treatment Act of 1974

h. public health statutes

Case Study

Use your critical-thinking skills to answer the questions that follow the case study.
Barbara, a medical assistant, noticed that her aunt, who suffered chronic pain from a neck injury, carried two bottles of Percodan in her purse. "Two doctors write prescriptions for me," Barbara's aunt confided, "but neither knows about the other. That's the only way I can get enough medication to control my pain."

29. In Barbara's place, would you report your aunt's deception to the physicians named on her prescriptions? Explain your answer

_____

_____

30. What would you tell your aunt?

_____

_____

31. How can physicians guard against such abuses by patients?

_____

_____

One of a physician's patients, a well-respected citizen in a small community, saw the doctor with a complaint of blood in his urine (hematuria). The physician asked the patient if he'd had any new sexual partners recently, and the patient admitted that he had. The physician explained to the patient that his urine specimen had been positive for the STD chlamydia. The physician urged the patient to discuss his medical condition with his wife, who was also the physician's patient, but the man seemed reluctant.

32. If the patient refuses to confide in the wife, what should the physician do?

_____

_____

33. What are the issues in this case?

_____

_____

_____

34. If the physician is undecided about a course of action, where might he or she seek guidance?

_____

_____

_____

Internet Activities

Complete the activities and answer the questions that follow.

35. Visit the Web site for federal statistics at www.fedstats.gov. For what year are the most recent statistics available? What is the birth rate for the United States for that year?

_____

_____

36. What was the death rate? What were the three leading causes of death in the United States?

_____

_____

37. Visit the Web site for the National Vaccine Injury Compensation Program (VICP) at www.hrsa.gov/vaccinecompensation/. Who is eligible to file a claim? Is the vaccine for the human papilloma virus covered under the VICP?

_____

_____

_____

38. Find the Web site for your state's Department of Health. Which communicable diseases must be reported in your state? To whom must you report communicable diseases? What is the process involved? At this Web site, can you tell which diseases are prevalent in your state? How?

_____

_____

_____

_____

Workplace Legalities

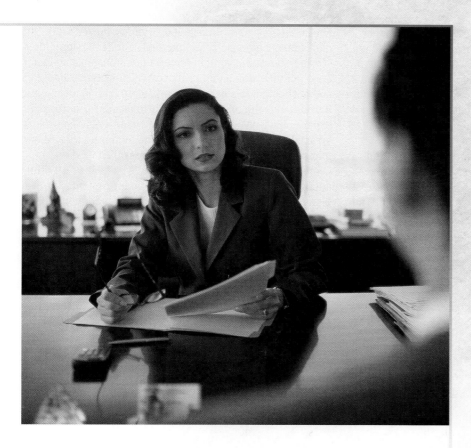

Learning Outcomes

After studying this chapter, you should be able to:

1. Identify how the workplace is affected by federal laws regarding hiring and firing, discrimination, and other workplace regulations.

2. Identify four areas for which standards are mandated by the Occupational Safety and Health Administration (OSHA) for work done in a clinical setting.

3. Discuss the role of health care practitioners in following OSHA standards for infection control in the medical office.

4. Define the role of the Clinical Laboratory Improvement Act of 1988 (CLIA) in quality laboratory testing.

5. State the purpose of workers' compensation laws and unemployment insurance.

6. Determine the appropriate legal process for hiring employees and maintaining the required paperwork while the person is employed.

Key Terms

affirmative action

Chemical Hygiene Plan

Clinical Laboratory Improvement Act (CLIA)

discrimination

employment-at-will

General Duty Clause

Hazard Communication Standard (HCS)

just cause

Medical Waste Tracking Act

Occupational Exposure to Bloodborne Pathogen Standard

Occupational Safety and Health Administration (OSHA)

public policy

right-to-know laws

surety bond

workers' compensation

wrongful discharge

Voice of Experience
Lab Supervisor Emphasizes Importance of Documentation

As the supervisor of a state medical laboratory in the Midwest, Marie has been responsible for hiring employees to fill 11 positions. Since Marie's lab does microbiology tests for the state, including bacteriology, parasitology, serology, virology, and immunology, she is keenly aware of the importance of accuracy in test results.

"We have a litigious public," Marie remarks, "and we can be sued if a laboratory test is not right. We are dependent on machines for test results, but we [the lab director and lab supervisor] are responsible for the errors of laboratory employees. The federal guidelines for a technical supervisor say that that person is responsible for every test result signed out."

Once, Marie recalls, a false positive test result led to potential damage to a patient. "She was pregnant and was given a certain medication as the result of a reported test result of 'positive' for a sexually transmitted disease. The result reported should have been 'negative.' The drug was not contraindicated for a pregnant woman, but she should

not have had to take it. Plus, she had the emotional distress of receiving a false positive STD test result." The error was reported to the woman's treating physician, and Marie was never informed of any ill effects.

The laboratory employee who committed the error had a two-year work history of certain behavior problems. The employee had often failed to show up for work and had been counseled for alcohol and drug problems. Marie had carefully documented the employee's behavior. She had also documented that she consistently checked and rechecked this person's work, often finding errors, and had met with the employee weekly to discuss progress and expectations. When the STD test result was reported in error, she felt the employee could no longer be trusted and that she had ample grounds for dismissal.

The employee was fired. Because of Marie's careful documentation, the employee had scant grounds for protesting the action and did not. "Good documentation is essential for those responsible for hiring and firing employees," Marie reiterates.

HOW THE LAW AFFECTS THE WORKPLACE

This chapter provides an overview of workplace law, but it does not cover every employment statute and situation. For more detail, consult U.S. and state codes and/or an attorney specializing in employment law.

Many federal and state laws govern the workplace. Federal laws may apply only to those businesses with a certain number of employees (such as 15, 20, or 50) who work for a minimum number of weeks during the year. State laws may apply to those areas not covered by federal law, or they may extend or overlap existing federal law.

Traditionally, employment followed the principle of **employment-at-will.** This meant that employees could be refused employment and could be disciplined or fired for any or no reason. In fact, either the employer or the employee could end the employment at any time. Now employment-at-will is affected not only by federal and state statutes, executive orders, and case law, but also by contracts between a worker and an employer, collective bargaining agreements between companies and unions, and civil service rules for government workers.

employment-at-will A concept of employment whereby either the employer or the employee can end the employment at any time, for any reason.

wrongful discharge A concept established by precedent that says an employer risks litigation if he or she does not have just cause for firing an employee.

just cause An employer's legal reason for firing an employee.

Hiring and Firing

Employees generally cannot sue their employers simply because they have been fired, but an employer cannot fire an employee for an illegal reason. When no law exists that prohibits a specific reason for firing an employee, the discharged worker may have cause for litigation under precedent for **wrongful discharge.** Generally, in such cases the employer must have documentation that shows **just cause** (a legal reason) for dismissing the

public policy The common law concept of wrongful discharge when an employee has acted for the "common good."

discrimination Prejudiced or prejudicial outlook, action, or treatment.

employee. Promises made to the employee orally, in a written contract, or in a company handbook may be used as evidence should a suit involving wrongful discharge be filed against his or her employer.

State courts vary in their willingness to accept the common law concept of wrongful discharge, but most recognize **public policy** or "common good" reasons for lawsuits brought by fired employees, such as refusing to commit an illegal act, whistleblowing, performing a legal duty, or exercising a private right.

Discrimination

Discrimination in the workplace, or treating employees differently in hiring, firing, work assignments, or other aspects of employment because of personal traits or practices, is illegal. Federal laws prohibit employers from firing or otherwise discriminating against employees for any of the following reasons:

- Belonging to a particular race or religion, being one sex or another, or having a particular age or disability.
- Joining a union or engaging in political activity.
- Preventing the collection of retirement benefits.
- Reporting company safety violations.
- Exercising the right to free speech.
- Refusing to take drug or lie detector tests (with some exceptions).

Most states have passed laws that add to the federal list of prohibited discriminatory employment practices. Title VII of the Civil Rights Act makes sexual discrimination illegal, and sexual harassment is considered a form of sexual discrimination. In 1980 the Equal Employment Opportunity Commission (EEOC) defined sexual harassment as follows:

Unwelcome sexual advances, requests for sexual favors, and other verbal or physical conduct of a sexual nature constitute sexual harassment when (1) submission to such conduct is made either explicitly or implicitly a term or condition of an individual's employment; (2) submission to or rejection of such conduct by an individual is used as a basis for employment decisions affecting such individual; or (3) such conduct has the purpose or effect of unreasonably interfering with an individual's work performance or creating an intimidating, hostile, or offensive working environment.

Parts 1 and 2 of this definition prohibit what is known as *quid pro quo* (from Latin, meaning "something for something") sexual harassment. Part 3 prohibits conduct that interferes with an employee's work performance or creates a hostile working environment.

Court decisions have affirmed that sexual harassment of employees, either male or female, is cause for legal action. Employers may be found liable even though an employee actually committed the offense. For example, if the offending employee is a supervisor, the employer is usually automatically held liable. If a nonsupervisory employee sexually harasses another worker, the employer is held liable only if he or she knew or should have known about the offense and did nothing to stop it. See Figure 9-1.

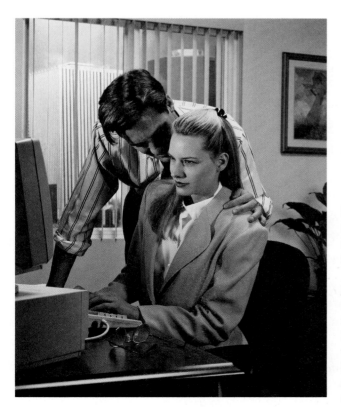

FIGURE 9-1 Sexual harassment in the workplace.

CHECK YOUR PROGRESS

1. Define *employment-at-will*.

_____

_____

2. Define *wrongful discharge*.

_____

_____

3. Define *just cause*.

_____

_____

4. Define *public policy*.

_____

_____

CLASSIC
Court Case

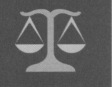

Fired Employee Sues and Wins

A discharged radiology technologist brought suit for breach of employment contract. Her complaint alleged that termination of employment-at-will was in retaliation for her refusal to perform catheterizations which were illegal for her to perform since she was not trained to do the procedure.

After the technician's dismissal, the New Jersey Board of Medical Examiners concluded that such an act performed by her would violate the state's medical practice act. The New Jersey Board of Nursing issued a cease-and-desist order to the defendants to stop ordering unqualified personnel to perform catheterizations.

The court ruled that public policy was an issue, since the public has a "foremost interest" in the administration of medical care. The technician won her suit.

O'Sullivan v. Mallon, 390 Atl.2d 149 (1987).

CHECK YOUR PROGRESS

5. Who is liable if sexual harassment in the workplace occurs?

_____

6. Sexual harassment may involve any of the following types of interaction:

_____

7. A federal law called _____ prohibits sexual harassment in the workplace.

8. The demand for sexual favors in exchange for employment benefits is called _____.

9. Sexual harassment can include unwanted physical advances, explicit sexual propositions, and _____.

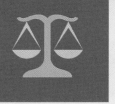

CLASSIC
Court Case

A History-Making Sexual Harassment Case

A bank employee worked for Meritor Savings for more than four years. During that time she claimed that her supervisor continued to make sexual propositions. She finally complied, fearing for her job. She also claimed that her supervisor publicly fondled her and forcibly raped her. When she was fired after an indefinite sick leave, she sued for sexual harassment.

A trial court ruled for the bank, finding no *quid pro quo* discrimination, but the employee appealed, and the appellate court found in her favor. The bank appealed, but the U.S. Supreme Court upheld the appellate court's decision in the plaintiff's favor. In a precedent-setting pronouncement, the Court said, "A plaintiff may establish a violation of Title VII by proving that discrimination based on sex has created a hostile or abusive work environment. . . ." The Court remanded the case to the district court for further proceedings.

Meritor Savings Bank, FSB v. Vinson, 106 S.C. 2399, 91 L.Ed.2d 49, 447 U.S. 57 (U.S. Sup. Ct., 1986).

LABOR AND EMPLOYMENT LAWS

The following federal laws cover discrimination in hiring and firing, workers' wages and hours, worker safety, and other workplace issues.

Employment Discrimination Laws

These laws address discrimination in hiring and firing.

Wagner Act of 1935. This act makes it illegal to discriminate in hiring or firing because of union membership or organizational activities.

Title VII of the Civil Rights Act of 1964. This act applies to businesses with 15 or more employees working at least 20 weeks of the year. The law prevents employers from discriminating in hiring or firing on the basis of race, color, religion, sex, or national origin. Some states have laws that also prohibit discrimination based on marital status, parenthood, mental health, mental retardation, sexual orientation, personal appearance, or political affiliation.

affirmative action Programs that use goals and quotas to provide preferential treatment for minority persons determined to have been underutilized in the past.

Title VII also specifically prevents federal judges from using **affirmative action** plans—programs intended to remedy the effects of past discrimination—just to correct an imbalance between the percentage of minority persons working for a specific employer and the percentage of qualified minority members in the workplace. Federal judges can order affirmative action plans only when they decide an employer has intentionally discriminated against a minority group.

Title VII created the U.S. Equal Employment Opportunity Commission (EEOC). The EEOC enforces Title VII provisions, the Age Discrimination in Employment Act, the Equal Pay Act, and Section 501 of the Rehabilitation Act. EEOC field offices handle charges or complaints of employment discrimination.

Age Discrimination in Employment Act (ADEA) of 1967. This act applies to businesses with 20 or more employees working at least 20 weeks of the year. It prohibits discrimination in hiring or firing based on age, for persons aged 40 or older.

Rehabilitation Act of 1973. This act applies to employers with federal contracts of $2,500 or more. It prohibits discrimination in employment practices based on physical disabilities or mental health. It also requires federal contractors to implement affirmative action plans in hiring and promoting disabled employees.

1976 Pregnancy Discrimination Act. This is an amendment to Title VII of the Civil Rights Act that makes it illegal to fire an employee based on pregnancy, childbirth, or related medical conditions.

Titles I and V of the Americans With Disabilities Act of 1990. This act applies to all employers with 15 or more employees working at least 20 weeks during the year. Titles I and III of the act ban discrimination against disabled persons in the workplace, mandate equal access for the disabled to certain public facilities, and require all commercial firms to make existing facilities and grounds more accessible to the disabled.

The Civil Rights Act of 1991. This act, among other things, provides monetary damages in cases of intentional employment discrimination.

Wage and Hour Laws

The following laws address wages and hours of work.

1935 Social Security Act. Funded by the Federal Insurance Contribution Act (FICA), the act now encompasses "old age" and survivors insurance (OASI), public disability insurance, unemployment insurance (through the Federal Unemployment Tax Act), and the hospital insurance program (Medicare).

1938 Fair Labor Standards Act. This act prohibits child labor and the firing of employees for exercising their rights under the act's wage and hour standards. It also provides for overtime pay and a minimum wage. New FairPay regulations under the act went into effect on August 23, 2004. The new rules guarantee overtime protection to workers earning less than $23,660 annually and continue exemptions of the overtime rule for certain "learned professional employees." Some nurses may receive overtime pay, depending on how they are paid—hourly or by salary—and licensed practical nurses "and other similar health care employees" are guaranteed overtime pay under the FairPay regulations.

Equal Pay Act of 1963. As an amendment to the Fair Labor Standards Act, this act requires equal pay for men and women doing equal work.

Employee Retirement Income Security Act of 1974 (ERISA). This act regulates private pension funds and employer benefit programs. As part of its provisions, employers cannot prevent employees from collecting retirement benefits from plans covered by the act.

Workplace Safety Laws

There is one important law that addresses health and safety in the workplace.

Occupational Safety and Health Act of 1970. This act ensures the safety of workers and prohibits firing an employee for reporting workplace safety hazards or violations.

Other Terms of Employment

Labor and employment laws may also address employees' family emergencies and other family situations.

Family Leave Act of 1991. This act applies to employers with 50 or more employees. It mandates allowing employees to take unpaid leave time for maternity, for adoption, or for caring for ill family members.

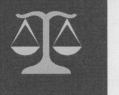

Court Case

Criminal Background Check Leads to Loss of License for Home Health Care Provider

A state agency licensed a woman to provide home health care services to Medicaid recipients. Seven years later, the woman applied to renew her license and was asked to undergo a criminal background check. Although the woman did not admit to committing a major crime, the state agency's background check found within its own records that as a juvenile the woman had admitted to and been convicted of murder. Her license was suspended, and the woman sued the agency for invasion of privacy.

A court granted the state agency summary judgment, holding that the woman had failed to prove invasion of privacy. The woman appealed, but a higher court upheld the judgment, and the woman's license remained suspended.

Jane Doe v. State of Idaho, Dept. of Health and Welfare, 72 P.3d 897, 2003 Ida. LEXIS 107.

CHECK YOUR PROGRESS

10. What federal act makes it illegal for employers to discriminate against employees or potential employees on the basis of race, color, religion, sex, or national origin?

_____

_____

11. Which act protects the rights of pregnant employees?

_____

_____

12. Social Security benefits are disbursed under the authority of which act?

_____

_____

EMPLOYEE SAFETY AND WELFARE

Certain federal and state laws provide specifically for employee safety and welfare. Major areas covered include workplace safety, including medical hazards, job-related injuries and illnesses, and unemployment or reemployment.

Occupational Safety and Health Administration (OSHA)
Established by the Occupational Safety and Health Act of 1970, the organization that is charged with writing and enforcing compulsory standards for health and safety in the workplace.

Occupational Safety and Health Administration (OSHA)

In the 1960s job-related disabilities and injuries caused more lost workdays in U.S. companies than did strikes. As a result of increasing concern over such statistics, in 1970 Congress passed the Occupational Safety and Health Act. The act established the **Occupational Safety and Health Administration (OSHA),** charged with writing and enforcing compulsory standards for health and safety in the workplace.

Workplace Legalities   **239**

The act covers all employers and employees, with few exceptions. Standards cover four areas of employment—general industry, maritime, construction, and agriculture—and include regulations for the physical workplace, machinery and equipment, materials, power sources, processing, protective clothing, first aid, and workplace administration.

All employers must know those standards that apply to their business. The *Federal Register,* a U.S. government publication that contains all administrative laws, is the primary source of information for OSHA standards.

Under the authority of the U.S. Secretary of Labor, Occupational Safety and Health Administration inspectors may conduct workplace inspections unannounced; issue citations to employers for violations of the act; and, in some cases, levy fines. All 111 million workplaces covered by the Occupation Safety and Health Act cannot be inspected at one time; therefore priorities have been established for inspecting the worst situations first. The priority of workplace inspectionsis as follows:

1. Imminent danger situations receive top priority. An imminent danger is any condition where there is reasonable certainty that a danger exists that can be expected to cause death or serious physical harm immediately or before the danger can be eliminated through normal enforcement procedures.

   If an OSHA inspector finds an imminent danger situation, he or she will ask the employer to voluntarily remedy the situation so that employees are no longer exposed to the dangerous situation. If the employer fails to do this, an OSHA compliance officer may apply to the federal district court for an injunction to stop work until unsafe conditions are corrected.

2. Second priority goes to the investigation of fatalities and accidents resulting in a death or hospitalization of three or more employees. The employer must report such catastrophes to OSHA within 8 hours. OSHA investigates to determine the cause of these accidents and whether existing OSHA standards were violated.

3. Third priority goes to formal employee complaints of unsafe or unhealthful working conditions and to referrals from any source about a workplace hazard. The Act gives each employee the right to request an OSHA inspection when the employee believes he or she is in imminent danger from a hazard or when he or she thinks that there is a violation of an OSHA standard that threatens physical harm. OSHA will maintain confidentiality if requested, and will inform the employee of any action taken.

4. Fourth in priority are programmed inspections aimed at specific high-hazard industries, workplaces, occupations, or health substances, or other industries identified in OSHA's current inspection procedures. OSHA selects industries for inspection on the basis of factors such as the injury incidence rates, previous citation history, employee exposure to toxic substances, or random selection.

5. Last on the list of priorities for OSHA inspections are follow-up inspections. A follow-up inspection determines if the employer has corrected previously cited violations. If an employer has failed to abate a violation, the OSHA compliance officer informs the employer that he or she is subject to "Failure to Abate" alleged violations. This involves proposed additional daily penalties until the employer corrects the violation.

Fines are imposed as penalties for violations. Employers and employees may appeal under some circumstances.

Under OSHA standards, both employers and employees have certain rights and responsibilities. Employers must provide a hazard-free workplace and comply with all applicable OSHA standards. Employers must also inform all employees about OSHA safety and health requirements, keep certain records, and compile and post an annual summary of work-related injuries and illnesses. It is the employer's responsibility to ensure that employees wear safety equipment when necessary, to provide safety training, and to discipline employees for violation of safety rules. The law prohibits employers from retaliating in any way against employees who file complaints under the act.

For their part, employees must comply with all applicable OSHA standards, report hazardous conditions, follow all safety and health rules established by the employer, and use protective equipment when necessary. Many states have employee **right-to-know laws,** which allow employees access to information about toxic or hazardous substances, employer duties, employee rights, and other health and safety issues.

Federal OSHA authority extends to all private sector employers with one or more employees, as well as to federal civilian employees. In addition, many states administer their own occupational safety and health programs through plans approved under section 18(b) of the federal OSHA act.

right-to-know laws State laws that allow employees access to information about toxic or hazardous substances, employer duties, employee rights, and other workplace health and safety issues.

Hazard Communication Standard (HCS) An OSHA standard intended to increase health care practitioners' awareness of risks, improve work practices and appropriate use of personal protective equipment, and reduce injuries and illnesses in the workplace.

OSHA Health Standards and CDC Guidelines

OSHA standards for medical settings and health care workers often are influenced by and/or closely associated with guidelines issued by the Centers for Disease Control and Prevention (CDC). Listed below are a few of the OSHA standards and CDC guidelines that most often affect health care practitioners working in medical settings.

Medical Hazard Regulations

The **Hazard Communication Standard (HCS)** is an OSHA standard that is intended to increase health care practitioners' awareness of risk, improve work practices and appropriate use of personal protective equipment, and reduce injuries and illnesses. See Figure 9-2.

Under the HCS, medical offices must have a written hazard communication program. A list of all office hazards must be compiled, posted on bulletin boards, and placed in a hazard communication manual. The list must include hazardous chemicals, hazardous equipment, and hazardous wastes. Hazards often found in the medical office include disinfectant sprays and lab reagents, electrical and mechanical equipment, and blood and body fluids.

Employers must obtain a Material Safety Data Sheet (MSDS) for each hazardous chemical in use in the office. These sheets should be kept on file, and new ones should be posted where employees can readily see them. Manufacturers must supply MSDSs when requested. Each hazardous product in use must have a hazard label which is a condensed version of the MSDS.

Employees must determine what hazardous chemicals are used, initial and date new MSDSs as they are read, and initial and date records of safety training. Health care practitioners should see that a hazard communication manual is kept up to date

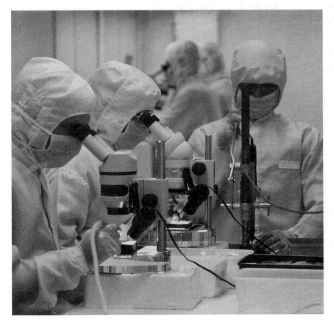

FIGURE 9-2 Medical laboratory personnel wearing biohazard suits. OSHA and CDC regulations govern safety in medical laboratories.

General Duty Clause A section of the Hazard Communication Standard stating that any equipment that may pose a health risk must be specified as a hazard.

Chemical Hygiene Plan The Standard for Occupational Exposures to Hazardous Chemicals in Laboratories, which clarifies the handling of hazardous chemicals in medical laboratories.

Occupational Exposure to Bloodborne Pathogen Standard An OSHA regulation designed to protect health care workers from the risk of exposure to bloodborne pathogens.

and is accessible to all coworkers. Under the **General Duty Clause** of the HCS, any equipment that may pose a health risk is included as a hazard. This clause covers all areas for which OSHA has not developed specific standards and holds the employer ultimately responsible for the safety of employees: "Each employer shall furnish a place of employment which is free from recognized hazards that are causing or are likely to cause death or serious physical harm to his/her employees."

Chemical Hygiene Plan

The Standard for Occupational Exposures to Hazardous Chemicals in Laboratories, or the **Chemical Hygiene Plan,** further clarifies the proper handling of hazardous chemicals in medical laboratories.

Occupational Exposure to Bloodborne Pathogen Standard

The **Occupational Exposure to Bloodborne Pathogen Standard** is an OSHA regulation passed in 1991. The standard is designed to protect workers in health care and related occupations from the risk of exposure to bloodborne *pathogens* (disease-causing organisms) such as the human immunodeficiency virus (HIV) and the hepatitis B virus (HBV). The standard requires posting of safety guidelines, exposure incident reporting, and formulation of a written exposure control plan that outlines the protective measures an employer will take to eliminate or minimize employee exposure to blood and other body fluids. The plan must be available to OSHA inspectors and to employees.

As mandated by the Needlestick Safety and Prevention Act, passed by Congress in 2000, the Occupational Exposure to Bloodborne Pathogen Standard, 29 CFR 1910.1030, was revised in 2001 to include new provisions requiring employers to maintain a sharps injury log and to involve non-managerial employees in selecting safer medical devices.

By authority of the Bloodborne Pathogen Standard, OSHA can levy fines for violations leading to employee exposure to bloodborne pathogens, based upon guidelines issued by the CDC. The CDC's Guidelines for Universal Precautions for Hospitals can apply to any laboratory and include the following:

- Do not contaminate the outside of containers when collecting specimens. All specimen containers should have secure lids.
- Wear gloves when processing patients' specimens, including blood, body fluids containing blood, and other fluids. Masks and goggles should be worn if splashing or aerosolization may occur. Change gloves and wash hands after handling each specimen.
- Use biological safety cabinets for blending and vigorous mixing whenever there is a potential for droplets.
- Do not pipette fluids by mouth. Use mechanical pipetting devices.
- Use extreme caution when handling needles. Do not bend, recap, or remove needles from disposable syringes. Place entire needle assembly in a clearly marked puncture-resistant container.
- Decontaminate work surfaces with a chemical germicide after spills and daily when work is completed.
- Clearly and permanently label tissue or serum specimens to be stored as potentially hazardous.
- Never eat, drink, or smoke in the laboratory.
- Remove protective clothing, and wash hands before leaving the laboratory.

Medical Waste Tracking Act
The federal law that authorizes OSHA to inspect hazardous medical wastes and to cite offices for unsafe or unhealthy practices regarding these wastes.

Medical Waste Tracking Act

By authority of the **Medical Waste Tracking Act,** OSHA may inspect hazardous medical wastes and will cite medical facilities for unsafe or unhealthy practices regarding these wastes. Hazardous medical wastes include blood products, body fluids, tissues, cultures, vaccines (live and weakened), sharps, table paper (with body fluids on them), gloves, speculums, cotton swabs, and inoculating loops.

A puncture-proof, approved sharps container must be provided for the disposal of sharp objects. Chemicals should be discarded in a glass or metal container. Flushable chemicals can be washed down the drain with large quantities of water. Other hazardous medical wastes must be contained in plastic, leak-proof biohazard bags. Incineration is often used to dispose of medical wastes. Reputable, licensed waste handlers should be used to handle this material.

Training and Accident Report Documentation

Under OSHA standards, each employer must have a written training program detailing how employees will be provided with information and training regarding hazards in the workplace. Training should include information about hazards in the work area, the location of the list of hazards and MSDSs, explanations of MSDSs and the hazardous chemical labeling system, and any measures that employees can take to protect themselves against these hazards. Training logs should be kept, and employees who complete training should sign and date the log.

Accidents occurring in the office must be reported. Reports should include

I Employer's name and address.

I Employee's name, address, and phone number.

I Specific information about the accident—when, where, what, and how it occurred.

I Nature of the injury.

I Follow-up information, such as medical treatment or hospitalization.

Each employer who is subject to OSHA record-keeping requirements must maintain a log of all occupational injuries and illnesses. Logs must be kept for five years following the end of the calendar year to which they relate and must be available for inspection by representatives of the U.S. Department of Labor, the U.S. Department of Health and Human Services, and state officials.

OSHA standards for health care settings may be obtained from U.S. Department of Labor, Occupational Safety and Health Administration, Directorate of Health Standards Programs, 200 Constitution Ave. NW, Washington, DC 20210, from state or regional OSHA offices, and from the OSHA Web site at www.osha.gov.

Centers for Disease Control and Prevention (CDC) Guidelines

CDC guidelines divide tasks for health care practitioners into two groups. Category I tasks include those that involve potential contact of mucous membranes or skin with blood, body fluids, or tissue. This category also includes potential for spills or splashes. Gloves, eye masks, gowns, and other protective equipment are required for these tasks. Such tasks include capillary puncture, phlebotomy, pelvic exams, minor suturing, and throat culture.

Category II tasks do not involve direct contact with blood, body fluids, or tissue. Because unplanned exposure may occur, however, protective equipment should be worn by health care practitioners who perform these tasks, which include urinalysis; examination of fecal occult blood; X-rays; ultrasound; ECG; injections; and the examination of sweat, tears, saliva, and nasal secretions.

The CDC maintains an online database of universal precautions guidelines that includes more specific information on a variety of disease and exposure topics. It can be accessed at www.cdc.gov/ncidod/dhqp/bp_universal_precautions.html.

Clinical Laboratory Improvement Act (CLIA) of 1988

Clinical Laboratory Improvement Act (CLIA) Also called Clinical Laboratory Improvement Amendments. Federal statute passed in 1988 that established minimum quality standards for all laboratory testing.

The **Clinical Laboratory Improvement Act (CLIA)** of 1988, also called the Clinical Laboratory Improvement Amendments, replaced 1967 laboratory testing legislation that established standards for Medicare and Medicaid. The act established minimum quality standards for all laboratory testing and has been extensively amended since it was first written. The regulations define a laboratory as any facility that performs laboratory testing on specimens derived from humans for diagnosing, preventing, or treating disease or for assessing health. The law requires that laboratories obtain certification, pay applicable fees, and follow regulations concerning testing, personnel, inspections, test management, quality control, and quality assurance.

The Centers for Medicare and Medicaid Services (CMS), formerly the Health Care Finance Administration (HCFA), has responsibility for financial management operations of the CLIA program. The FDA has responsibility for some CLIA functions.

More information about Clinical Laboratory Improvement Act/Amendments is available online at www.fda.gov/cdrh/clia/.

Workers' Compensation

workers' compensation A form of insurance established by federal and state statutes that provides reimbursement for workers who are injured on the job.

Federal and state **workers' compensation** laws establish procedures for compensating workers who are injured on the job. The employer pays the cost of the insurance premium for the employee. These laws allow the injured worker to file a claim for compensation with the state or the federal government instead of suing. However, the laws require workers to accept workers' compensation as the exclusive remedy for on-the-job injuries. Federal laws cover the following employees: workers in Washington, DC; coal miners; maritime workers; and federal employees. State laws cover those workers not protected under federal statutes.

Workers who are injured on the job or who contract an occupational disease may apply for five types of state compensation benefits:

I Medical treatment, including hospital, medical and surgical services, medications, and prosthetic devices.

I Temporary disability indemnity, in the form of weekly cash payments made directly to the injured or ill employee.

I Permanent disability indemnity, which can be a lump sum award or a weekly or monthly cash payment.

I Death benefits for survivors, which consist of cash payments to dependents of employees killed on the job.

I Rehabilitation benefits, which are paid for medical or vocational rehabilitation.

Employees who are injured on the job or become ill due to work-related causes must immediately report the injury or illness to a supervisor. An injury

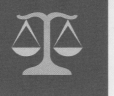
report and claim for compensation are then filed with the appropriate state workers' compensation agency. Forms from the attending or designated workers' compensation physician who examines and treats the employee must also be filed with the appropriate agency as proof of the employee's injury or illness.

A medical office employee may be responsible for filing the physician's report with the state workers' compensation agency. Requirements concerning waiting periods and other filing specifics vary with each state. When a claim is filed, all questions must be answered in full and as thoroughly as possible.

Unemployment Insurance

Unemployment insurance (sometimes called reemployment insurance) funds are managed jointly by state and federal governments. Under the Federal Unemployment Tax Act (FUTA), employers contribute to a fund that is paid out to eligible unemployed workers. Each state also provides unemployment insurance, and credit is given employers against the FUTA tax for amounts paid to the state unemployment fund. The total cost is borne by the employer in all but a few states.

Out-of-work employees should contact a state unemployment office to determine whether they qualify for unemployment benefits. Former employees are denied unemployment compensation for three main reasons: (1) they quit their jobs without cause, (2) they were fired for misconduct, or (3) they are unemployed because of a labor dispute. Independent contractors and self-employed individuals usually do not qualify for unemployment compensation.

Individuals may file for unemployment benefits at state unemployment offices. A claimant needs

- A Social Security card.
- W-2 statements for the past one to two years.
- Other wage records for the past 18 months.
- Employers' names and addresses for the past 18-month employment period.
- A statement of the reasons for leaving the job.
- The employer's unemployment insurance account number, if available.

13. List three OSHA standards that deal specifically with health care workers' safety.

_____

_____

14. Distinguish between workers' compensation and unemployment insurance.

_____

_____

HIRING AND THE NEW EMPLOYEE

When interviewing for a position or when asked to interview a job applicant, the health care practitioner must know legal boundaries.

Interviews

Because of federal and state laws against discrimination in hiring, inquiries cannot be made concerning an applicant's

- Race or color.
- Religion or creed.
- Gender.
- Family.
- Marital status.
- Method of birth control.
- Age, birth date, or birthplace.
- Disability.
- Arrest record (with some exceptions in many states).
- Residency duration.
- National origin. (However, the Immigration Reform and Control Act of 1986 requires new employees to complete an I-9 form, intended to prevent the employment of illegal aliens.)
- General military experience or discharge.
- Membership in organizations.

Questions concerning one's Social Security number, qualifications (including license or certificate), and job experience are proper, and they should be answered as thoroughly and truthfully as possible. As part of the hiring process, applicants may be asked to take a physical examination.

During a job interview, applicants may refuse to answer a question that is clearly improper or not job-related, but this could cost them the job. The question, "May I ask how this relates to the position?" is generally more acceptable than a blunt, "That question is illegal, and I don't have to answer it." Furthermore, the mere asking of an improper preemployment interview question does not in itself give an applicant grounds for a legal challenge if he or she is not hired.

15. Place a check mark beside those questions that are considered to be illegal if asked in a pre-employment interview.

_____ Why are you leaving your present position?

_____ Do you belong to a church?

_____ What do you hope to achieve over the next five years?

_____ How many children do you have, and how old are they?

_____ Who will watch your children while you work?

_____ Why do you want to work for us?

_____ How many years' experience do you have as a medical assistant?

_____ What nationality are you?

The following guidelines can help those employees who are responsible for conducting pre-employment interviews:

- Make a list of questions that relate specifically to the job description of the position to be filled, and stick to them.
- Do not rush the interview, nor let it drag on beyond reasonable time limits.
- General questions that may prove helpful include these: What are your qualifications for this position? Why are you leaving your present position? Why do you want this job? What salary do you expect? When can you begin work? What are your professional strengths? What are your professional goals?
- Remain objective and listen well.
- End the interview on a positive note. Indicate when a decision will be made, and follow through on your promise to inform the applicant of your decision, one way or the other.

Bonding

surety bond A type of insurance that allows employers, if covered, to collect up to the specified amount of the bond if an employee embezzles or otherwise absconds with business funds.

In some medical offices and other workplace locations where employees are responsible for collecting fees and handling financial matters, prospective employees may be asked whether they are bondable. An employer can purchase a **surety bond** for a specific amount from an insurance carrier. If a bonded employee should embezzle or otherwise abscond with funds, the employer can collect from the insurance carrier up to the amount of the bond. However, the employer must have filed a complaint against the alleged dishonest employee in order to collect on the bond. If the insurance company pays the bond, it will then seek to recover the amount from the offending employee.

Employment Paperwork

Once employed, the new worker will be asked to provide certain information so that the employer may comply with federal and state regulations. Complete records for every employee must include

- Social Security number.
- Number of exemptions claimed.
- Gross salary.

- Deductions for Social Security; Medicare; and federal, state, and city taxes.
- Withholding for state disability insurance, state unemployment tax, and health care plans, if applicable.

The law requires employers to withhold specified amounts from employees' pay and to keep records of and send these sums to the proper income tax center. The amount to be withheld is based upon the employee's total salary, the number of exemptions he or she claims, marital status, and the length of the pay period involved.

Health care practitioners who are self-employed do not have to deduct withholding, but they must make quarterly city, state, and federal income tax payments. Self-employed individuals must also pay Social Security taxes (FICA), via a self-employment tax percentage that is higher than the rate paid by individuals who are not self-employed. The difference lies in the fact that a self-employed individual is making both the employer and the employee contribution.

Employers must provide each employee with a Form W-2, Wage and Tax Statement, by January 31 of each year. The W-2 shows the following information:

- Employer's tax identification number.
- Employee's Social Security number.
- Total earnings (wages and other compensation) paid by the employer.
- Amounts deducted for income tax and Social Security.
- Amount of advance earned income credit payment, if any.

Most employers want the workplace to be as pleasant and safe for employees as it can possibly be. However, it is still the employee's responsibility to know the employment legalities most likely to affect him or her and to work within this legal framework to help ensure a satisfying and productive employer-employee relationship.

Ethics Issues

Workplace Legalities

ETHICS ISSUE 1: All ethical guidelines for health care practitioners remind them to be aware that, even though sexually suggestive behavior may not have crossed the line legally, any form of sexual harassment or exploitation between medical supervisors and trainees, employers and employees, coworkers, or medical practitioners and patients is unethical.

DISCUSSION QUESTIONS

1. You are a surgical technologist in a large hospital. Whenever you work with a certain surgeon she tells off-color jokes to you and your coworkers and makes suggestive comments to workers of the opposite sex. One coworker tells you that he might quit his job because he is married, and the surgeon's behavior makes him so uncomfortable that he dreads coming to work. Is the surgeon's behavior illegal or simply in bad taste? Explain your answer.

_____

_____

2. Do you or your coworkers have grounds for a sexual harassment complaint? Explain your answer.

_____

_____

3. If you have determined that you do have a complaint, how would you proceed?

_____

_____

ETHICS ISSUE 2: Patients are often accompanied by third parties who play an important part in the health care practitioner–patient relationship. The health care practitioner interacts and communicates with these individuals and often is in a position to offer them information, advice, and emotional support. The more deeply involved the individual is in the clinical encounter and in medical decision making, the more troubling sexual or romantic contact with the health care practitioner would be. Key third parties include, but are not limited to, spouses or partners, parents, guardians, and proxies.

DISCUSSION QUESTIONS

1. As a medical assistant, you have been present when a young, single father brings his infant in for check-ups. The child is seriously ill, and the father begins consulting you about his emotional anguish. You are also single and sense an attraction. When the young man asks you out, should you accept? Explain your answer.

_____

_____

2. Do you believe ethical standards governing such relationships are stricter for health care practitioners than for other professions, such as law professors and students? In your view, is this as it should be? Explain your answer.

_____

_____

_____

ETHICS ISSUE 3: Racial bias can be subtle and difficult to recognize, but in health care situations it is unethical.

DISCUSSION QUESTION

1. You are a dental hygienist who has a relative fighting in Iraq. A patient of Middle Eastern ethnicity makes an appointment and your negative emotions are overwhelming. In your opinion, is it ethical for you to refuse to treat this patient? Explain your answer.

_____

_____

 Go to www.mhhe.com/judson5e to practice your case review skills. Then read on for more information.

CHAPTER 9 REVIEW

Applying Knowledge

Answer the following questions or complete the following statements in the spaces provided.

1. Under the concept of employment-at-will, who has the right to terminate employment?

_____

2. What evidence may be produced to substantiate a wrongful discharge claim?

_____

3. List three federal laws that protect employees from potential discrimination.

_____

_____

_____

4. Title VII of the _____ Act makes sexual discrimination illegal. _____ is considered a form of sexual discrimination.

5. What federal office can be contacted to report any charges or complaints of employment discrimination?

_____

6. _____, "something for something," is a form of sexual harassment. Another form of sexual harassment is behavior toward an employee that creates a(n) _____ that interferes with an employee's work performance.

7. _____ laws allow an injured employee to file a claim with the state or federal government instead of _____. However, employees are required to accept this compensation as a(n) _____ for on-the-job illness or injury.

8. For what three reasons may an ex-employee be denied unemployment compensation?

_____

_____

_____

9. What information is given on the employee's Form W-2?

_____

_____

_____

10. What government publication is the primary source for locating OSHA standards?

_____

11. _____ standards require an employer to provide a safe workplace, to inform employees about hazards, to keep certain records, and to post an annual summary of accidents.

12. Who has the primary responsibility for providing safety training or appropriate safety equipment for employees?

_____

13. _____ laws are state laws that allow employees access to information about toxic or hazardous substances, employer duties, employee rights, and other workplace health and safety issues.

14. CDC guidelines divide tasks for health care workers into which two groups?

_____

_____

15. Under OSHA standards, accidents occurring in the office must be reported. What five facts should be included?

_____

_____

_____

_____

_____

16. Manufacturers of potentially hazardous chemicals must supply which document, upon request, for a specific product?

_____

17. This federal agency issues universal precautions for safe practices in the hospital or medical office.

_____

Match each description that follows with the correct term by writing the appropriate letter in the space provided.

_____ 18. Established the EEOC.

_____ 19. Makes it illegal to discriminate because of pregnancy, childbirth, or related medical conditions.

_____ 20. Protects employees aged 40 or older.

_____ 21. Protects employees who engage in union or other organizational activities,

_____ 22. Regulates private pension funds and employer benefit programs.

_____ 23. Requires equal pay for equal work.

_____ 24. Ensures a safe work environment.

_____ 25. Regulates child labor, and provides for minimum wages and overtime pay.

_____ 26. Provides for Medicare, unemployment insurance, disability, and OASI, through FICA funding.

_____ 27. Protects the disabled and mentally ill.

_____ 28. Provides minimum federal standards for quality laboratory testing.

a. Wagner Act

b. Social Security Act

c. Fair Labor Standards Act

d. Equal Pay Act

e. Civil Rights Act of 1964

f. Age in Discrimination in Employment Act

g. Occupational Safety and Health Act

h. Rehabilitation Act

i. Employee Retirement Income Security Act

j. Pregnancy Discrimination Act

k. Clinical Laboratory Improvement Act/Amendments

Case Study

Use your critical-thinking skills to answer the questions that follow the case study.

You have recently graduated from a two-year medical assistant program, have earned certification, and want to apply for the following advertised positions: (1) a CMA in a pediatrics clinic and (2) a CMA/receptionist for a physician in private practice.

29. Write letters of application for each position and a résumé to be included with the cover letters. Consider the following questions:

30. What information will you give about your educational, employment, and personal background?

_____

_____

_____

31. If interviewed for the position, how will you follow up?

_____

_____

_____

The relationship between cleanliness and disease has been established, over time, within the medical community. Despite the conclusive evidence that "germs" cause disease and clean hands help stop the spread of germs, a recent study suggests that many doctors and other health care practitioners are not as careful as they should be to wash hands between patient contacts. In one intensive care unit surveyed, only about 17 percent of physicians complied with the recommended regimen, which includes lathering hands with germicidal soap, rinsing twice for at least 30 seconds, then thorough drying.

Studies have revealed that 20,000 people die each year in the United States as the result of infections contracted in hospitals. Hand-washing alone won't solve the problem, but hand-to-hand and glove-to-glove contact between health care provider and patient is still a major route of disease transmission.

Some hospitals and other medical facilities are suggesting that patients remind doctors, nurses, and other health care practitioners to wash their hands before beginning an examination or treatment.

32. In your opinion, is this a reasonable approach to the problem? Explain your answer.

_____

_____

33. What other methods might be used in addition to or instead of patient involvement to encourage proper hygiene among health care practitioners?

_____

_____

34. Do you believe hygiene is a moral obligation for health care practitioners? Explain your answer.

_____

_____

Internet Activities

Complete the activities and answer the questions that follow.

35. Visit the Web site for the Equal Employment Opportunity Commission (EEOC) at www.eeoc.gov/index. html. List those laws enforced by the EEOC.

_____

_____

_____

36. Visit the Web site for OSHA's bloodborne pathogen site at www.osha.gov/SLTC/bloodbornepathogens/. Summarize what should be done following exposure to blood. List at least three other topics covered at this Web site.

_____

_____

_____

_____

37. Visit the Web site for OSHA's whistleblowing regulations at www.osha.gov/dep/oia/whistleblower/ index.html. What types of discrimination does the regulation prohibit? Summarize how one would file a complaint with OSHA under the whistleblowing regulations.

_____

_____

_____

CHAPTER 10

The Beginning of Life and Childhood

Learning Outcomes

After studying this chapter, you should be able to:

1. Define genetics and heredity.

2. List several situations in which genetic testing might be appropriate and explain how it might lead to genetic discrimination.

3. Define cloning, and explain why it is a controversial issue.

4. Discuss the different types of stem cells used in research.

5. Distinguish between mature and emancipated minors, and discuss those situations where such minors might legally make their own health care decisions.

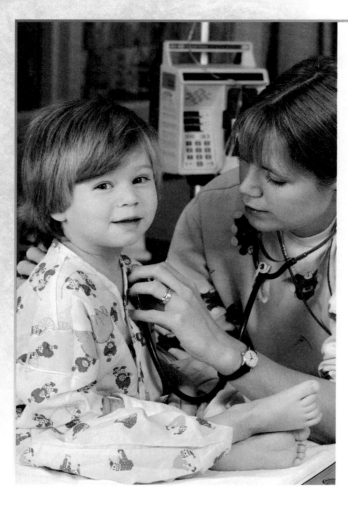

Key Terms

amniocentesis

chromosome

clone

cloning

DNA (deoxyribonucleic acid)

emancipated minors

gene

genetic counselor

genetic discrimination

genetic engineering

genetics

genome

heredity

heterologous artificial insemination

homologous artificial insemination

Human Genome Project

infertility

in vitro fertilization (IVF)

mature minors

parens patriae

safe haven laws

stem cells

surrogate mother

xenotransplantation

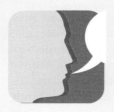

Voice of Experience
Genetic Research: Checks and Balances

Carma is an oncology-certified RN with a master's degree in Health Administration. She is also the research administrator for the Human Gene Therapy Department of a Midwestern health system. The Human Gene Therapy Department where Carma works is a private facility funded by grants and the sponsoring health system. According to Carma, the mission of her department is "to advance and apply the science of gene therapy for cancer." The department does laboratory research and performs clinical trials for the use of gene therapy.

In one clinical trial, scientists at Carma's department genetically altered a virus to be used in targeting ovarian cancer cells. Two additional projects deal with breast cancer. One involves developing a breast cancer vaccine and the other uses radioactive iodine to target breast cancer cells, much as radioactive iodine is used to treat thyroid cancer.

Carma says that data provided by the Human Genome Project has helped further the work of her department.

"We still don't know, though, how genes are linked," she emphasizes. "For example, two of the genes that cause breast cancer have been identified, but since we are not sure how genes interact, if we alter those genes to not cause cancer, there could be a cascade of other effects."

Carma's facility does not do genetic testing, but she stresses that such testing should not be done without genetic counseling. Carma also emphasizes that many checks and balances exist for gene therapy research and clinical trials. "Gene therapy protocols within our department must be approved by the Institutional Review Board (IRB), a local group composed of scientific and medical personnel as well as chaplains and other laypeople. Any research project involving humans in any way (physically as well as psychologically) needs approval from the IRB." Any gene therapy protocol is also subject to FDA approval.

An ethical concern in genetic research, Carma adds, is to question whether a project should be done just because it is possible. "Just because we can do it doesn't always mean we should do it," she emphasizes.

THE INFLUENCE OF TECHNOLOGY ON THE BEGINNING OF LIFE

Health care practitioners have always had to make informed decisions based on legal and ethical principles and on personal values. But in today's technological world the task becomes even more difficult, perhaps especially when those decisions apply to the beginning of life and to childhood.

GENETICS

genetics The science that accounts for natural differences and resemblances among organisms related by descent.

heredity The process by which organisms pass genetic traits on to their offspring.

DNA (deoxyribonucleic acid) The combination of proteins, called nucleotides, that is arranged to make up an organism's chromosomes.

Genetics was often in the news from the mid-1990s into the twenty-first century, as scientists published the results of experiments in genetics research. **Genetics,** as you probably remember from earlier science courses, is the study of **heredity,** or how traits are passed from one generation to the next.

As a result of genetics research, improved science education, and extensive media coverage of genetics procedures and issues, health care practitioners and members of the general public have become familiar with the term **DNA (deoxyribonucleic acid).** DNA is the combination of proteins called nucleotides that are arranged to make up each human **chromosome.** See Figure 10-1.

Forty-six chromosomes (23 pairs) are found inside the nucleus of every human cell, except egg and sperm cells, which have 23 chromosomes each. We inherit half of our chromosome complement from our mother and half from our father. These 46 chromosomes carry the genes responsible for all our human characteristics, from eye, skin, and hair color to height, body type,

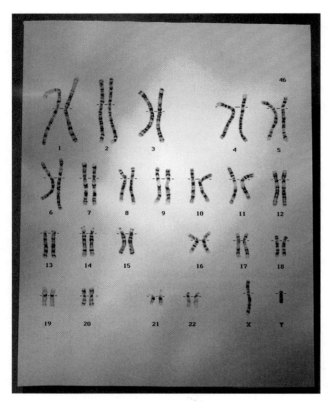

FIGURE 10-1 Comparison of chromosomes to check for disease.

📖 **chromosome** A microscopic structure found within the nucleus of a plant or animal cell that carries genes responsible for the organism's characteristics.

and intelligence. Each **gene** is a tiny segment of DNA that holds the formula for making a specific molecule.

The genes that make up the human **genome**—all the genetic information necessary to create a human being—are responsible for all the cells, organs, tissues, and traits that make up each individual. Some of these genes are also responsible for the more than 4,000 genetic diseases that can afflict human beings, including cystic fibrosis, sickle cell anemia, hemophilia, Huntington's disease, Down syndrome, Tay-Sachs disease, multiple sclerosis, some forms of cancer, and other diseases.

The Human Genome Project

The **Human Genome Project,** funded by the U.S. government, was started in 1990 to analyze the entire human genome. A genome is all the DNA in an organism, including its genes. Scientists around the world who worked on the project set out to map the 80,000 to 100,000 genes they believed existed within the 23 pairs of human chromosomes. The project was scheduled for completion in 2003 but was finished ahead of time, in mid-2000. One surprising finding was that instead of the suspected 100,000 genes, humans have approximately 20,000 to 25,000 genes.

Goals of the Human Genome Project that have largely been accomplished were to locate and map the location of each gene on all 46 chromosomes and to create a data bank of the information that would be available to all scientists or physicians who could use it. The scientists involved in the project also vowed to continue to examine the ethical, legal, and social issues originating with human genetics research, and to train other scientists to use the technologies developed in order to improve human health.

CHECK YOUR PROGRESS

Give the term that is defined by each phrase.

1. The science that studies inherited traits (heredity).

_____

2. The thread-like structures inside cell nuclei that are composed of DNA and carry an organism's genes. _____

3. A tiny segment of DNA that holds instructions for making a specific molecule.

_____

4. All the genes necessary to replicate a human being.

_____

5. A worldwide project to locate and map the location of all human genes.

_____

gene A tiny segment of DNA found on a chromosome in a cell. Each gene holds the formula for making a specific molecule.

genome All the DNA in an organism, including its genes.

Human Genome Project A scientific project funded by the U.S. government, begun in 1990 and successfully completed in 2000, for the purpose of mapping all of a human's genes. This Web site is an excellent resource: www. ornl.gov/sci/techresources/ HumanGenome/home.shtml.

amniocentesis A test whereby the physician withdraws a sample of amniotic fluid (the fluid surrounding the developing fetus inside the mother's womb) from the uterus of a pregnant woman. The fluid is then tested for genetic or other conditions that may lead to abnormal development of the fetus.

genetic counselor An expert in human genetics who is qualified to counsel individuals who may have inherited genes for certain diseases or conditions.

Genetic Testing

Since, like fingerprints, each individual's DNA is unique to that person, DNA testing has become a reliable method of identifying the source of body fluids and tissues left at crime scenes, determining parentage, and testing for other genetic information. Specially trained technicians perform DNA tests. The tests are conducted from samples of solid tissues such as hair roots, skin, or bone, and from body fluids such as blood, semen, or saliva.

In addition to forensic use and tracing lineage, genetic testing has made it possible for individuals to determine whether or not they carry a gene for an inherited disease and for expectant parents to determine, through **amniocentesis,** whether or not a developing fetus shows signs of abnormalities. During amniocentesis, the physician withdraws a sample of amniotic fluid (the fluid surrounding the developing fetus inside the mother's womb) from the uterus of a pregnant woman. The fluid is then tested for genetic or other conditions that may lead to abnormal development of the fetus. Down syndrome is one inherited condition that is often detected through amniocentesis

Individuals who come from families where certain inherited diseases have appeared may opt for genetic testing to confirm or rule out the presence of a disease-causing gene. For example, Huntington's disease (formerly known as Huntington's chorea) runs in families, but symptoms typically do not develop until individuals reach middle age. Since the disease is incurable, debilitating, and fatal, affecting the brain and the nervous system, adults who have relatives who have developed the disease may opt to be tested in order to plan for any eventuality.

On the other hand, individuals with a family history of incurable inherited diseases may opt not to be tested simply to preserve peace of mind. Health care practitioners should refer any patient who wants to undergo genetic testing to a **genetic counselor.** Genetic counselors can explain test results and help patients deal with difficult questions concerning those results.

Some inherited diseases (Figure 10-2) for which genetic tests are available include

- Cystic fibrosis, a disease that affects the mucus glands of the lungs, liver, pancreas, and intestines, causing progressive disability due to multisystem failure. There is no cure and many individuals with the disease die young, often in their 20s and 30s.

- Down syndrome, a disease that causes mental retardation and other physical problems.

- Fragile X syndrome, a rare disease that causes mental retardation.

- Gaucher's disease, a condition affecting fat metabolism.

- Hemochromatosis, an iron storage disorder and the most commonly occurring inherited disease.

- Huntington's disease, also called Huntington's chorea, an untreatable, ultimately fatal disease of the brain and nervous system.

- Mucopolysaccharidosis (MPS), a metabolic disorder that causes skeletal deformities and usually mental retardation.

- Phenylketonuria (PKU), a metabolic disorder for which all newborns are tested. It results in mental retardation if left untreated.

- Sickle-cell anemia, a malformation of the red blood cells most often diagnosed in African Americans.

- Some forms of breast, ovarian, and colon cancer.

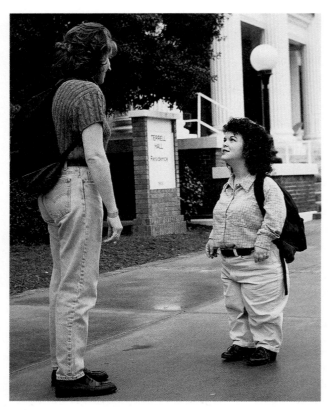

FIGURE 10-2 Two students, one of normal height, and the other an achondroplastic dwarf. Mutations in the fibroblast growth factor receptor 3 gene (FGFR3) cause achondroplasia.

■ Spinocerebellar ataxia, a rare disorder that eventually destroys the brain's cerebellum.

■ Tay-Sachs disease, a lipid metabolism disorder that affects some people of Jewish descent. Children with the disease seldom survive childhood.

As genetic testing has become more widely available and more reliable, use of test results has become an important issue. For example, if a couple learns through amniocentesis that the fetus the mother is carrying will be born with Down syndrome, should they consider aborting the fetus? Should the young man who learns he has the gene for Huntington's disease opt not to marry, to avoid taking the chance of passing the gene on to offspring? And will the woman who learns she has one of two genes known to predispose her to breast cancer live her life any differently than she would have had she not been tested?

Genetic testing has also raised the issue of privacy. For instance, should employers and health and life insurance companies have access to genetic test results? How can individuals be certain that information about their genetic makeup is not shared with unknown sources?

Clearly, advances in genetics and genetic testing have led to difficult ethical, social, and medical questions for patients and their families and for health care practitioners.

Genetic Testing and Discrimination

With the increased ability to identify genetic differences comes increasing concern for the proper use of such information. The term **genetic discrimination** describes the differential treatment of individuals based on their actual or presumed genetic differences.

genetic discrimination
Differential treatment of individuals based on their actual or presumed genetic differences.

Harvard Medical School's Lisa N. Geller and her colleagues conducted a comprehensive and often-quoted study of genetic discrimination throughout the 1990s. The study found that a number of institutions were reported to have engaged in genetic discrimination, including health and life insurance companies, health care providers, blood banks, adoption agencies, the military, and schools. Geller's study included individuals at risk for or related to people with hemochromatosis, phenylketonuria (PKU), mucopolysaccharidosis (MPS), and Huntington's disease.

Four hundred and fifty-five respondents out of 917 who returned questionnaires for Geller's study said they had experienced genetic discrimination. In one case, a health maintenance organization had covered the medical expenses of a child since birth but refused to pay for occupational therapy after she was diagnosed with mucopolysaccharidosis, claiming that the condition was preexisting.

In another case, a 24-year-old woman was denied life insurance due to her family history of Huntington's disease and the fact that she had not been tested for the presence of the gene. If she agreed to be tested and was found not to carry the gene, the insurance company would issue her a policy.

Geller also reported that in several cases, medical professionals reportedly pressured patients at risk for having children with serious genetic conditions to undergo prenatal diagnostic testing or to decide against having children.

There are now laws in place to prevent genetic discrimination. As of July 2004, 41 states had laws prohibiting discrimination in health insurance based on genetic tests. Laws in 27 states addressed genetic discrimination in employment. In addition, the Health Insurance Portability and Accountability Act (HIPAA) passed in 1996 prevents health insurers from denying coverage based on genetic information. HIPAA, however, applies only to individuals moving between group health insurance plans. (Chapter 7, "Privacy Law and HIPAA," discusses HIPAA in detail.)

The Americans with Disabilities Act (ADA) of 1990, discussed in Chapter 9, "Workplace Legalities," also offers some protection against genetic discrimination in the workplace. It protects those who have a genetic condition or disease, or are regarded as having a disability, against discrimination. Under a 1995 ruling by the Equal Employment Opportunities Commission, the ADA applies to anyone who is discriminated against on the basis of genetic information relating to illness, disease, condition, or other disorders. Furthermore, under the ADA, a person with a disability cannot be denied insurance or be subject to different terms or conditions of insurance based on disability alone, if the disability does not pose increased risks. Most recently, the Genetic Information Nondiscrimination Act (GINA), passed in May 2008, prohibits employers and insurers from discriminating against individuals based on DNA that may affect their health.

In February 2000, then President Bill Clinton signed an executive order banning the federal government from using genetic data in employment decisions. Under the order, the government cannot request or require job applicants or employees to take genetic tests. The government is also prohibited from using information from genetic tests in hiring or promotion decisions.

Genetic Engineering

Our increased body of knowledge about DNA, chromosome structure, and the basis of heredity has allowed scientists to manipulate DNA within the cells of plants and animals to ensure that certain traits will appear and be passed on, or that certain undesirable characteristics are eliminated. This is called **genetic engineering.** Because the chemical composition of DNA is nearly identical throughout the plant and animal kingdoms, genes can often be interchanged among plants and animals to transfer desirable characteristics to different species. Through this process, for example, genes from a species of Arctic flounder have been added to strawberry plants to make them better able to withstand cold temperatures. Genetic engineering has also created corn and soybean crops that are resistant to insect-borne diseases, "golden" rice with increased beta-carotene content, and bacteria that can devour oil spilled into oceans.

However beneficial a genetic engineering plan may sound, controversy is almost guaranteed as a new project is announced. Objections may be raised on the religious or moral grounds that humans simply should not tamper with the time-honored progression of life as dictated by nature. Or opponents may fear that the process will harm the environment by releasing genetically engineered super-species that may crowd out naturally occurring species and lead to the eventual disappearance of many original organisms. Critics may also fear that the undisclosed addition of genes to plants or animals ingested by humans can have unforeseen effects. For instance, some fear that genes from peanut plants added to a product might cause harmful reactions in unsuspecting consumers who are allergic to peanuts.

Clearly, if genetic engineering is to truly benefit society, scientists and governments must consider the objections and fears of concerned individuals and proceed with research in a manner that takes these concerns into account.

genetic engineering
Manipulation of DNA within the cells of plants and animals, through synthesis, alteration, or repair, to ensure that certain harmful traits will be eliminated in offspring and that desirable traits will appear and be passed on.

clone An organism produced asexually, usually from a single cell of the parent.

cloning The process by which organisms are created asexually, usually from a single cell of the parent organism.

xenotransplantation Transplantation of animal tissues and organs into humans.

stem cells Cells that have the potential to become any type of body cell.

Cloning

One type of genetic engineering that is extremely controversial is cloning. The word **clone** comes from the Latin root meaning "to cut from." A clone is an organism grown from a single cell of the parent, and so it is genetically identical to the parent. In other words, the genes and chromosomes found in each cell's nucleus are the same in clone and parent. Identical twins are clones. So are all the cells in our bodies except for eggs and sperm: Somatic (body) cells divide to produce clones or exact replicas of themselves. Therefore, cells within the liver and other organs, within walls of blood vessels and arteries, within the skin, and so on, are exactly like the cells that divided to produce them.

The term **cloning** was thrust into the public consciousness with the birth of Dolly, a Finn Dorset sheep, in July 1996. Dolly was the product of scientists at the Roslin Institute near Edinburgh, Scotland. Her birth was controversial because she was the world's first mammal cloned from an adult parent cell. That is, Dolly was not the product of union of egg and sperm, but was created from a single cell scraped from the inside of her six-year-old mother's udder. Scientists used a process called nuclear transfer to clone Dolly from the udder cell.

Since Dolly's birth, scientists have cloned cattle, goats, mice, monkeys, and pigs. One objective of the cloning of farm and laboratory animals is to breed genetically identical animals that can produce substances useful in medicine, such as insulin and growth hormone. Another objective in cloning farm animals is the consistent production of prime, low-fat meat.

A third objective of animal cloning is to clone animal tissues and organs for human medical use. Because pigs are similar to humans in organ size and other biological aspects, an objective in cloning them is to grow a potential source of organs and tissue for transplanting into human patients. Transplanting animal tissues and organs into humans is called **xenotransplantation.** Research in this area is continuing, but at least two major difficulties make the process problematic. Animal cells produce a sugar that human cells do not, causing a severe immune rejection reaction in humans when animal tissues are transplanted. In addition, scientists have found that human cells can be infected with some viruses that exist in animals.

Many animal rights proponents object on ethical grounds to using animals in this way. They argue that animals should be allowed to exist in nature without being subjected to experiments for the benefit of humankind. Furthermore, other groups object to introducing animal cells into humans on ethical grounds and on grounds that the animal tissue can harm people.

By 2000, the United States and other countries had either banned human cloning outright or had established ethical guidelines that limited or prohibited it. In 2001, however, British lawmakers passed legislation making it legal in Great Britain to clone human embryos for research only.

Human Stem Cell Research

Early-stage human embryos, called blastocysts, consist of about 20 cells and are considered valuable for research because they are composed of **stem cells.** These early embryonic cells have the potential to become any type of body cell. Interest in this type of research—the *therapeutic* use of stem cells—remains intense because stem cells have shown promise for treating patients with a wide variety of medical problems. For example, stem cells that develop into neuronal tissue could be used to treat patients with Parkinson's and Alzheimer's diseases, as well as patients with strokes, spinal cord injuries, and other neurological disorders. Stem cells that become pancreatic islet cells might help those with diabetes. Skin tissue grown from stem cells could replace burned tissue, and cultivated cardiac tissue might help damaged arteries and hearts.

The use of embryonic stem cells to research human *reproductive* cycles and traits, however, is widely criticized as unethical. It is already possible for parents to choose the sex of their offspring—by in vitro fertilization of eggs by X or Y sperm cells to create the desired XX or XY combination—but this raises the issue of the desirability of creating "designer babies."

Most embryos used in stem cell research in the United States are the frozen products of in vitro fertilization that were not used to produce a pregnancy and are destined to eventually be destroyed. In 2001, President George W. Bush ordered that federal financing could be allowed only for stem cell research using cells grown from human embryos destroyed before August 9, 2001. By 2004, in contrast, England, Australia, Israel, and Portugal actively supported stem cell research without such restrictions.

Opponents to human embryonic stem cell research of any kind argue that regardless of how the embryos were created, they are human beings with inherent rights to ethical and legal protection. Others argue that since the embryos are not growing within a uterus, they are not subject to the same protection as fetuses, and since most would be destroyed anyway, the good that could come from such research far outweighs any downside. To date, the United States government has limited funding for human embryonic stem cell research according to the terms mentioned above, which means that scientists who wish to do research using embryonic stem cells must find private funding. Some state governments such as California, Connecticut, Illinois, Maryland, Massachusetts, New Jersey, New York, and Wisconsin have begun funding embryonic stem cell research.

Because of the controversy over using human embryonic cells in research, scientists are searching for other sources of stem cells. They have discovered that some adult human body tissues, such as bone marrow and fat, also contain cells that can function as stem cells. Adult stem cells are multipotent, however, which means that they can become only a limited number of types of tissues and cells in the body. For example, adult blood-forming stem cells (found in bone marrow) have been used successfully to treat only blood-based diseases such as leukemia and lymphoma. Embryonic stem cells have greater potential to treat a wider variety of diseases because they are pluripotent—they can become almost all types of tissues and cells in the body.

Adult stem cells are found in small quantities in adult tissues and umbilical cord blood, and scientists have found they do not have the same capacity to produce diverse tissues or to multiply as embryonic stem cells. If a patient receives an adult stem cell transplant from a donor, the patient's body might reject it—a problem that researchers anticipate could be overcome with therapeutic cloning. Furthermore, adult stem cells may have more genetic abnormalities, which occur naturally during the aging process and with exposure to harmful agents.

Some scientists are exploring the possibility that adult stem cells are more flexible than previously thought, but many questions remain about the potential of adult stem cells, and much more research is required to answer them.

Amniotic stem cells are another possibility as a source for researchers. Amniotic stem cells are found in the fluid that surrounds a fetus. Scientists recently showed that they can be induced to create more cell types than was previously thought. However, the research is not intended as a replacement for embryonic stem cell research.

Some individuals within the scientific community agree that both adult and embryonic stem cell research show great potential to revolutionize the practice of medicine and that both types of research should be pursued.

Gene Therapy

gene therapy Treating harmful genetic diseases or traits by eliminating or modifying the harmful gene.

Gene therapy is rapidly becoming an effective tool for correcting and preventing certain diseases. In fact, therapy for genetic disease is often very similar to therapy for other types of disorders, as in the following cases:

- Special diets can eliminate compounds that are toxic to patients. This applies to such diseases as phenylketonuria and homocystinuria.
- Vitamins or other agents can improve a biochemical pathway and thus reduce toxic levels of a compound. For example, folic acid reduces homocysteine levels in a person who carries the 5, 10-methylene tetrahydrofolate reductase polymorphism gene.

Gene therapy may involve replacing a deficiency or blocking an overactive pathway. For instance, a fetus can sometimes be treated by treating the mother (e.g., corticosteroids for congenital virilizing adrenal hypoplasia) or by using in utero (inside the uterus) cellular therapy (e.g., bone marrow transplantation). Similarly, a newborn with a genetic disease may be a candidate for treatment with bone marrow or organ transplantation.

Genetic therapy may also involve the insertion of normal copies of a gene into the cells of persons with a specific genetic disease. (This is called somatic gene therapy.) Such somatic gene therapy has been undertaken for severe genetic disorders such as adenosine deaminase deficiency, an immunodeficiency that usually results in death during the first few months of life.

CHECK YOUR PROGRESS

6. The process of manipulating the DNA of organisms to produce desired results is called _____.

7. Define *genetic discrimination*.

_____

_____

8. Define *cloning*.

_____

_____

9. Name and briefly define five methods of gene therapy.

_____

_____

_____

_____

_____

Germ-line gene therapy involves the correction of an abnormality in the genes of sperm or egg but is presently considered an inappropriate way to deal with genetic diseases because of ethical issues, cost, lack of research in humans, lack of knowledge about whether or not changes would be maintained in the growing embryo, and the relative ease of treating the pertinent conditions somatically when needed.

Gene therapy could also involve turning off genes before their harmful properties can be expressed. For example, if the gene for Huntington's disease could be turned off before carriers reached adulthood, theoretically the disease could not develop.

CONCEPTION AND THE BEGINNING OF LIFE

Fortunately, most couples who decide to have a child are able to conceive naturally, and most pregnancies proceed without problems. However, a 2007 survey conducted by the makers of Fertell, the first at-home fertility screening test for couples, revealed that one in seven adults between the ages of 25 and 45, or six million Americans, will have difficulty conceiving. Of this number, either husband or wife will experience **infertility,** that is, the failure to conceive for a period of 12 months or longer due to a deviation from or interruption of the normal structure or function of any reproductive part, organ, or system.

Infertility

When couples have reproductive difficulties and consult physicians who specialize in infertility problems, diagnoses are made and appropriate treatment recommended. Several options for infertile couples exist, depending on the type of fertility problem:

- **In vitro fertilization (IVF).** In this process, eggs and sperm are brought together outside of the body in a test tube or petri dish. When fertilization takes place, the resulting embryo can then be frozen in liquid nitrogen for future use or implanted in the female uterus for pregnancy to occur.
- **Artificial insemination.** This process involves the mechanical injection of viable semen into the vagina. If the husband's sperm cells are used to fertilize the wife's eggs, the process is called **homologous artificial insemination.** If the husband's sperm cells are not viable, a donor's sperm may be used to fertilize the wife's eggs. This is called **heterologous artificial insemination.**
- Surrogacy. If a woman cannot carry an embryo to term, the couple may elect to contract with a surrogate mother.

Surrogacy

A **surrogate mother** is a woman who agrees to carry a child to term for a couple, often for a fee. If the surrogate is not genetically related to the embryo, the type of surrogacy is called *gestational* surrogacy. If the surrogate contributes eggs to produce the embryo or is related to either husband or wife, the type of surrogacy is called *traditional* surrogacy. (In one much-publicized case in the United States, a woman carried her own grandchild to term for her married daughter who was born without a uterus.) Traditional surrogacy differs from gestational surrogacy in that a traditional surrogate is genetically related to the fetus she carries.

infertility The failure to conceive for a period of 12 months or longer due to a deviation from or interruption of the normal structure or function of any reproductive part, organ, or system.

in vitro fertilization (IVF) Fertilization that takes place outside a woman's body, literally, "in glass," as in a test tube.

artificial insemination The mechanical injection of viable semen into the vagina.

homologous artificial insemination The process in which a husband's sperm is mechanically injected into his wife's vagina to fertilize her eggs.

heterologous artificial insemination The process in which donor sperm is mechanically injected into a woman's vagina to fertilize her eggs.

surrogate mother A woman who becomes pregnant, usually by artificial insemination or surgical implantation of a fertilized egg, and bears a child for another woman.

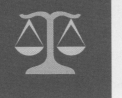

Baby M—A Traditional Surrogacy Case

In 1985, a woman signed a contract agreeing to serve as a surrogate for a couple who could not conceive. She was then medically inseminated with the husband's sperm and a pregnancy resulted. When the child was born in March 1986, the surrogate mother refused to give up the infant. The genetic father sued for violation of the surrogacy contract. The contract specified that the genetic father and his wife held custody and that the surrogate would terminate her parental rights. The trial court, considering the best interests of the child, affirmed the validity of the contract. In March 1987, an appellate court terminated the surrogate mother's parental rights and gave full custody of the then one-year-old Baby M to her genetic father and his wife. The genetic father's wife legally adopted the baby.

In re Baby M, 537 A.2d 1227 (N.J., 1988).

Infertility treatments can cost several thousand dollars, with no guarantee of success. Most insurance plans do not cover expenses for infertility treatments or for contracting with a surrogate mother to bear a child. The law has been slow to catch up with technology, but many states have passed legislation regulating infertility clinics and surrogacy. Health care practitioners dealing with infertility should check state laws for current regulations.

Surrogacy is a relatively new concept in reproductive technology; thus, there is not a large volume of case law. The two cases on this page, however, have contributed to establishing precedent for legal decisions.

Adoption

Adoption is also an option for those couples who want to raise children. All 50 states have laws regulating adoption. Certain areas of federal law may also affect some aspects of the parent-child relationship established by

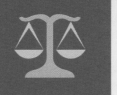

Gestational Surrogacy Contract Held Valid

A married couple was unable to have a child because the wife had undergone a hysterectomy. The wife's ovaries had not been removed, however, and could still produce eggs, so the couple opted for gestational surrogacy. They entered into a surrogacy contract with a woman who agreed to relinquish her parental rights after the child was born in exchange for a $10,000 fee and a paid life insurance policy. The wife's eggs were fertilized in vitro with the husband's sperm, and the resulting embryo was implanted into the surrogate's uterus. While she was still pregnant, the surrogate demanded immediate payment and threatened not to relinquish the child when it was born. The couple who had contracted with the surrogate filed a lawsuit seeking a legal determination that the surrogate had no parental rights to the baby. The surrogate countersued and the court consolidated the two cases.

A trial court found for the married couple. It determined that the couple was the child's "natural parents" and held that the surrogate had no parental rights to the child. An appellate court and the state supreme court upheld this decision.

Johnson v. Calvert, 851 P.2d 776 (Cal., 1993).

adoption. For example, the Adoption Assistance and Child Welfare Act of 1980, the Child Abuse Prevention and Treatment and Adoption Reform Act, and the Indian Child Welfare Act all contain provisions that pertain to adoptive parents and their children.

Typically, any adult who shows the desire to be a fit parent may adopt a child. Depending upon state law, both married and unmarried couples may adopt, and single people may adopt through a process called single-parent adoption. Some states list special requirements for adoptive parents, such as requiring an adoptive parent to be a specified number of years older than the child. There may also be state requirements concerning residency, or the marital state of the prospective parent. Any adult who wishes to adopt will need to check state law before proceeding, and if potential adoptive parents use an adoption agency, they will also have to meet any agency requirements.

Some single individuals or couples may have a more difficult time qualifying as adoptive parents than others. For example, single men, gay singles, and homosexual couples may not specifically be prevented from adopting by state law, but they may have a more difficult time meeting state and agency requirements than married couples would. All states strive to find placements that meet the best interest of the child, so in some cases potential adoptive parents may be asked additional questions about lifestyle and why they want to adopt. (See below for a more thorough explanation of "best interest of the child.")

Generally, couples can adopt a child of a different race. Adoptions of Native American children, however, are governed by the Indian Child Welfare Act, and the act's provisions outline specific rules and procedures that must be followed if the adoption of a Native American child is to be approved.

There are several different types of adoptions, depending upon services used and whether or not a blood or marital relationship exists between adoptive parents and children

▮ Agency adoptions occur when state-licensed and/or state-regulated public or private adoption agencies place children with adoptive parents. Charities or religious or social service organizations often operate private agencies. Adoption agencies usually place those children who have been orphaned or whose parents have lost or relinquished parental rights through abuse, abandonment, or inability to support.

▮ Independent or private adoptions are arranged without the involvement of adoption agencies. Potential adoptive parents may hear of a mother who wants to give up her child, or they may advertise in newspapers or on the Internet to find such a mother. At some point in the process, an attorney must be involved to ensure the legality of the adoption. A few states prohibit independent adoptions. In those states where independent adoptions are allowed, they are usually strictly regulated.

▮ Identified adoptions are those in which adopting parents locate a birth mother, or vice versa, and then ask an agency to take over the adoption process. Prospective parents who find a birth mother willing to give up her child can bypass the long waiting lists that most agencies maintain for adoptions and can perhaps be better assured that the adoption will proceed in an orderly and legal fashion.

▮ International adoptions occur when couples adopt children who are citizens of foreign countries. In these procedures, adoptive parents must not only meet requirements of the foreign country where the child resides; they must also meet all U.S. state requirements and U.S. Immigration and Naturalization Service rules for international adoptions.

■ Relative adoptions are those in which the child is related to the adoptive parent by blood or marriage. Stepparent and grandparent/grandchildren adoptions fall within this category.

RIGHTS OF CHILDREN

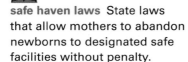

parens patriae A legal doctrine that gives the state the authority to act in a child's best interest.

Common law has established the rights of parents to make health care decisions for minor children. In some circumstances, under the doctrine of **parens patriae,** the state may act as the parental authority. This doctrine is the legal principle that grants the state the broad authority to act in the child's *best interest. Parenspatriae*—literally, "father of the people"—in practice the doctrine allows the state to override parental decisions alleged to go against the best interests of children. It also allows the state to remove abused or neglected children from the custody of offending parents.

Best Interest of the Child Concept

When alternatives are available for child placement or for determining medical treatment for minor children, the common standard is the "best interest of the child." In other words, which alternative will best safeguard the child's growth, development, and health? This standard is used in child placement situations. It is also used when legal authorities must work with health care practitioners to determine the least harmful and most appropriate treatment for an ailing child.

Rights of the Newborn

Legally, the legal rights of newborns are the same as those of any other American citizen of any age. For severely disabled newborns, however, existing law provides for several treatment options. Under the federal Child Abuse Amendments (U.S. Code, Title 42, Section 5106g), if the parents agree, physicians may legally withhold treatment, including food and water, from infants who

■ Are chronically and irreversibly comatose.

■ Will most certainly die and for whom treatment is considered futile.

■ Would suffer inhumanely if treatment were provided.

Treatment of severely disabled newborns raises many ethical questions. Should the federal government intrude into physicians' and parents' decisions with imposed regulations? Is it ever in an infant's "best interest" to die, or should medical treatment be administered regardless of the probable outcome? Is quality of life an issue that can ethically be considered? Who should decide among treatment options for disabled newborns if the parents are unwilling or unable to make such decisions?

Abandoned Infants

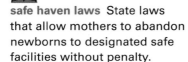

safe haven laws State laws that allow mothers to abandon newborns to designated safe facilities without penalty.

Throughout the 1990s, newborn babies abandoned and left to die in dumpsters, public bathrooms, and other locations led to legislation allowing a parent to abandon a newborn at a safe location without legal prosecution or with reduced legal prosecution. By 2008, 46 states had enacted such **safe haven laws,** allowing abandonment at a fire station, police station, or hospital. State laws vary greatly:

- In some states, the baby can be handed to a doctor or police officer, or left at a fire station or hospital.
- Some states allow either reduction or elimination of prosecution.
- In some states, the parent can remain anonymous, while in others he or she must reveal identity and give a medical history. In some states, medical histories can also be dropped off anonymously.
- Some states place a limit on the age of a baby that can be abandoned. This is to encourage a parent to abandon the baby early, so it can receive adequate nutrition and medical care, rather than hiding the baby and letting it become malnourished or otherwise unhealthy.
- Nebraska is one state that did not specify that its safe haven law, passed in July 2008, applied to infants only, and within a short time 16 children, including teenagers, had been abandoned to the care of the state. Nebraska legislators considered a special session to change the word "child" in the state's safe haven law to "infant."

(See www.childwelfare.gov/systemwide/laws_policies/statutes/safehavenall. pdf for state-specific information about safe haven laws.)

Reports by the National Conference of State Legislatures and the national Evan B. Donaldson Adoption Institute indicate that the problem of abandonment of newborns has not been resolved and that, in fact, the laws have caused some undesirable results:

- The "no hassle" provisions discourage mothers from using established adoption and child welfare policies, while encouraging irresponsible and destructive behavior.

CHECK YOUR PROGRESS

10. Define *infertility*.

_____

11. List and define three medical procedures that might be available to infertile couples.

_____

_____

_____

12. Adoptions are regulated primarily by

_____.

13. Name four types of adoptions.

_____

_____

14. Under existing Child Abuse Amendments, physicians may, with the consent of parents, withhold treatment for those infants who

_____

_____

_____

15. What are "safe haven" laws designed to prevent?

_____

- The laws seem to some to be government statements that it's OK to abandon a baby.
- The abandoned children have little hope of learning family medical histories.
- The laws allow one parent to abandon a child, thus stripping the other parent of all rights.

The issue of abandonment also raises many ethical questions for society and for health care practitioners. Is the "safe haven" concept ethical, since prosecution is usually waived for parental abandonment—a form of child abuse and neglect? Should abandoned infants be eventually returned to the parent(s) who abandoned them, or should such parents be forced to relinquish parental rights? What public health measures might help prevent such events from occurring?

Teenagers

While common law has dictated that parents have a right to decide what medical care their young children receive, laws for newborns differ from those for older children. For example, states recognize that some older minors have the capacity to consent to their own medical care. For instance, teenagers considered mature or emancipated minors may give consent for medical treatment.

Mature minors are individuals in their mid- to late teens who are considered mature enough to comprehend a physician's recommendations and give informed consent. Most states allow mature minors to seek medical treatment without the consent of a parent or guardian in certain critical areas, such as mental health, drug and/or alcohol addiction, treatment for sexually transmitted diseases, pregnancy, and contraceptive services.

Emancipated minors legally live outside of their parents' or guardians' control. A judge may issue an emancipation order at the request of parents or a minor child after certain important factors have been considered:

- Does the minor live at home with parents or other supervising adults, or is he or she living independently? If living at home, does he or she pay for room and board?
- Does the minor have a job, and does he or she spend his or her earnings without parental supervision?
- Does the minor pay his or her own debts?
- Is the minor claimed as a dependent on the parents' tax return?

The court may declare minors emancipated if one or more of the following criteria are met:

- They are self-supporting.
- They are married, provided the marriage is legal. In most states, persons must be at least 16 to marry and those under the age of 18 must have parental consent. Emancipation is not forfeited if the minor divorces or is separated or widowed.
- They are serving in the armed forces.

Emancipated minors do not usually gain all the rights of adults. Some limits, such as the legal age for purchasing alcohol or tobacco products, voting age, mandatory school attendance age (unless married), and other legal age restrictions, still apply.

mature minors Individuals in their mid- to late teens who, for health care purposes, are considered mature enough to comprehend a physician's recommendations and give informed consent.

emancipated minors Individuals in their mid- to late teens who legally live outside of parents' or guardians' control.

Minors have the same constitutional rights as adults, including the right to privacy. This is especially relevant for the increasing numbers of adolescents in the United States who are sexually active. Many hesitate to seek birth control or family planning counseling if they must inform or seek consent from their parents.

No state explicitly requires parental involvement for a minor to obtain any of the services listed above. In some states, however, laws leave the decision about whether or not to inform parents that minor sons and daughters have received or are seeking contraceptives, prenatal care, or STD services to the discretion of the treating physician, based on the best interest of the minor.

In addition to the ability to consent to these specific services, laws in some states give minors the right to consent to general medical and surgical care under some circumstances, such as being a parent themselves, being pregnant, or reaching a certain age.

Several states also allow minors who are parents to consent to medical care for their children. In many states, mothers who are minors may also legally place their children for adoption without the consent or knowledge of the mothers' parents.

In many states, minors seeking an abortion must involve at least one parent in the decision. This means that teenagers who do not tell their parents about a pregnancy must either travel out of state or obtain approval from a judge—a process known as *judicial bypass*—in order to obtain an abortion. Currently, the trend is toward state and federal legislation making it increasingly difficult for minors to obtain an abortion without parental involvement.

For exact legal restrictions regarding minors, health care practitioners should check statutes in the states where they practice.

In certain cases, the legal right of a minor to decline medical treatment has been upheld.

CHECK YOUR PROGRESS

16. Define the term *mature minor*.

_____

_____

17. Name three criteria that may be considered to determine if a minor is to be declared *emancipated*.

_____

_____

_____

18. What effect do the above designations have upon a minor's health care decisions?

_____

_____

19. In what treatment areas are minors most likely to make their own health care decisions?

_____

_____

Court Case

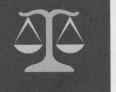

Judge Rules That Minor May Consent to Her Own Medical Treatment

Nancy, a 17-year-old Kansas girl, gave permission for a doctor to transplant some skin from her wrist to her finger. Her mother later sued on Nancy's behalf, on the grounds that Nancy was a minor.

Nancy's mother had been hospitalized for major surgery. After the operation, Nancy accompanied her mother to her hospital room. A nurse asked Nancy to wait in the hallway. She didn't notice that Nancy's hand was resting on the wall near the door jamb, with her right ring finger in the space between the door and the jamb. As the nurse closed the door, Nancy cried out in pain. The door had closed on her finger, severing the tip.

Nancy was taken to the emergency room, where a doctor decided to graft a small piece of skin from Nancy's wrist over the raw tip of her finger. Nancy's mother was still recovering from her surgery, and it would be hours before she could give consent for her daughter's treatment. Nancy's parents were divorced, and her father lived in another city. To spare Nancy a long, uncomfortable wait, the emergency room physician called the girl's family physician and received his agreement that he should treat Nancy.

When Nancy's mother recovered, she sued the hospital, claiming that the nurse had been negligent in causing her daughter's injury and that the doctor had not obtained proper consent to treat her minor daughter.

The nurse was not found negligent. Regarding the question of consent, the Kansas Supreme Court ruled that Nancy "was of sufficient age and maturity to know and understand the nature and consequences of the 'pinch graft' utilized in the repair of her finger."

Younts v. St. Francis Hosp. and School of Nursing, 205 Kan. 292, 469 P.2d 330, 338 (1970).

Court Case

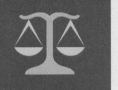

Minor Says No to Surgery

Believing they were acting in the best interests of a minor, a county health department in New York State tried to obtain the court's permission to seek surgery for a 14-year-old boy who had a cleft palate and upper lip.

The boy's father would not consent to surgery for his son because he believed that forces in the universe would heal all ailments. Influenced by his father, the boy refused the offer of surgery for his condition.

The court ruled that the boy could not be forced to have surgery. He could turn down the procedure, because his cooperation would be needed for the speech therapy that would follow. A majority of the judges saw less harm in letting him wait until he was an adult and could make the choice for himself than in pursuing surgery.

In the Matter of S., 309 N.Y. 80, 127 N.E. 2d 820 (1955).

Ethics Issues   The Beginning of Life and Childhood

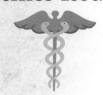

ETHICS ISSUE 1: Reproductive science has progressed so rapidly that laws have not kept pace. For example, in 1996, a couple lost their adult, single daughter, Julie, to leukemia. Before her death, Julie had paid a fertility clinic to harvest and freeze several of her eggs. When Julie died, her parents inherited the frozen eggs, along with Julie's furniture and other material possessions. Julie's parents then paid a surrogate mother to carry one of Julie's implanted eggs, fertilized by a sperm donor. Julie's parents did not plan to raise their grandchild themselves.

"This field [reproductive medicine] is screaming for oversight, regulation and control," Arthur Caplan, director of the Center for Bioethics at the University of Pennsylvania, told *The Washington Post* in 1998 when asked about the above scenario. "If you are going to make babies in new and novel ways, you have to be sure it's in the interest of the baby."

DISCUSSION QUESTIONS

1. Although no laws prevented the parents in the above situation from paying a surrogate mother to carry one of their deceased daughter's fertilized eggs, in your opinion, did they act ethically? Why or why not? What values are involved in your answer?

_____

_____

2. In your opinion, how should the child's parents have been determined in the above scenario? (The surrogate mother miscarried.)

_____

_____

According to the American Academy of Pediatrics, health care practitioners and parents should share the responsibility for decision making involving the medical care of young patients. Practitioners should seek the informed permission of parents before medical interventions (except in emergencies when parents cannot be contacted), and the informed permission of parents should include all of the elements of standard informed consent.

However, the Academy acknowledges that in our pluralistic society, the many religious, social, cultural, and philosophical positions on what constitutes acceptable child rearing and child welfare often makes this shared decision making difficult. The law generally provides parents with wide discretionary authority in raising their children, but health care practitioners know that parents are sometimes guilty of child abuse and neglect. Therefore, providers of health care services to children have to carefully balance the rights of their young patients with the family's rights to raise their children as they see fit.

ETHICS ISSUE 2: At four, Bobby had had two bone marrow transplants to treat a genetic metabolic disorder called Hurler syndrome. Back in the hospital, his kidneys were failing, and his body was painfully swollen from an accumulation of fluids. Steroids had turned the boy's skin bright pink, and multisystem organ failure required the use of machines to keep him somewhat stable. Clearly, aggressive medical care was keeping Bobby alive. Bobby's mother proudly remarked often that he was "a fighter."

DISCUSSION QUESTIONS

1. In your opinion, does Bobby have the right to be taken off the machines that are keeping him alive? Explain your answer.

_____

_____

2. If the parents seem unable to make the decision to take Bobby off the life-sustaining machines, what would you do, as a health care practitioner involved in Bobby's care?

_____

_____

3. The hospital ethics advisor who consulted in the above case said of Bobby, "It's an example of a child's basic interests being held hostage. What were they [the parents] hoping for? [Bobby] had given it all he had." Do you agree or disagree with the ethics advisor's remarks? Explain your answer.

_____

_____

4. Above all, what should health care practitioners bear in mind when treating children?

_____

_____

Minors should be strongly encouraged to discuss pregnancies with parents. Health care practitioners should know the law in their states on parental involvement to ensure that procedures are consistent with legal obligations. Health care practitioners can explain how parental involvement may be helpful and that most parents are understanding and supportive. When a minor seems especially concerned about involving parents, health care practitioners should determine whether or not the minor's reluctance is due to misperceptions about the consequences of parental involvement.

Health care practitioners should not feel compelled to require minors to involve their parents. Minors should be encouraged to seek the counsel of those adults they trust, if parents are not going to be involved.

ETHICS ISSUE 3. Your neighbor's daughter, who is 16, has made an appointment to see a physician in the clinic where you work as a medical assistant. You have assisted the physician with the examination of the girl, and he has determined that she is pregnant.

DISCUSSION QUESTIONS

1. The patient's mother telephones you at home, demanding to know why her daughter saw the physician. What do you tell her?

_____

_____

2. When the patient learns she is pregnant, she tearfully requests information about an abortion. What are you and the girl's physician allowed to tell her—both legally and ethically? Based on your personal values, what would you tell the girl?

_____

_____

Go to www.mhhe.com/judson5e to practice your case review skills. Then read on for more information.

Applying Knowledge

Answer the following questions in the spaces provided.

1. Define *genetics.*

_____

2. Define *DNA.*

_____

3. List three situations in which DNA testing might be indicated.

_____

_____

_____

4. Name two federal laws that help prevent genetic discrimination in employment and among health insurers.

_____

_____

5. Name two goals of the Human Genome Project.

_____

_____

Match the following definitions with the terms they define:

_____6. An experimental treatment for hereditary diseases.

_____7. A procedure used to reveal the presence of a disease-causing gene or genes.

_____8. The manipulation of DNA to produce desired results in organisms.

_____9. A person's being treated differently than others because of his or her genetic makeup.

a. genetic discrimination

b. gene therapy

c. genetic engineering

d. genetic testing

10. Define cloning.

_____

11. Define xenotransplantation.

_____

12. Cloning is a form of

_____

13. Why, in your opinion, do many people object to the prospect of cloning?

_____

_____

14. Explain why stem cells are valued for certain types of scientific research.

_____

_____

15. What is the purpose of "safe haven" laws?

_____

_____

Match the following terms with their correct definitions:

_____ **16.** The use of a husband's sperm to
fertilize his wife's eggs.

_____ **17.** An arrangement between an infertile couple and
a woman who agrees to carry their child to term.

_____ **18.** The union of eggs and sperm outside
of the body, in a test tube or petri dish.

_____ **19.** The mechanical injection of viable
semen into a woman's vagina.

_____ **20.** A surrogate arrangement in which the surrogate mother
is genetically related to the child she will carry.

_____ **21.** The use of a sperm donor to fertilize a woman's eggs.

_____ **22.** A surrogate arrangement in which the surrogate
mother is not genetically related to the child she will carry.

a. homologous artificial
insemination

b. traditional surrogacy

c. artificial insemination

d. heterologous artificial
insemination

e. gestational surrogacy

f. in vitro fertilization

g. surrogacy

23. Define the doctrine of *parens patriae*.

_____

24. *Parens patriae* is the basis for the _____ consideration.

25. Federal regulations concerning severely disabled newborns take their authority from which federal
regulation?

_____

_____

26. Teenagers classified as _____ or _____ can
generally make their own health care decisions.

27. A physician or other health care practitioner who treats a minor without parental consent risks being
charged with _____.

Case Study

Use your critical-thinking skills to answer the questions that follow each of the case studies.

In 1984 John Moore, an Alaskan businessman, was treated at the University of California at Los Angeles (UCLA) for a rare cancer. During his treatment, a doctor and researcher discovered that tissue from Moore's spleen produced a blood protein that encourages the growth of cancer-fighting white blood cells.

Without Moore's knowledge or consent, university scientists created a cell line from his tissue. They obtained a patent on their invention, which was estimated to be worth about $3 billion in potential profits. Moore later learned that his tissue had been used in this way, and he sued UCLA, claiming that only he could own his tissue. The California Supreme Court ruled against Moore in 1990, saying that he had no property right over his own body tissues. This court's decision paved the way for other researchers to patent genes and tissues.

Since Moore's suit, some states have passed laws defining DNA ownership. For example, a 1995 Oregon law declared that a person owned his or her DNA and that of any children. In 2001, however, Oregon legislators reversed the 1995 law, holding that genetic information would no longer be considered private property once it was separated from a person's identity through encryption or anonymous research.

28. In your opinion, should genes be considered private property? Why or why not?

_____

_____

29. Should individuals receive payment if they turn over ownership of genes to researchers? Why or why not?

_____

_____

30. Should scientists or drug companies be allowed to patent genes as they do other discoveries and inventions? Why or why not?

_____

_____

As reproductive technology advanced, headlines announcing "Couple Battles over Frozen Embryos" became more and more commonplace. For example, in the 1980s a man went to court and succeeded in preventing his ex-wife from using their frozen embryos to become pregnant. He maintained that after he and his wife had divorced, he no longer wanted to become a parent, and should not be forced to do so against his will.

In 1998, a divorced woman in New Jersey won a legal battle with her ex-husband over custody of seven frozen embryos the couple had created in vitro while still married. The wife wanted to have the embryos destroyed, while the ex-husband argued his right to adopt his own embryos to be implanted in a future partner or donated to an infertile couple.

31. In your opinion, should frozen embryos be considered property to be awarded during a divorce? Why or why not?

_____

_____

32. Should a man who loses custody of frozen embryos in a lawsuit be responsible for child support if his ex-wife is implanted with the embryos and becomes pregnant at a later date? Explain your answer.

_____

_____

33. Should the husband or wife who wins custody of frozen embryos be allowed to destroy them, against the wishes of the ex-husband or ex-wife? Why or why not?

_____

_____

Internet Activities

Complete the activities and answer the questions that follow.

34. Visit the Web site for the Human Genome Project at www.ornl.gov/sci/techresources/Human_Genome/project/about.shtml. What are three of the medical applications expected to result from the project or presently in use as a result of the project?

_____

_____

_____

35. Visit the patients' Web site for the American Society for Reproductive Medicine (ASRM) at www.asrm.org/Patients/mainpati.html. Under "Frequently Asked Questions" (FAQ), how does the ASRM define *infertility*? List two other frequently asked questions and their answers.

_____

_____

_____

36. Visit the Planned Parenthood Federation of America's Web site for teens at www.teenwire.com. Briefly summarize the topics available there. In your opinion, does the site promote valid health care issues? Why or why not? The site is controversial. Comment on why you think this is so.

_____

_____

Death and Dying

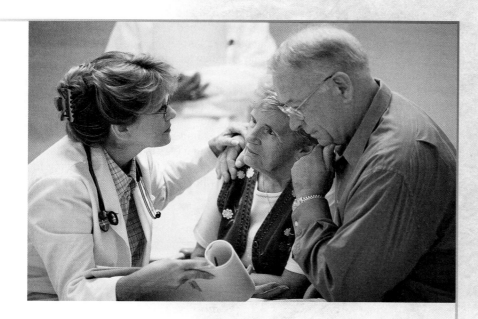

Learning Outcomes

After studying this chapter, you should be able to:

1. Discuss accepted criteria for determining death.

2. Determine the health care professional's role in caring for the dying.

3. Explain differences between a living will, a health care proxy, and durable power of attorney.

4. Discuss the various stages of grief.

5. Begin to form a knowledge base for assisting dying patients and their family members through the grieving process, as well as forming a personal philosophy concerning death and dying.

6. Identify the major features of organ donation in the United States.

Key Terms

active euthanasia

brain death

coma

curative care

durable power of attorney

health care proxy

hospice

involuntary euthanasia

living will

National Organ Transplant Act

palliative care

passive euthanasia

Patient Self-Determination Act

persistent vegetative state (PVS)

terminally ill

thanatology

Uniform Anatomical Gift Act

Uniform Determination of Death Act

Uniform Rights of the Terminally Ill Act

voluntary euthanasia

Voice of Experience
Nurse Tends Dying Patients

Angela has been a registered nurse for 14 years. Just as some hospital nurses are drawn to surgery, the emergency room, or the intensive care unit, Angela prefers hospice and palliative care. "Broadly speaking," Angela explains, "medicine is about repairing, extending, and medicating, while end-of-life care is more about the patient as an individual, about basic human needs. In addition, it isn't just the patient you are caring for; you are caring for the entire family group—everybody needs you.

"We live in a time when death has been removed from family and home for the most part," Angela continues, "and people generally have less understanding of the process than a hundred years ago.... The family most often feels helpless and confused. The hospice nurse is able to help not just the patient, but the family, too, through a sad and often frightening time."

Sometimes family members are hesitant about approaching a dying loved one. For example, Angela remembers a situation where the mother of two siblings in their 30s was dying. "When I arrived they were practically plastered against the walls of the room, clearly unsure of what they should be doing." Angela encouraged the two family members to come to their mother's bedside and comfort her. "The son pulled a chair to the side of the bed and held his mother's hand. The daughter climbed onto the bed and cradled her mother.... I like to think that because I urged them to take a more active part in her passing that they found comfort after their mother was gone."

Angela also recalls a patient in his 80s whose 32 family members joined him in his hospice room. "It was almost a living wake. They talked for hours about his life and the experiences they had each shared with him. They laughed and they cried and it was wonderful. This sharing in their loved one's death was a beautiful experience for those left behind, and I hope it helped him in some way as well."

ATTITUDES TOWARD DEATH AND DYING

Prior to the twentieth century, death was an intimate experience for most families. Antibiotics and chemotherapies had not yet been discovered; genetically engineered drugs, organ transplantation, and life-support machines were still science fiction; and infectious diseases periodically decimated populations. Nearly every husband and wife, mother and father, brother and sister had lost a loved one. Loved ones customarily died at home, surrounded by family members who bade them good-bye and then mourned their passing with funeral rituals and rites, including the following:

- Black has long been worn by undertakers, mourners, and pallbearers to show grief. In ancient times it was also used as a disguise to protect against malevolent spirits that might be lurking nearby.

- An early custom for mourners was to go barefoot and to wear sackcloth and ashes. This was said to discourage the dead from becoming envious as they might be if mourners appeared at funerals wearing new clothes and shoes.

- Pagan tribes began the custom of covering the face of the deceased with a sheet, since they believed that the spirit of the deceased escaped through the mouth. They often held the mouth and nose of a sick person shut, hoping to retain the spirit and thus delay death.

- In earlier times, traffic was halted for a funeral procession because any delay in transporting a soul might turn it into a restless ghost, reluctant to pass over into the next world.

- Wakes held today come from the ancient custom of keeping watch over the deceased, hoping that life would return. In England the dead were always carried out of the house feet first; otherwise, their spirits might look back into the house and beckon family members to come with them.

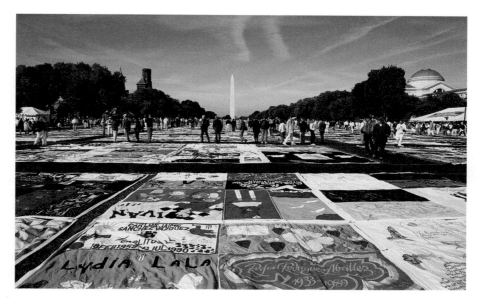

FIGURE 11-1   Individuals around the United States contributed to the AIDS memorial quilt, shown here in Washington, DC.

- Pagan beliefs concerning funeral wreaths held that the circle formed by the wreath would keep the dead person's spirit within bounds.
- The firing of a rifle volley over the deceased is similar to the tribal practice of throwing spears into the air to ward off spirits hovering over the deceased.
- In the past, holy water was sprinkled on the body to protect it from demons.

By the late twentieth century, individuals were more likely to die in the hospital, at least in the Western world. Once admitted to hospitals, the dying were isolated from family members and surrounded by machines designed to prolong life as long as possible. Consequently, modern technology has effectively hidden death from view, but in so doing it has also made the end of life a fearful prospect.

Attitudes toward death and dying vary with individuals, of course, but as each of us ages, we will likely begin to think of our own mortality and perhaps to wonder how the end will come. Will I die alone, in an impersonal, clinical hospital environment? Will my health care providers be so committed to preserving life that they prolong my dying to an irrational degree? Will I suffer in pain? Will I feel a sense of tasks left unfinished and goals left unrealized, or will I experience a peaceful letting go?

Because the fears associated with death and dying are universal, health care practitioners should evaluate their own attitudes in order to effectively and compassionately respond to dying patients and their families (Figure 11-1).

DETERMINATION OF DEATH

Uniform Determination of Death Act A proposal that established uniform guidelines for determining when death has occurred.

Modern medical technology and life-support equipment may keep a person's body "alive"—the heart may beat and blood may circulate—long after the brain ceases to function. This makes it difficult in some cases to determine the moment when death actually occurs. For this reason, in 1981 a **Uniform Determination of Death Act** was proposed by the President's Commission for the Study of Ethical Problems in Medicine and Biomedical

brain death Final cessation of bodily activity, used to determine when death actually occurs; circulatory and respiratory functions have irreversibly ceased, and the entire brain (including the brain stem) has irreversibly ceased to function.

coma A condition of deep stupor from which the patient cannot be roused by external stimuli.

persistent vegetative state (PVS) Severe mental impairment characterized by irreversible cessation of the higher functions of the brain, most often caused by damage to the cerebral cortex.

Research working in cooperation with the American Bar Association, the American Medical Association, and the National Conference of Commissioners on Uniform State Laws. The National Conference of Commissioners on Uniform State Laws has no legislative authority. Acts the commissioners propose must still be approved by state legislatures, and that is sometimes difficult to accomplish. States have their own criteria for determining when death actually occurs, but most have adopted the act's definition of **brain death** as a means of determining when death actually occurs:

- Circulatory and respiratory functions have irreversibly ceased.
- The entire brain, including the brain stem, has irreversibly ceased to function.

When the brain is injured or shuts down due to lack of oxygen, a patient may appear near death when, in fact, he or she is in a **coma,** which is a condition of deep stupor from which a patient cannot be roused by external stimuli. Patients can and do recover from comas, as opposed to a persistent vegetative state. **Persistent vegetative state (PVS)** exists as a result of severe mental impairment, characterized by irreversible cessation of the higher functions of the brain, most often caused by damage to the cerebral cortex. In PVS, only involuntary bodily functions are present, and there exists no reasonable expectation of regaining significant mental function.

Before pronouncing an unresponsive and unconscious patient dead, physicians may perform a series of tests to determine whether death has occurred. Death is indicated if the following signs are present. The patient

- Cannot breathe without assistance.
- Has no coughing or gagging reflex.
- Has no pupil response to light.
- Has no blinking reflex when the cornea is touched.
- Has no grimace reflex when the head is rotated or ears are flushed with ice water.
- Has no response to pain.

Today the declaration of death occurs only when the last signs of brain and respiratory activity are gone. Technically, death results from lack of oxygen. When deprived of oxygen, cells cannot maintain metabolic function and soon begin to deteriorate.

Autopsies

After a patient is declared dead, family members (next of kin) may be asked to consent to an autopsy. An autopsy is a postmortem examination to determine cause of death and/or to obtain physiological evidence when necessary. Autopsies performed in hospitals may confirm or correct clinical diagnoses, thus providing a measure of quality assurance. Autopsy results can also highlight those cases in which diagnoses tend to be incorrect, or treatments tend to be ineffective, thereby adding to scientific knowledge and revealing areas that need further study. In cases of suspicious deaths, autopsy results can provide information to help law enforcement authorities, such as cause and time of death. (Legal requirements concerning autopsies are discussed in Chapter 8.)

While autopsies must be performed in cases in which the death is suspicious or due to homicide, the number of autopsies performed in all other deaths each year has steadily declined. One reason that fewer autopsies are performed today is cost—insurance companies and government health care

1. Briefly explain how attitudes toward death and dying in the United States have changed over the years.

_____

_____

2. The _____,
while not a law, was proposed as a universal means of determining when death actually occurs.

3. Distinguish between *comatose* and *persistent vegetative state*.

_____

_____

4. Define *brain death*.

_____

_____

5. Name six signs for which physicians may test that indicate death has occurred.

_____ _____

_____ _____

_____ _____

programs usually do not pay for autopsies. (However, when patients die in hospitals, often an autopsy can be performed free of charge.) Some clinicians argue that technological advances have made clinical diagnoses more accurate, so that postmortem diagnoses are less essential. Another reason for the decline in autopsies is that in many smaller hospitals, pathologists are not readily available.

Furthermore, even though autopsies can yield information that may clarify causes of death, reveal genetic disease that runs in families, or reassure survivors that their loved ones could not have been saved, when an autopsy is not mandated by law, family members are often reluctant to give consent. They may feel that their loved one has "suffered enough," that the physician already knows the cause of death, or that the procedure would interfere with viewing of the body during funeral rites. Health care practitioners may believe that these perceptions of autopsies are inaccurate, but they must remain sensitive to the beliefs and emotions of surviving family members.

TEACHING HEALTH CARE PRACTITIONERS TO CARE FOR DYING PATIENTS

terminally ill Referring to patients who are expected to die within six months.

While modern medicine has effectively prolonged the moment of death, in many cases it has dealt less conscientiously with compassionate, comfort care for **terminally ill** patients: those who are not expected to live beyond six months, usually because of a chronic illness that has progressed beyond effective treatment or for which there is no cure.

Studies published within the last two decades have shown the need for educating health care practitioners in end-of-life care:

■ A 1995 study published in the *Journal of the American Medical Association* (JAMA) found that nearly 4 out of every 10 terminally ill patients spend at least 10 days in intensive care connected to life-sustaining machines. The same study found that half of patients who die in hospitals experience moderate to severe pain.

■ In November 1996, the Robert Wood Johnson Foundation published results of the largest study ever conducted on patients near death. The six-year Study to Understand Prognoses and Preferences for Outcomes and Risks of Treatment (SUPPORT) showed that more than 50 percent of people dying in hospitals suffered from uncontrolled pain, and that decisions to medicate were inappropriately timed. The study of 9,100 hospitalized patients also showed that most physicians did not know their patients' end-of-life wishes or did not follow them, and that half of those patients who were conscious during the last three days of life died in pain.

■ A survey by the Association of American Medical Colleges in 1998 found that 122 medical schools (96.1 percent) included information about death and dying as part of an existing course, but just 6 schools (4.7 percent) featured the subject as a separate required course. Fifty schools (39.4 percent) offered a course in death and dying as an elective.

■ A survey of medical textbooks, published in the February 9, 2001, issue of the *Journal of American Medicine* (JAMA) showed that most "don't deal with the end of life," according to the article's lead author, Michael Rabow of the University of California at San Francisco medical school. Of the 50 top-selling textbooks that were reviewed, 56.9 percent did not discuss end-of-life care at all. The remaining books either covered the topic minimally (19.1 percent) or did include some helpful information on end-of-life care (24.1 percent).

■ A report by the National Research Council and the Institute of Medicine issued in June 2001 states that U.S. physicians and hospitals are not prepared to handle the suffering of dying cancer patients. The report, *Improving Palliative Care for Cancer: Summary and Recommendations,* says that federal research and training efforts have focused largely on treatment and finding cures, while neglecting symptom control measures that could relieve a patient's suffering.

■ In 2001, the American Medical Association (AMA), an organization for physicians, first implemented a program called Education for Physicians on End of Life Care (EPEC). The project, now funded by Northwestern University Medical School, is designed to educate all health care practitioners on the essential clinical competencies required to provide quality end-of-life care.

■ In 2004, the American Medical Students Association (AMSA) formed a death and dying interest group, in response to medical students' consensus that medical school leaves students inadequately prepared to communicate with terminally ill patients, as well as poorly equipped emotionally to deal with matters of death and dying. The AMSA interest group continues to provide guidance, support, and resources for students who wish to supplement their medical education in the area of death and dying.

Fortunately, the need to teach end-of-life care to physicians and other health care practitioners has been recognized. Increasingly, schools that train health care providers are offering courses in **thanatology**—the study of death and of the psychological methods of coping with death. In addition, many organizations exist that list their primary mission as advocacy

thanatology The study of death and of the psychological methods of coping with it.

for improved care for the dying and educating health professionals and the public about end-of-life issues. A sampling of such groups includes Americans for Better Care of the Dying (ABCD) (www.abcd-caring.org/), Compassion & Choices (www.compassionandchoices.org/), Finding Our Way (FOW) (www.findingourway.net/), Partnership for Caring (www. partnershipforcaring.com/), Growth House (www.growthhouse.org/), and the American Institute of Life-Threatening Illness and Loss (www.lifethreat. org). An Internet search titled "death and dying" will provide URLs for many more organizations. Many of these organizations provide living will and medical power of attorney forms, and all provide useful information to the public. Some routinely file *amicus curiae* (friend of the court) briefs in legal cases addressing end-of-life issues. Others are engaged in research, public advocacy, and education activities to improve the care of the dying and their families.

Despite a conscious effort to improve training and attitudes regarding dying patients, end-of-life care remains one of the most emotional issues for health care practitioners.

THE RIGHT TO DIE MOVEMENT

Americans have long been concerned that advancing medical technology may allow health care practitioners to prolong death beyond the point where any quality of life can be maintained or a cure realized, thus depriving individuals of the right to die as they wish. This concern led to the first living will, created and made available to the public by attorney Luis Kutner, who founded the Euthanasia Society. Kutner's goal was to help dying people exercise their rights to control end-of-life medical care.

The right to die first became a matter for the courts to deliberate in 1976, with the death of Karen Ann Quinlan.

The Quinlan case raised important questions in bioethics, euthanasia, and the legal rights of guardians. The case resulted in the development of formal ethics committees in hospitals, long-term care facilities, and hospices. It also called attention to the need for advance health directives.

Another landmark case in the right to die movement involved a 26-year-old woman who was severely injured in a car crash.

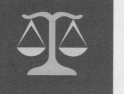

CLASSIC
Court Case

Right to Die Precedent

In 1976, the parents of Karen Ann Quinlan, then 22, obtained permission from a New Jersey court to remove their daughter from a respirator. Karen Ann had been in a persistent vegetative state for several months, after allegedly ingesting an unknown combination of alcohol and drugs. Karen Ann's father, as her legal guardian, had asked her physicians to remove the respirator believed to be sustaining her life. The physicians refused, and the Quinlans sued for their daughter's right to die. A lower court held for the physicians, but on appeal, judges allowed Karen Ann's respirator to be disconnected. She continued to live via a feeding tube, but died in June 1985 of pneumonia, at the age of 31.

In re Quinlan, 70 N.J. 10, 49, 355 A.2d 647, 668 (1976).

Court Case

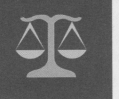

Legal Struggle to Remove Feeding Tube

On January 11, 1983, Nancy Beth Cruzan was driving alone when she lost control of her older model car that had no seat belts. Nancy was thrown from the car and landed face down in a water-filled ditch. When emergency medical technicians arrived Nancy had no vital signs, but the EMTs resuscitated her. After about two weeks Nancy had not awakened and her condition was diagnosed as persistent vegetative state, following irreversible brain damage. Physicians inserted a feeding tube for Nancy's long-term care.

After four years with no improvement, Nancy's parents asked to have the feeding tube removed. The hospital demanded a court order, and a three-year legal battle ensued. The trial court ruled that the feeding tube could be removed, based on testimony given by one of Nancy's friends that she would not want to live on artificial life support. The Missouri State Supreme Court reversed the trial court's ruling, holding that the lower court did not meet the *clear and convincing evidence* standard. The case reached the United States Supreme Court, where justices affirmed the Missouri State Supreme Court ruling and recognized that the right to refuse medical treatment is guaranteed by the U.S. Constitution. The case was sent back to the trial court, for the purpose of gathering clear and convincing evidence that Nancy Cruzan would not have wanted to live in a persistent vegetative state. Three of Nancy's friends testified as to her wishes, and the court ruled that this met the clear and convincing evidence standard, and that the feeding tube could be removed. This decision was also appealed, but the appeal failed to change the court's ruling, and Nancy's feeding tube was removed in December 1990. She died 11 days later.

Cruzan v. Director, Missouri Department of Health, 497 US 261 (1990).

While the above landmark legal cases furthered certain right-to-die arguments, other events in the nation's history have also furthered the cause. Here is a timeline:

- 1946—Committee of 1776 Physicians for Legalizing Voluntary Euthanasia is formed in New York State.
- 1967—Attorney Luis Kutner and members of the Euthanasia Society (later called Choice in Dying and then Partnership for Caring, both organizations now defunct) devise the original living will.
- 1973—American Hospital Association creates the Patient's Bill of Rights.
- 1976—California's Natural Death Act, the nation's first right-to-die statute, is signed into law.
- 1977—Laws dealing with the refusal of treatment are passed in Arkansas, Idaho, Nevada, New Mexico, North Carolina, Oregon, and Texas.
- 1984—The District of Columbia and 22 states have statutes that recognize advance directives.
- 1989—The **Uniform Rights of the Terminally Ill Act** serves as a guideline for state legislatures in constructing laws addressing advance directives.
- 1990—Congress passes the Patient Self-Determination Act, the first federal act concerning advance directives.
- 1992—Pennsylvania becomes the fiftieth state to enact advance-directive legislation.

Uniform Rights of the Terminally Ill Act A federal statute passed in 1989 to guide state legislatures in constructing laws to address advance directives.

- 1997—The U.S. Supreme Court holds that state bans on physician-assisted suicide do not violate the U.S. Constitution. The Court leaves the decision up to each state on whether to ban physician-assisted suicide.
- 1997—Oregon's Death With Dignity Act is passed, making the state the first to permit physician-assisted suicide in certain circumstances.
- 1997—By this date, 35 states have enacted statutes expressly criminalizing assisted suicide; 9 states criminalize assisted suicide through common law.
- 2001—The California Supreme Court clarifies the right to die in a decision that states the right to die does not extend to people who are conscious and in a twilight state, are unable to communicate or care for themselves, and have not left formal written directions for health care.
- 2001—Attorney General John Ashcroft issues a directive stating that a doctor could lose his or her federal registration to prescribe controlled substances if the registration were used to prescribe federally controlled substances for assisted suicide. The Justice Department is seeking a judgment that would leave the Death With Dignity Act in force, but would prohibit Oregon's physicians from prescribing controlled substances for the purpose of assisted suicide. Attorney General Ashcroft's petition for a rehearing is denied.

CLASSIC
Court Case

Right to Die or the Right to Live?

In 1990, 27-year-old Terri Schindler Schiavo suffered an apparent heart attack at her home in Florida. Emergency medical technicians restored a heartbeat, but Terri remained comatose at first, then later semi-comatose. Terri's husband, Michael Schiavo, was appointed her guardian, and she was placed in a long-term care facility, where she was finally diagnosed as being in a persistent vegetative state (PVS).

In 1992, Michael Schiavo sued Terri's physician for malpractice, and was awarded $600,000. Terri was awarded $1.4 million and $250,000 in separate medical malpractice trials.

In 1993, Michael Schiavo refused medically recommended rehabilitative therapy for Terri, and her parents intervened. Bob and Mary Schindler, Terri's parents, petitioned the court to remove Michael Schiavo as Terri's guardian. A judge denied the guardianship petition. In 1997, a judge approved Michael Schiavo's petition to remove the tubes delivering Terri's hydration and nutrition. Terri seemed semiconscious, and her parents insisted she might be successfully rehabilitated.

In 1998 the court appointed a guardian ad litem to investigate Terri's case. The guardian ad litem recommended against removing Terri's feeding tubes and was dismissed for bias. In 2001, the court ordered the feeding tubes removed, despite physicians' testimonials that Terri was not in a PVS and could swallow. Many physicians also testified that Terri was in a PVS. In April of that year, Terri's feeding tubes were removed, but in light of new evidence, a new judge ordered feeding restored.

Court battles continued, with Michael Schiavo petitioning the court to end Terri's life and her parents counterpetitioning to keep Terri alive. Finally, in October 2003, the Florida legislature passed a law—"Terri's Law"—allowing then Governor Jeb Bush to issue an executive order to let Terri continue to receive nutrition and hydration. The law was repealed in September 2004.

In March 2005, Terri's husband, Michael Schiavo, won court approval to have his wife's feeding tube removed. Terri died 13 days later, on March 31, 2005, after having been in an apparent persistent vegetative state for 15 years. An autopsy performed in June 2005 confirmed that Schiavo was in a persistent vegetative state.

The list of citations is impossibly long. A complete list is available at www.terrisfight.org

6. Define *terminally ill.*

_____

_____

7. Define *thanatology.*

_____

_____

8. How were decisions in the *Quinlan, Cruzan,* and *Shiavo* cases significant in the right-to-die movement?

_____

_____

_____

_____

EUTHANASIA AND PHYSICIAN-ASSISTED SUICIDE

active euthanasia A conscious medical act that results in the death of a dying person.

passive euthanasia The act of allowing a dying patient to die naturally, without medical interference.

voluntary euthanasia The act of ending a dying patient's life by medical means with his or her permission.

involuntary euthanasia The act of ending a terminal patient's life by medical means without his or her permission.

In the United States, debate has raged over whether or not physicians should play a state-sanctioned role in ending a patient's life. *Euthanasia,* which in Greek means "good death," refers to mercy killing of the hopelessly ill. Physicians may be involved in a variety of ways:

- **Active euthanasia** is a conscious medical act that results in the death of a dying person.
- **Passive euthanasia** is the act of allowing a patient to die naturally, without medical interference.
- **Voluntary euthanasia** requires the patient's consent, or that of his or her designated representative, to use medical means to end the patient's life.
- **Involuntary euthanasia** is the act of ending a patient's life by medical means without the consent of the patient or his or her representative.
- *Physician-assisted suicide* loosely refers to any of these euthanasia situations in which a doctor takes part in a patient's suicide.

Most states have laws against physician-assisted suicide, but many have been challenged in court. All states have some form of right-to-die law that allows patients to decide whether they want to receive medical treatment when they are no longer competent to make decisions. Physician-assisted suicide is legal in several countries, including Germany and the Netherlands.

In the United States, only Oregon has passed a law that allows physician-assisted suicide. Oregon's Death With Dignity Act was first passed in 1994. It did not go into effect until November 1997, however, when voters rejected an initiative to repeal the act by a 60 percent to 40 percent margin. The law was the first in the United States to permit physician-assisted suicide and in 2007 remained the only state law to legalize physician-assisted suicide.

Opponents to the Oregon law, including the National Right to Life organization, the federal Drug Enforcement Administration, and the Oregon Medical Association, have challenged the law. In January 2006 the United States Supreme Court upheld Oregon's Death With Dignity Act.

9. Define *euthanasia*.

_____

_____

10. How does passive euthanasia differ from active euthanasia? Is either process legal in the United States?

_____

_____

11. How does voluntary euthanasia differ from involuntary euthanasia? Is either process legal in the United States?

_____

_____

12. In your opinion, is Oregon's Death With Dignity Act ethical? Explain your answer.

_____

_____

There are many sides to the debate over physician-assisted suicide. Some advocates believe a person has the right to control his or her own life, including choosing to end it. Others see the question from a quality-of-life perspective. That is, when one suffers from an incurable, debilitating, and/or painful disease, he or she should have the right to end the suffering. Another group argues that physician-assisted suicide should be permissible only if a person is nearly brain-dead with no chance of recovery.

Those who argue against physician-assisted suicide also hold a variety of opinions. Some simply say that killing a human being is always wrong. Others cite the Hippocratic oath as evidence that physicians are always bound to protect life and, therefore, should not be asked to assist a suicide. Opponents also claim that the potential for abuse is too great. For example, if physician-assisted suicide is sanctioned, will relatives of wealthy patients advocate for their deaths? Does serious illness alter mental states so that these patients cannot be trusted to make such decisions rationally? Will quality-of-life issues take precedence in deciding who should take advantage of statues that regulate physician-assisted suicide?

The debate over physician-assisted suicide will continue for years to come, but until legal issues are settled, health care practitioners are reminded that, legally and ethically, they are bound to consider existing law and the welfare of patients.

CARING FOR DYING PATIENTS

palliative care Treatment of a terminally ill patient's symptoms in order to make dying more comfortable; also called comfort care.

When it becomes evident that a patient's disease is incurable and death is imminent, **palliative care** may serve the dying patient better than **curative care.** Curative care consists of treatments and procedures directed toward curing a patient's disease. Palliative care, also called comfort care, is directed toward providing relief to terminally ill patients through symptom and pain

curative care Treatment directed toward curing a patient's disease.

management. The goal is not to cure, but to provide comfort and maintain the highest possible quality of life. Going beyond relief of disease symptoms, palliative care includes relief of emotional distress and other problems, so that a patient's last months and days may be as comfortable as possible.

Traditionally, in educational programs for health care practitioners, courses of study have placed more emphasis on curative care than on palliative care. Treatments included in curative care include surgery, chemotherapy, radiation therapy, and other treatments and procedures, and may be used more aggressively as a patient's disease progresses. Since most physicians are taught to fight disease with every product and technique at their command, it is sometimes difficult for them to recognize or admit that curative care has failed or is no longer effective in treating a patient's disease. Through use of palliative care, health care providers can help relieve a dying patient's pain and emotional distress and ease the journey toward life's end.

Hospice Care

hospice A facility or program (often carried out in a patient's home) in which teams of health care practitioners and volunteers provide a continuing environment that focuses on the physical, emotional, and psychological needs of the dying patient.

Terminally ill patients are often referred to facilities or agencies that provide **hospice** care (Figure 11-2). A hospice in medieval times was a way station for travelers. The first modern hospice facilities were established in England in the 1960s as places where patients could go to die in comfort.

In the United States, hospice care may be provided in facilities built especially for that purpose, in hospitals and nursing homes, or at home. Hospice care focuses on relieving pain, controlling symptoms, and meeting emotional needs and personal values of the terminally ill, instead of targeting the underlying disease process. The hospice philosophy also recognizes that family members and other caregivers deserve care and support, continuing after the death of the patient. Hospice programs ease dying; they do not support active euthanasia or assisted suicide.

Bereavement services are also available through hospice care to help patients discuss such issues as preparing a will and planning a funeral, and to help surviving family members cope with grief and loss after the patient dies. Hospice programs generally provide bereavement services through

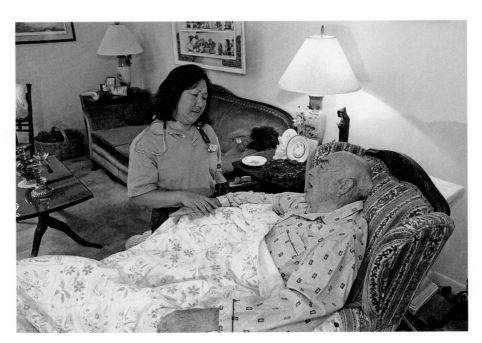

FIGURE 11-2 A nurse with an elderly man receiving hospice care.

discussion groups, follow-up visits from hospice personnel, and sometimes referral to appropriate mental health professionals.

Most in-home hospice programs are independently run in a fashion similar to visiting nurse or home health care agencies. Patients receive coordinated care at home by multidisciplinary teams composed of physicians, nurses, social workers, home health aides, pharmacists, physical therapists, clergy, volunteers, and family members. Hospice teams meet regularly to work on patients' needs concerning pain and other serious symptoms, depression, family problems, inadequate housing, financial problems, or lack of transportation. The team then expands, amends, or otherwise revises each patient's care plan, as necessary.

For patients to be eligible for hospice care, physicians usually must certify that they are not expected to live beyond six months. Hospice care is generally reimbursed by Medicare, Medicaid, and many private insurance companies and managed care programs.

PLANNING AHEAD

Patient Self-Determination Act
A federal law passed in 1990 that requires hospitals and other health care providers to provide written information to patients regarding their rights under state law to make medical decisions and execute advance directives.

In today's health care environment, individuals are well advised to be prepared for the time when they or their legal representatives may have to make decisions about medical treatment, including the use of life-sustaining measures. To address this concern, the federal **Patient Self-Determination Act** was passed in 1990 and took effect December 1, 1991. The act requires hospitals and other health care providers to provide written information to patients regarding their rights under state law to make medical decisions and execute advance directives. (Advance directives include the living will;

CHECK YOUR PROGRESS

13. Distinguish between *palliative care* and *curative care*.

_____

_____

14. Define *hospice*.

_____

_____

Indicate with a "C" or a "P" whether each of the following actions constitutes a form of curative care or palliative care.

_____ **15.** Allowing a patient who is terminally ill with lung and stomach cancer to self-administer morphine patches as needed for pain relief.

_____ **16.** Administering radiation treatments after breast cancer surgery.

_____ **17.** Surgical severing of certain nerves to relieve suffering for a patient terminally ill with cancer of the spine.

_____ **18.** Counseling a terminally ill patient and his or her family concerning funeral arrangements and other end-of-life decisions.

_____ **19.** Administering antibiotics to cure an infected tooth.

_____ **20.** Cosmetic surgery for a teenaged patient whose face was burned in a fire.

durable power of attorney; and the health care proxy, which is simply a durable power of attorney for medical care.) The act also provides that

- Health care providers will document in the patient's medical record whether he or she has executed an advance directive.
- Providers may not discriminate against an individual based on whether or not he or she has executed an advance directive.
- Providers must comply with state laws respecting advance directives.
- Providers must have a policy for educating staff and the community regarding advance directives.

Congress's action in passing this law was due, in large part, to the Nancy Cruzan case, decided by the U.S. Supreme Court in June 1990.

As a result of the Patient Self-Determination Act, patients are encouraged to execute living wills or durable powers of attorney while still able to do so and before life-sustaining measures become necessary for life to continue.

Living Will

living will An advance directive that specifies an individual's end-of-life wishes.

A **living will** directly provides instructions to physicians, hospitals, and other health care providers involved in a patient's treatment. It may detail circumstances under which treatment should be discontinued, such as coma, brain death, or a terminal condition. It may also detail which treatments or medications to suspend (for example, invasive surgery, artificial nutrition or hydration, and measures that serve no purpose except to delay death) and which to maintain (for example, kidney dialysis and drugs for pain). In addition, it may list which "heroic measures" (for example, emergency surgery and CPR) should and should not be used. A living will may also indicate preferences regarding organ donation, autopsy, and alternative treatments. Living wills may designate an agent to carry out these wishes if the patient is incapable of making decisions.

All 50 states accept the validity of living wills, although they also specify various requirements that must be met. Standard state forms may be obtained from a number of sources for completion by individuals and their attorneys.

Generic living will forms may also be obtained from various sources, but users should be aware of any state-specific requirements. Copies of completed forms should be given to designated family members or agents and may be filed with medical records upon a patient's admission to the hospital. See Figure 11-3.

If the time comes when I am incapacitated to the point when I can on longer actively take part in decisions for my own life, and am unable to direct my physician as to my own medical care, I wish this statement to stand as a testament of my wishes. I _____ (name) request that I be allowed to die and not be kept alive through life-support systems if my condition is deemed terminal. I do not intend any direct taking of my life, but only that my dying not be unreasonably prolonged. This request is made, after careful reflection, while I am of sound mind.

_____
(signature)

_____
(date)

FIGURE 11-3   Sample Living Will

Durable Power of Attorney

durable power of attorney An advance directive that confers upon a designee the authority to make a variety of legal decisions on behalf of the grantor, usually including health care decisions.

The **durable power of attorney** is not specifically a medical document, but it may serve that purpose. It confers upon a designee the authority to make a variety of legal decisions on behalf of the grantor. It takes effect when the grantor loses the capacity to make decisions, through either unconsciousness or mental incompetence. The document may place limits on the rights and responsibilities of the designee (usually an attorney or a spouse), and it may give specific instructions regarding the grantor's medical and other preferences. Standard forms are available and are governed by state law.

Health Care Proxy

health care proxy A durable power of attorney issued for purposes of health care decisions only.

A **health care proxy,** or *health care power of attorney,* is a state-specific, end-of-life document. The health care proxy or health care power of attorney differs from the durable power of attorney in that it pertains just to health care decisions and not to other legal decisions. With it, individuals specify their wishes and designate an agent to make medical decisions for them in the event that they lose the ability to reason or communicate. As with the living will, this document outlines specific types of care and treatment that should be permitted or excluded. It also carefully outlines the specific responsibilities and authority of the proxy. Some states prohibit attending physicians, hospital employees, or other health care providers from serving as proxies, unless related to the patient by blood. Patients should name one or more alternates in case the primary proxy cannot serve when called. See Figure 11-4.

Do-Not-Resuscitate (DNR) Order

When admitted to a hospital, most patients are allowed by state law to specify that they are not to be revived if their heart stops. The request can be made via a standard do-not-resuscitate (DNR) order which is then placed

CHECK YOUR PROGRESS

21. What purpose do advance directives serve?

_____

_____

22. Distinguish between a living will and a durable power of attorney.

_____

_____

23. Distinguish between a health care proxy and a durable power of attorney.

_____

_____

24. How must health care practitioners proceed if a patient has a do-not-resuscitate order in place?

_____

_____

25. Generic living will forms are acceptable, legal documents, with what caveat?

_____

_____

I, _____ , designate and appoint:

Name: _____

Address: _____

Telephone Number: _____

to be my agent for health care decisions and pursuant to the language stated below, on my behalf to:

(1) Consent, refuse consent, or withdraw consent to any care, treatment, service or procedure to maintain, diagnose or treat a physical or mental condition, and to make decisions about organ donation, autopsy and disposition of the body;

(2) make all necessary arrangements at any hospital, psychiatric hospital or psychiatric treatment facility, hospice, nursing home or similar institution; to employ or discharge health care personnel to include physicians, psychiatrists, psychologists, dentists, nurses, therapists or any other person who is licensed, certified or otherwise authorized or permitted by the laws of this state to administer health care as the agent shall deem necessary for my physical, mental and emotional well-being; and

(3) request, receive and review any information, verbal or written, regarding my personal affairs or physical or mental health including medical and hospital records and to execute any releases of other documents that may be required in order to obtain such information.

In exercising the grant of authority set forth above my agent for health care decisions shall:

_____

The powers of the agent herein shall be limited to the extent set out in writing in this durable power of attorney for health care decisions, and shall not include the power to revoke or invalidate any previously existing declaration made in accordance with the natural death act.

The agent shall be prohibited from authorizing consent for the following items:

_____

The durable power of attorney for health care decisions shall be subject to these additional limitations:

_____

This power of attorney for health care decisions shall become effective immediately and shall not be affected by my subsequent disability or incapacity or upon the occurrence of my disability or incapacity.

Any durable power of attorney for health care decisions I have previously made is hereby revoked. This durable power of attorney for health care decisions shall be revoked in writing, executed and witnessed or acknowledged in the same manner as required herein.

Executed this _____ , at _____

_____
(Signature of principal)

State _____ County _____ S.S. No. _____

This instrument was acknowledged before me _____ (date) by _____ (name)

_____
(Signature of notary public)

FIGURE 11-4　Sample Health Care Proxy

with the patient's chart. In some hospitals patients may also wear a bracelet alerting medical personnel to the existence of a DNR order.

THE NATIONAL ORGAN TRANSPLANT ACT

National Organ Transplant Act
Passed in 1984, a statute that provides grants to qualified organ procurement organizations and established an Organ Procurement and Transplantation Network.

Passed in 1984, the **National Organ Transplant Act** addresses the severe shortage of organs available for transplantation. It provides funds for (1) grants to qualified organ procurement organizations (OPOs) and (2) the establishment of an Organ Procurement and Transplantation Network (OPTN) to assist OPOs in the distribution of unused organs outside their geographical area.

The Organ Procurement and Transplantation Network maintains the only national patient waiting list. It is a unique public/private organization that links all the professionals involved in the organ donation and transplantation system. OPTN goals are to

- Increase the effectiveness and efficiency of organ sharing and equity in the national system of organ allocation.
- Increase the supply of donated organs available for transplantation.

The United Network for Organ Sharing (UNOS), based in Richmond, Virginia, administers the OPTN under contract with the Health Resources and Services Administration of the U.S. Department of Health and Human Services.

Studies conducted by UNOS in 2004 found the increasing need for more donor organs a recurring theme, especially for pancreas, liver, and kidney transplants. Over the decade from 1992 to 2002, the organ transplant waiting list increased by 150 percent, and long wait times for transplant candidates also indicated that supply was not meeting demand.

At the beginning of 2008 there were over 98,000 people waiting for transplants. The number of transplants from January through October 2007 was 12,026. Of those transplants, 6,713 were from deceased donors and 5,313 were from live donors.

In February 2002, UNOS made a significant change to policy for determining the order for liver transplants, based on studies that showed that U.S. surgeons were transplanting livers into their own patients first, even when those patients were not as sick as others. Changes to the UNOS liver policy addressed the equitable allocation of human livers for transplant based on two formulas that put sickest transplant candidates on the waiting list ahead of others: one for adults, known as the Model for End-State Liver Disease (MELD), and one for children, known as the Pediatric End-State Liver Disease Model (PELD). Higher MELD and PELD scores (and thus greater priority for a transplant) are associated with a higher risk of death while awaiting a transplant. In 2004, however, transplant officials said that despite the new UNOS rule, federal regulations governing transplants may need changing so that the sickest patients receive organ transplants ahead of others on the waiting list who are not as sick.

Although there is a national coordinated effort to maintain a list of people in need of an organ transplant, there is no national registry for donors. There are coordinated efforts through organ procurement organizations nationwide to coordinate donor information through OPTN. The Association of Organ Procurement Organizations (www.aopo.org) provides a list of organizations at the local level in each state.

The Organ Donation and Recovery Improvement Act, passed in 2004, established programs to increase organ donation through public awareness campaigns and education projects, and provided grants programs for individual states supporting use of hospital-based organ procurement coordinators, research and demonstration projects, and reimbursement to living donors for travel-related expenses.

Organ Donor Directives

Patients may also want to make clear to hospital personnel that they wish to donate organs for transplantation or medical research in the event of their death. This can be accomplished in several ways:

- Some states allow licensed drivers to fill out organ donation forms on the back of their licenses.
- Nondrivers or residents of states where drivers' licenses do not include this information may carry an organ donor card in their wallets, specifying their desire to donate organs.
- Organizations such as the National Kidney Foundation, the United Network for Organ Sharing (UNOS), and the Living Bank provide donor registration materials in response to requests.
- In addition to having an organ donor card, patients should make clear to family members their wishes regarding organ donation in the event of their death.

Uniform Anatomical Gift Act

Uniform Anatomical Gift Act
A national statute allowing individuals to donate their bodies or body parts, after death, for use in transplant surgery, tissue banks, or medical research or education.

In 1968 the **Uniform Anatomical Gift Act** was approved by the National Conference of Commissioners on Uniform State Laws for the purpose of allowing individuals to donate their bodies or body parts, after death, for use in transplant surgery, tissue banks, or medical research or education. The act was not officially enacted as law, but states accepted it because it made certain provisions uniform throughout all states. Major provisions include the following:

- Any person 18 years of age or older who is of sound mind may make a gift of his or her body, or certain bodily organs, to be used in medical research or for transplantation or storage in a tissue bank.
- Donations made through a legal will are not to be held up by probate.
- Except in autopsies, the donor's rights override those of others.
- Survivors may speak for the deceased if arrangements were not made prior to his or her death (provided the deceased did not express an objection to donation before his or her dëath).
- Physicians who rely on donation documents for the acceptance of bodies or organs are immune from civil or criminal prosecution. However, if the physician (or hospital) knows the deceased was opposed to donation or if, in the absence of prior arrangements, survivors express an objection, then the donation should be refused.
- Hospitals, surgeons, physicians, accredited medical or dental schools, colleges and universities, and tissue banks or storage facilities may accept anatomical gifts for research, advancement of medical or dental science, therapy, or transplantation.
- Time of death of the donor must be established by a physician who is not involved in transplanting the donor's designated organs, and the donor's attending physician cannot be a member of the transplant team.
- Donors may revoke the gift, and gifts may be rejected.

FIGURE 11-5 A Sample
Uniform Donor Card

UNIFORM DONOR CARD

Of _____
          Print or type name of donor
in the hope that I may help others, I hereby make this anatomical
gift, if medically acceptable, to take effect upon my death. The
words and marks below indicate my desires.
I give: (a) ☐ any needed organs or parts
      (b) ☐ only the following organs or parts

_____
          Specify the organ(s) or part(s)

for the purposes of transplantation, therapy, medical research or
education:
      (c) ☐ my body for anatomical study if needed.
Limitations or special wishes, if any: _____

Front of card

**Signed by the donor and the following two witnesses in
the presence of each other:**

Signature of Donor _____
Date of Birth of Donor _____
Date Signed _____
City and State _____
Witness _____
Witness _____
THIS IS A LEGAL DOCUMENT UNDER THE UNIFORM
ANATOMICAL GIFT ACT OR SIMILAR LAWS.

Back of card

Some states provide for prospective donors to indicate their wish to
donate on the back of their driver's licenses. Alternatively, donors may carry
signed and witnessed Uniform Donor Cards (Figure 11-5).

Frequently Asked Questions about Organ Donation

Since there are more people waiting for organ transplants than there are
organs available, individuals are encouraged to designate their willingness
to become donors. One way to increase the numbers of possible organ
donors is to make sure that potential donors understand the process. Here
are a few of the most commonly asked questions about organ donation, followed by summarized answers from the experts:

Q: What organs and tissues can be transplanted?
A: Organs that can be transplanted include heart, kidney, pancreas,
   lung, stomach, and small and large intestines. Other tissues often
   transplanted include bone, corneas, skin, heart valves, veins, cartilage,
   and other connective tissues.

Q: Is the donor or the donor's family responsible for paying for
   transplantation of donated organs?
A: No. Costs are borne by the recipient or his or her insurance plan, when
   applicable.

Q: If a prospective, designated donor is injured in an accident, will the attending doctors allow that person to die in order to harvest donated organs?

A: Absolutely not. A willingness to donate organs in no way compromises the medical care provided to accident victims. The organ procurement organization (OPO) is notified that organs are available only after a patient is declared dead, and the transplant team is not notified until surviving family members have consented to donation.

Q: How old or young can a donor be?

A: Donors range from newborns to persons about the age of 70.

Q: If a person donated an organ, would the recipient and/or the recipient's family learn the donor's identity and contact the donor or his or her family?

A: A donor's name is released to recipients only if the recipient asks for the information and the donor's family agrees.

Q: Are organs transplanted only after a prospective donor has died?

A: Not necessarily. Voluntary transplants from living donors to living recipients may also take place. For example, kidneys, lungs, skin, and other tissues are successfully transplanted from compatible living donors to recipients.

Q: May a family member who is an acceptable medical match for a recipient refuse to donate an organ to a relative in need of a transplant?

A: Of course. No laws exist that would compel a person to donate an organ against his or her will, regardless of relationship to the intended recipient.

CHECK YOUR PROGRESS

26. What law made organ donation possible in the United States?

_____

_____

27. In your opinion, why is there a shortage of transplant organs in the United States?

_____

_____

28. What suggestions do you have for alleviating the shortage of transplant organs?

_____

_____

29. What is UNOS, and what is its function?

_____

_____

30. A widely circulated urban legend tells of a person who has a sexual tryst with a stranger and awakens in a bathtub minus a kidney. Why do you know the story is untrue?

_____

_____

Q: If I, as a willing organ donor, sign the back of my driver's license indicating that I am a donor, and then die, can my relatives legally "undo" my wishes?

A: No. A signed declaration on the back of a driver's license still is legally effective to authorize donation in every state in the United States. Moreover, the relevant laws specify that the consent of the donor's relatives is not needed in such circumstances. However, prospective organ donors should also make their wishes known to family members while they are able, because in spite of their having signed a card, if relatives protest the donation, fear of bad publicity regarding organ donation will likely prevent the donation from occurring.

THE GRIEVING PROCESS

Regardless of our personal philosophy and belief system concerning death and dying, we are all destined to experience the loss of an acquaintance, a friend, or a loved one. At that time, we need to grieve. Unfortunately, in our modern-day culture we are often uncertain of how to deal with grief in our own lives or how to help someone else who is grieving. The following facts and guidelines can help us respond helpfully to others.

What Is Grief?

Grief is the human reaction to loss. Individuals may grieve over a divorce, the loss of a job, or relocation, but grief after the death of a loved one is undoubtedly the most painful. Patients who are diagnosed with a terminal illness also experience profound grief. The grieving process is necessary, in both instances, in order for healing or resolution to take place.

CHECK YOUR PROGRESS

The following questionnaire is intended to generate discussion. Check each statement that tells how you feel. There are no correct or incorrect answers.

_____ 31. I feel uncomfortable talking to someone who is dying.

_____ 32. I do not know what to say to a person who is dying.

_____ 33. I would not want to tell a patient that he or she has a terminal condition.

_____ 34. I think I can help a dying patient be more comfortable with his or her impending death.

_____ 35. I am afraid of becoming too attached to a dying patient, and as a result I will not be able to control my feelings.

_____ 36. I do not think a person should be told that his or her condition is terminal, because doing so adds to his or her suffering.

_____ 37. I do not think death should be discussed in the presence of children.

_____ 38. The thought of being around a dying person makes me uncomfortable.

_____ 39. I think elderly people are the most fearful of death.

_____ 40. Being around a dying person reminds me that someday I, too, will die.

The above questionnaire has been adapted from a book by W. Worden, *Grief Counseling and Grief Therapy* (New York: Springer Publishing Co., 1982).

Stages of Grief

Dr. Elisabeth Kübler-Ross, recognized for many years as an authority in the field of death and dying, was the first to list and describe the coping mechanisms of people who grieve. Such individuals experience five stages of grief, she maintained, not necessarily in any particular order, before coming to terms with the death of a loved one or the prospect of imminent death.

Stage 1. This first stage is identified with feelings of denial and isolation. This is the it-can't-be-true stage, in which patients believe the physician's diagnosis must be a mistake, or relatives informed of a loved one's death deny that the person is gone. They may suggest that X-rays or results of blood tests were somehow mixed up or that identities of accident victims were somehow mistaken. Denial is usually a temporary state, claims Kübler-Ross, and is soon replaced by partial acceptance. A terminally ill patient seldom continues to deny his or her disease until death comes, and grieving relatives realize all too soon that a loved one has, in fact, died.

Stage 2. When denial can no longer be maintained, the patient or grieving relative progresses to anger, rage, and resentment. "Why me?" is the typical reaction. Patients are angry over the "betrayal" of once-healthy bodies and the loss of control over their lives. Grieving relatives may feel anger toward a God that took the loved one away. Even the terminally ill family member may feel the same anger at God for leaving others behind to bear the pain of loss. Anger is a normal reaction to death and may be expressed in different ways. For example, a bereaved person may yell at others or withdraw in sullen silence.

Stage 3. Grieving individuals next respond with attempts at bargaining and guilt. Just as children continue to ask for a favor after parents have said no, patients may ask for "just enough time to see my daughter married" or "one more week at work before I have to quit." Something in the human psyche seems to believe, if only for a short time, that if we are "good," the "bad" will be taken away or postponed.

A corresponding experience for individuals grieving the loss of a loved one is guilt. The bereaved person may somehow feel responsible for the death, especially if the relationship with the deceased was not good. He or she might be tortured by thoughts of how things might have been different if only the loved one had lived.

Stage 4. The fourth stage involves depression or sadness, which is the most expected reaction to loss. Patients coping with terminal illness may face not only physical pain and debilitation but also loss of financial security and inevitable changes in lifestyle—all of which can cause them to feel that their situation is hopeless. Individuals grieving the loss of a loved one may see no point in going on.

During this state bereaved persons may cry frequently or may be unable to cry at all, expressing their grief in body language—downcast eyes, shuffling steps, and stooped shoulders. Daily routines may be difficult or impossible to maintain. If depression continues for a prolonged period of time, health care providers, family members, or friends should help the bereaved person seek professional counseling.

Stage 5. Finally, those experiencing the grieving process reach a stage of acceptance. At this point the person has finally accepted his or her loss. Terminally ill patients have come to terms with dying, and bereaved persons have accepted that the loved one is gone. For example, patients may write wills, complete advance directives, or plan funerals. A grieving spouse may finally decide to remove a deceased partner's clothing from a shared closet or to convert his or her office to a spare bedroom. Grieving family members can now move on to the growth stage, in which they adjust daily routines or become involved in new activities and relationships.

Although the stages of grief have been universally observed, each person dealing with loss grieves differently. Bereaved persons may not show their grief. A stage may be skipped or returned to repeatedly during the grieving process. A combination of all of the emotions just described may be felt at the same time.

Finding Support

People who are grieving can find support from a variety of sources. They can read books on the subject, attend a bereavement support group sponsored by a hospital or hospice, visit a counselor, talk with a member of the clergy, or talk with family members and friends (Figure 11-6).

Health care practitioners can be excellent sources of support for terminally ill patients and their families. Talking and listening are the most helpful activities others can perform, the experts advise. Do not force a conversation, but make yourself available to talk. Do not respond in kind if patients are angry and resentful. Talking about distress helps relieve it, and sensitive listening is effective in itself. The following list of recommendations for talking to a dying patient is adapted from *"I Don't Know What to Say . . .": How to Help and Support Someone Who Is Dying* (Little, Brown and Company, 1989), by oncologist Dr. Robert Buckman:

- Pay attention to setting. Sit down, relax, do not appear rushed, and act as though you are ready to listen.
- Determine whether or not the patient wants to talk. Ask, "Do you feel like talking?" before plunging into conversation.
- Listen well, and show that you are listening. Pay attention to the patient's words, without the distraction of planning your next remark.
- Encourage the patient to talk by saying, "What do you mean?" or "Tell me more."

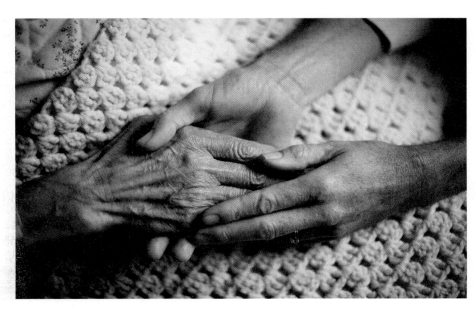

FIGURE 11-6 Health care practitioners can be caring sources of support for grieving patients and for family members.

- Remember that silence and nonverbal communication, such as grasping a hand or touching a shoulder, are also effective.

- Do not be afraid to describe your own feelings. It is permissible to say, "I find this difficult to talk about" or even, "I don't know what to say."

- Make sure you haven't misunderstood. You can ask, "How did it feel?" or say, "You seem angry."

- Do not change the subject. If you are uncomfortable, admit it. Don't try to distract the patient by changing the subject to something less threatening, such as the weather.

- Do not give advice early. The time may come when the patient asks your advice, but it is usually not prudent to offer unsolicited advice, because it stops the dialogue.

- Encourage reminiscence. Sharing memories can be a wrenching experience, but it can also encourage patients to look positively at the past.

- Respond to humor. Humor allows patients to express fears in a nonthreatening way. Do not try to cheer someone up with your own jokes, but if patients want to tell jokes or funny stories, humor them.

In short, the more you try to understand the feelings of others, the more support you will be able to give.

Ethics Issues

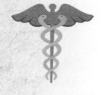

Death and Dying

ETHICS ISSUE 1: Don Lundy, EMS Director for Charleston County, South Carolina, says that DNR requests continue to be an ethical issue for EMTs. "The legal question has been answered," Lundy says, "but is it right or wrong [for EMTs] to support a DNR?" Most EMTs, Lundy explains, "would rather do too much than not enough."

DISCUSSION QUESTIONS

1. Assume you are an emergency medical technician (EMT) responding to a 911 call at a grocery store. An elderly shopper has collapsed, and she is unconscious on the floor when you arrive. Her vital signs are weak. The woman is placed in the ambulance, where she arrests. You notice that the woman is wearing a bracelet that says "DNR," and a quick check of her purse reveals a signed and witnessed DNR order. What do you do?

_____

_____

2. EMTs reach the hospital with a patient who then arrests. The patient has been hospitalized before, and a DNR order is in place. The patient is middle-aged, and when his family arrives his wife says, "I don't care what he says. Do everything to keep him alive." As a health care practitioner on the team assigned to care for this patient, what will you do?

_____

_____

ETHICS ISSUE 2: In Maryland, according to EMS Director Lundy, state law allows EMTs to do what is right for the patient when transporting them for care. In other states, the law may say you must obey the patient's instructions, regardless of what those instructions are.

DISCUSSION QUESTIONS

1. As an EMT in Maryland, you are transporting a patient with chest pain, and you decide to transport her to a hospital with heart catheterization capabilities, even though the patient has expressed a desire to go to a less well equipped hospital in the area. Legally and ethically, how will you respond?

_____

_____

2. You are an EMT in South Carolina, where state law says the patient has the last word. The patient has been injured in a car accident, and you want to take him to a hospital with a level 1 trauma center, but he says no, take him to a different hospital, without a level 1 trauma center. Legally and ethically, what will you do?

_____

_____

ETHICS ISSUE 3: As a health care practitioner you are committed to acting in the patient's best interest, and you believe that the wishes of patients in end-of-life situations should be followed. Furthermore, professional codes of ethics generally state that the social commitment of health care practitioners is to sustain life and relieve suffering, and that when the performance of one duty conflicts with the other, the preferences of the patient should prevail.

DISCUSSION QUESTIONS

1. A young mother who was severely injured in a car accident is brought into the hospital trauma center where you work. She belongs to the Jehovah's Witnesses church, and emphatically states that she refuses to have a blood transfusion. You know she risks death without a transfusion, but she believes her decision is a matter of her salvation. As a member of the patient's health care team, what will you do?

_____

_____

2. The patient in the above car accident scenario is an elderly Jehovah's Witness and has no family. What will you do?

_____

_____

3. The female patient in the above car accident scenario is unconscious, but her husband makes her wishes known regarding blood transfusions. Can you accept the husband's decision on the patient's behalf? Explain your answer.

_____

_____

ETHICS ISSUE 4. Health care practitioners are ethically bound to respond to the needs of the patient at the end of life, but they are also ethically bound to preserve a patient's autonomy whenever possible.

DISCUSSION QUESTION

1. A mentally competent, elderly patient suffering from congestive heart failure presents a DNR order when admitted to the hospital. He also talks with his attending physician about his end-of-life care, asking for comfort care only. The physician concurs and records the patient's wishes on his chart. The patient's daughter arrives from out of state and loudly overrides her father's wishes. As a member of the man's health care team, what do you and others on the team do?

_____

_____

ETHICS ISSUE 5: Your elderly aunt has asked you to take on her health care power of attorney. She makes the request while she is healthy and able to make her own decisions. You agree and sign the appropriate legal papers. She tells you at this time that she never wants "heroic measures" to be undertaken to save her life, if her quality of life would suffer.

DISCUSSION QUESTIONS

1. Five years later your aunt is 86 and suffering from diabetes, coronary problems, and dementia. While in a long-term care facility, your aunt suffers a severe heart attack and is transported to the local hospital's emergency room. She is conscious when she reaches the emergency room, and when the attending physician asks her if she wants "all measures taken to preserve her life," she says yes. When you arrive at the hospital, your aunt is comatose and has been placed in the intensive care unit. Her physician says she cannot recover, but he could transport her to a larger hospital where physicians could "try" a pacemaker. How will you respond?

_____

_____

2. What ethical issues will influence your decision?

_____

_____

ETHICS ISSUE 6: You are one of the health care practitioners involved in the care of a recently divorced, 55-year-old man with severe rheumatoid arthritis. He comes to the clinic where you work for a routine visit, complaining of insomnia. He requests a specific barbiturate, Seconal, as a sleep aid, asking for a month's supply. He says he wakes up every morning at four, tired but unable to go back to sleep. He admits that he rarely leaves his house during the day and says he has no interest in his previous enjoyable activities.

DISCUSSION QUESTION

1. What is an ethically appropriate course of action?

_____

_____

ETHICS ISSUE 7: A terminally ill patient you help care for in a hospice situation seems alienated from family members. The patient talks to you about her family situation, and asks you to intervene. You are uncomfortable with the request but do not know how to reply.

DISCUSSION QUESTION

1. What, in your opinion, is the ethically appropriate course of action?

_____

_____

ETHICS ISSUE 8: A Jewish family wants to perform a *tarhara*—ceremony for washing a body—and bury a family member within 24 hours of his death in accordance with their religious beliefs.

DISCUSSION QUESTION

1. Should health care practitioners who treated the recently deceased help to accommodate his family's wishes? If so, how?

_____

_____

Go to www.mhhe.com/judson5e to practice your case review skills. Then read on for more information.

11 REVIEW

Applying Knowledge

Match each definition that follows with the correct term by writing the appropriate letter in the space provided.

_____1. One who has six months or less to live.

_____2. An irreversible condition that determines when death has occurred.

_____3. Care provided to relieve pain and make a patient's last days as comfortable as possible.

_____4. The range of emotions one feels in response to loss.

_____5. Care provided in an attempt to halt the disease process.

_____6. The study of death and its accompanying psychological aspects.

_____7. Greek for "good death."

a. grief

b. terminally ill

c. euthanasia

d. thanatology

e. palliative care

f. brain death

g. curative care

Answer the following questions in the spaces provided.

8. Do advance directives preserve a patient's autonomy? Explain your answer.

_____

_____

9. Technically, death results from what basic, biological cause?

_____

10. What is the accepted criteria for brain death?

_____

11. Does a diagnosis of persistent vegetative state offer hope for a complete recovery? Explain your answer.

_____

_____

12. Physician-assisted suicide occurs when

_____

13. Would you be in favor of national legislation that permits euthanasia in certain, highly regulated situations? Explain your answer.

_____

_____

_____

14. What is the philosophy behind the hospice movement?

_____

_____

15. If an autopsy is not required by law, for what other reasons might the procedure be performed?

_____

_____

16. In your opinion, why was there so much public interest in the Terry Schiavo case?

_____

_____

17. What is a simple definition of grief?

_____

_____

18. Briefly define the right-to-die movement in the United States.

_____

_____

19. Thus far in your education to become a health care practitioner, have you received any instruction regarding the care of the dying? If yes, to what extent? If no, what would you recommend?

_____

_____

20. List and repudiate five common myths concerning organ transplantation.

_____

_____

_____

_____

_____

_____

Select the correct answer from the choices provided.

_____ 21. Which of the following is *not* true of the Uniform Rights of the Terminally Ill Act?
   a.   A federal statute passed in 1989
   b.   Intended to guide state legislatures in constructing laws to address advance directives
   c.   Was repealed in 1994
   d.   None of the above are true

_____ 22. The Patient Self-Determination Act does *not* provide for
   a.   Documenting the existence of an advance directive in the patient's medical record
   b.   Nondiscrimination regarding whether or not a patient has an advance directive
   c.   Compliance with state laws respecting advance directives
   d.   Legal prosecution of health care practitioners who influence a patient's decision in preparing an advance directive

_____ 23. Landmark events in the right-to-die movement include
   a.   The Karen Ann Quinlan case
   b.   The Nancy Cruzan case
   c.   The Terry Shiavo case
   d.   All of the above

_____ 24. The Uniform Anatomical Gift Act does *not* include the provision(s) that
   a. Persons 18 and older and of sound mind may donate organs and tissues for transplantation.
   b. Donations made through a will are not to be held up in probate.
   c. Organs are not accepted from patients over 60 years of age.
   d. Except in autopsies, the donor's rights override the rights of others.

_____ 25. Dr. Elisabeth Kübler-Ross's five stages of coping with a death or with a terminal illness do *not* include which of the following:
   a. Acceptance
   b. Bargaining
   c. Depression
   d. All of the above are included

_____ 26. Which of the following is a modern-day custom regarding death?
   a. Holding a funeral
   b. As a survivor, wearing sackcloth and ashes for several days
   c. As a survivor, wailing loudly at certain times in public places
   d. None of the above

_____ 27. Recent reports indicate a decline in the number of nonmandatory autopsies performed in hospitals. Which of the following is a probable reason for the decline?
   a. Fewer patients are dying.
   b. Family members of deceased patients are often reluctant to give permission for an autopsy.
   c. No one wants to perform them.
   d. The law does not allow hospitals to perform autopsies.

_____ 28. Before pronouncing a nonresponsive and unconscious patient dead, physicians may perform certain tests. Which of the following is *not* a prescribed test for determining death?
   a. Cannot breathe without assistance
   b. Cannot stand unaided
   c. Has no coughing or gagging reflex
   d. Pupils do not respond to light

_____ 29. Which of the following is true of death in the United States in the twenty-first century?
   a. Most deaths are occurring among teenagers.
   b. Most deaths occur in hospitals.
   c. All deaths result in autopsies.
   d. Infants seldom die.

_____ 30. Recent reports indicate a continuing decline in the number of autopsies performed in the United States. Of what value is a nonmandatory autopsy performed after a hospital patient dies?
   a. Helps determine cause of death
   b. Helps advance medical knowledge about disease
   c. Helps reassure family members of the deceased that everything possible had been done for their loved one
   d. All of the above

Case Study

Use your critical-thinking skills to answer the questions that follow this case study.

31. You are the health care practitioner assigned to speak with a deceased patient's family about permission to do an autopsy, and you find yourself feeling reluctant to do so. What reasons can you think of that might make one feel reluctant in such a situation?

_____

_____

_____

Assume you are a home health care nurse, and you have been visiting Mrs. Smith for the past four years. She has tried to remain living at home but has had frequent falls and is not able to take care of herself. The family decides to place her in a long-term care facility. Though she is still alert and oriented, she has authorized her granddaughter to assume her health care power of attorney.

32. What are the granddaughter's legal and ethical obligations as her grandmother's agent with health care power of attorney?

_____

_____

_____

You are a member of a hospital resource allocation committee that must decide which three out of seven critical patients will receive immediate live-saving surgery. The hospital has resources to save just three of the seven, but without surgery, all seven patients will die. The situation is further complicated by the fact that a blizzard is raging outside, and none of the patients can be transferred to another hospital. All seven are too critically ill to be moved by snowmobile.

33. Working alone or in a group, decide what criteria will be used to make the decisions (consider age, social standing, benefit to society, lifestyle, degree of physical deterioration, etc.).

_____

_____

_____

34. Obtain a list of the seven patients from your instructor, and choose three patients to receive immediate life-saving surgery. Write your decisions, and/or discuss the rationale for your choices with the class.

_____

_____

_____

_____

_____

Internet Activities

Complete the activities and answer the questions that follow.

35. Visit the Web site for Caring Connections at www.caringinfo.org/. Download a living will and a health care power of attorney form, and compare the forms with those of a classmate from another state. Overall, how do the forms from another state differ from those for your state?

_____

_____

_____

36. Visit the Hospice Patients Alliance at www.hospicepatients.org/hospic4.html. List three recommendations offered at the site for choosing the right hospice for a dying family member.

_____

_____

_____

37. Visit the Web site for Healing Resources at www.webhealing.com. List three grief links found at the site that might help the bereaved. Why might these resources prove helpful?

_____

_____

_____

Health Care Trends and Forecasts

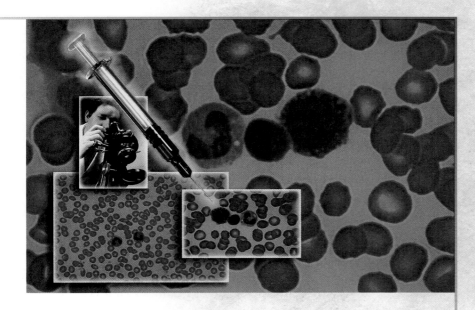

Learning Outcomes

After studying this chapter, you should be able to:

1. Identify the major stakeholders in the United States health care system.

2. Describe the major areas of concern to those stakeholders.

3. Explain the effect the baby boom generation will have on the U.S. health care system in the near future

4. Identify the major improvements in quality of care

5. Describe the major new trends that will affect health care in the U.S. in the next 20 years.

Key Terms

access

Agency for Healthcare Research and Quality (AHRQ)

baby boom generation

cost

genometrics

gross domestic product (GDP)

life expectancy

medical management

pharmacogenomics

quality

stakeholders

State Children's Health Initiative Program (SCHIP)

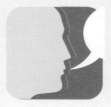

Voice of Experience
A Career for the Future

James, a physical therapist, says he feels secure in his profession, because he "can't be replaced by technology, and we [physical therapists] can't be outsourced overseas."

Not only does James have job security; seeing the United States is part of his job description, since he works for a national placement company for health care careers that sends him to facilities throughout the United States. Over the five years since graduating from his state university, James has worked in South Carolina, Arizona, Illinois, Texas, Maine, Alaska, and Montana. "I stay in one place as long as the facility needs me, or until I want to move on," he says. "Usually I can stay in one place as long as I want. I've never worked for a facility that no longer needed me."

The most rewarding aspect of his occupation, James says, is "seeing the progress with patients—the effect I have had." For example, James helped a patient in his 60s with chronic back pain to strengthen and stretch muscles. The exercises helped the patient so much that after treatment he was able to take a walking, sightseeing trip to China. James says the thank-you e-mail he received from the patient "made my day."

James says confidentiality is a constant concern in his work. "Often we have no private rooms where I work. There may be just curtains to pull, or patients might be together in a group on an exercise mat. I have to be careful what I say to a patient in front of other patients. Patients talk to each other and that's fine, but I have to be careful. A patient might ask, 'How is Mrs. Smith doing?' I might answer, 'I don't work with her,' or 'I don't know; check with her.'"

While frequent moves are tiring, and he is constantly finding new friends and learning new job routines, James likes the change of location his work provides: "It's a good way to see the country and get paid at the same time."

As you have progressed through *Law & Ethics for Medical Careers*, you have gained knowledge about legal issues affecting every health care practitioner. You have also learned that in addition to the law, ethics play a crucial role in health care decisions. This final chapter outlines major concerns all Americans have with the country's health care system, and offers a glimpse of possibilities for the future.

COST, ACCESS, AND QUALITY

stakeholders Those who have a vested interest in the health care industry in the United States, and in any efforts to reform the industry.

Key issues of concern to *stakeholders* within the American health care system are *cost*, *access*, and *quality*. **Stakeholders** are those who have a vested interest in the health care industry in the United States, and in any efforts to reform the industry. They include, but are not limited to, the following:

1. The public.
2. Employers.
3. Health care facilities.
4. Federal, state, and local governments.
5. Managed care organizations.
6. Private insurers.
7. Voluntary facilities and agencies that provide health care or influence health care policies.
8. Health care practitioner training institutions.
9. Professional associations and other health care industry organizations.
10. Medical research groups.

In the future, the continued interest of stakeholders in the health care industry will ensure that reform brought about through health care legislation will address cost, access, and quality of health care.

Cost refers to the amount individuals, employers, state and federal governments, managed care organizations, private insurers, and other stakeholders

cost The amount individuals, employers, state and federal governments, HMOs, and insurers spend on health care in the United States.

access The availability of health care and the means to purchase health care services.

quality The degree of excellence of health care services offered.

gross domestic product (GDP) America's total income for all goods and services.

spend on health care in the United States. As explained below in the section titled "Access," the number of people who have **access** to health care services—that is, the number of people for whom the services are available and for which they as consumers can pay—also helps determine cost. In addition, the cost of health care services also directly affects the **quality,** or degree of excellence, of health care services offered.

COST

Just as preparing a budget shows you how much of your income is spent on food (20 percent), housing (45 percent), clothing (15 percent), insurance (10 percent), and so on, the total cost of health care in the United States is often expressed as a percentage of the United States' gross domestic product. The **gross domestic product (GDP)** represents 100 percent of the country's income for all goods and services. The percentage of the GDP represented by health care spending was first determined in 1960, and it has been steadily increasing ever since. In 1960, health care spending accounted for slightly more than 5 percent of the GDP. In 2005 (the latest year for which statistics are available), health care spending had risen to 16 percent of the GDP, or $2 trillion—about $6,700 per person. The Health Care Financing Administration estimates that by 2010, if health care cost rises at 8 percent per year (the trend from 1960 to 1990), it will exceed 18 percent of the GDP. The National Coalition on Health Care predicts that by 2015, the United States could be spending 20 percent of the country's GDP on health care. By 2030, the Congressional Budget Office projects, health care spending could easily exceed 25 percent of the GDP—one dollar out of every four spent.

Dishonest medical providers also affect the cost of health care, as is evident in the following court case.

Why should health care stakeholders be concerned about the rising share of the GDP that health care expenditures consume? Because federal and state governments currently bear about 46 percent of the nation's health care costs, and higher health care spending is the main force expanding the federal budget. If the trend toward higher health care costs continues at the present rate of increase, the country could reach a point at which health care expenditures are so large that they overwhelm other important portions of government-spending allocations, such as schools, roads, parks, the environment, defense, and social welfare programs.

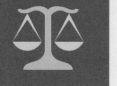

Court Case

Physician Accused of Soliciting Bribes

A physician accused of soliciting bribes in return for referring patients to a Medicaid provider moved to dismiss the indictment alleging mail fraud and violations of the Medicaid anti-kickback statue. The court denied the physician's motion to dismiss the indictment, noting that the physician's fiduciary duty under the "Referral of Patients" section of the AMA's *Code of Medical Ethics* supported an intangible rights mail fraud charge.

United States v. Neufeld, 908 F. Supp. 491, 500 (S.D. Ohio 1995).

Goverment Health Care Spending as a Percentage of Gross Domestic Product

Country	2002	2025	2050
Australia	6.4%	11.5%	21.1%
Austria	5.4	8.3	13.0
Canada	6.7	9.5	13.5
Germany	8.6	14.7	25.6
Japan	6.7	11.7	18.2
Norway	8.0	13.9	25.0
Spain	5.5	10.5	21.4
Sweden	7.9	10.2	12.9
United Kingdom	6.4	10.0	16.0
United States	6.6	13.8	32.7

Note: Numbers rounded.

Source: Authors' calculations based on Laurence Kotlikoff and Christian Hagist, "Who's Going Broke?" National Bureau of Economic Research, Working Paper No. 11833, December 2005, p. 29.

FIGURE 12-1 Health Care Spending Worldwide

Source: The National Center for Policy Analysis (NCPA), www.ncpa.org/pub/st/st286/st286c.html.

Figure 12-1 shows the government health care spending as a percentage of the GDP of the United States, as compared with other developed nations.

Other developed nations spend less for health care on a per capita basis than the United States, yet ensure wider access to health care for their citizens. The United States is the only nation on the above list that does not provide government-financed, universal health care to its citizens. (This is offered not as a judgment as to the desirability of universal health care, but simply as a matter of fact.)

American health care costs have continued to increase at alarming rates since 1960. See Figure 12-2 for the cost in 2004. Harry A. Sultz, DDS, MPH, and Kristina M. Young, MS, social and preventive medicine experts, attribute increases in the cost of health care to the following factors:

❚ Application of more advanced and more types of technology.

❚ Growth in the population of older adults.

❚ Emphasis on specialty medicine.

❚ Increasing numbers of uninsured and underinsured.

❚ Labor intensity of health care services.

❚ Reimbursement system incentives.[1]

Each of these factors is discussed below.

---

[1]Harry A. Sultz and Kristina M. Young, *Health Care USA, Understanding Its Organization and Delivery,* 5th ed. (Sudbury, MA: Jones & Bartlett, 2006), p. 243.

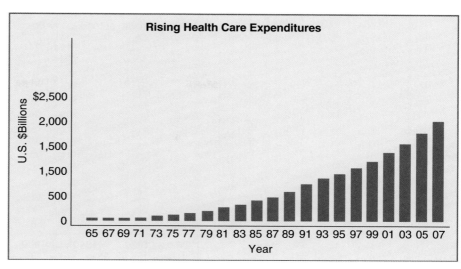

FIGURE 12-2 U.S. Health Care Spending Rises Yearly

Source: Harry A. Sultz and Kristina M. Young, *Health Care USA, Understanding Its Organization and Delivery,* 5th ed. (Sudbury, MA: Jones & Bartlett, 2006). Reprinted with permission.

New Health Care Technology

The availability of new computer-aided diagnostic and therapeutic tools, advanced surgical techniques and equipment, and an expanding array of medications are among many factors that have helped fuel the rise in health care costs.

Medical technologies currently in various stages of development that will be available, at a cost, in the future are discussed below, in the sections titled "Medical Technologies" and "Health Information Technologies." Because both the equipment and the employee training needed to implement new medical technologies are expensive, the expanded use of advanced technologies in the future will also add to the cost of health care services.

Widespread adoption of health information technology (HIT) in the future will also add to rising health care costs, since hardware, software, and personnel trained in HIT are costly.

Growth in the Population of Older Adults

baby boom generation Those individuals born between 1946 and 1964.

Much has been written about the effects of the baby boom generation on health care services in the United States. The **baby boom generation** is defined as those individuals born between 1946 and 1964. After American soldiers returned home from World War II in 1945 and 1946, the United States experienced an explosion of births (hence the name "baby boom") that continued for the next 18 years. In 1964, baby boomers made up 40 percent of all Americans. In the 1990s, about 76 million people were part of the baby boom generation, totaling 29 percent of the population in the United States. The baby boom population group is 70 percent larger than the generation born during the prior two decades, and baby boomers are expected to live longer than any previous generation. Baby boomers currently make up more than one-third of the U.S. population.

Because the baby boom generation is so large, its members have had a noticeable impact on all aspects of the nation's economy, including the health care industry, and as baby boomers age, they will continue to impact all health care services and costs.

Advances in medical technology have increased life spans for all Americans, including the baby boom generation. Consequently, there are more

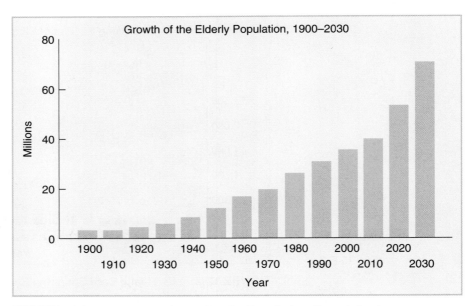

FIGURE 12-3 U.S Census Projection for Population Growth by Age
Source: U.S. Bureau of the Census.

Americans aged 65 and older than at any other time in history. In fact, the age group of those 85 years and older is growing faster than any other age group in the United States. Figure 12-3 below shows growth and projected growth of the U.S. population by age, from 1900 to 2030.

Not only do older people spend more on health care services than younger age groups, but they also use different services (Figure 12-4).

▌ Both older and younger health care consumers spend most of their health care dollars on hospital care and physician services, but health care expenses are greater for older Americans: $12,271 per person on average for people age 65 and older, versus $2,761 per person on average for people under age 65.

▌ Nursing home care takes a greater portion of the health care budget for the elderly: 22 percent of all health care spending per person over 65, versus 2 percent for people under 65.

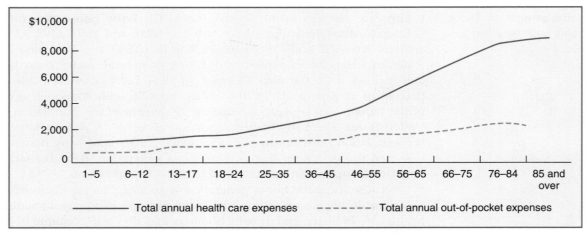

FIGURE 12-4 The Elderly Spend More on Health Care Services
Source: U.S. Dept. of HHS, Agency for Healthcare Research and Quality.

Emphasis on Specialty Medicine

Medical students in the United States are more than three times more likely to specialize than to remain generalists or primary physicians. Since specialists are paid at higher rates than primary physicians, the tendency of Americans to see specialists more often is also adding to the cost of health care. Managed care organizations have sought to control costs by instituting "gatekeepers" to restrict clients to primary physicians for initial diagnosis and treatment, and limiting referrals to specialists, but the practice has met with resistance from both physicians and patients. Because of this public outcry, many legislative initiatives at state and federal levels have sought to preserve patients' rights to insurance reimbursement for specialty treatment.

As medical technology advances, new specialties will arise, with the potential of further adding to the spiraling cost of health care services in the United States.

Increasing Numbers of Underinsured and Uninsured

As health care costs rise, so, too, does the number of people who cannot afford health insurance. According to the National Coalition on Health Care, nearly 47 million Americans, or 16 percent of the population, were without health insurance in 2005, the latest year for which government figures are available.

A recent Centers for Disease Control survey of uninsured Americans found that uninsured and underinsured people make more visits to emergency rooms than those who have health insurance, indicating that because of costs, a large percentage of the population is not receiving sufficient health care to protect them in the event of major illnesses or injuries. Since costs are higher for emergency room services than for care provided in physicians' offices or medical clinics, uninsured and underinsured patients add significantly to the cost of health care delivery.

Health care costs are also affected by the fact that uninsured individuals do not see physicians regularly and are, therefore, more likely to develop medical conditions that lead to costly complications or hospitalizations.

Labor Intensity of Health Care Services

The health care industry is the largest industry in the United States, employing about 13.4 million workers (2004 statistics from the U.S. Bureau of Labor Statistics) on a round-the-clock basis. Many of these workers have advanced educations and training, making labor an expensive component of total health care costs.

Technological advances and changing population demographics will contribute to the increasing health care services labor force, as new workers must be trained and new jobs created. In fact, U.S. Department of Labor forecasts for employment show that by 2012, 16 percent of all wage and salary jobs created will be in health services. It follows that an increasingly skilled health services labor force will further add to health care costs.

Reimbursement System Incentives

Dating back to the 1930s, health insurance has been the primary source of health care reimbursement in the United States. Historically, when insurance companies paid physicians, hospitals, and other health care providers, regardless of fees the providers charged, there was little incentive among

1. Who are the major stakeholders in the American health care system?

_____

_____

2. What three issues are of primary concern to stakeholders within the American health care system?

_____

_____

3. Discuss how the three factors identified in question 2 are interrelated.

_____

_____

4. How do increasing levels of medical and health care information technologies add to health care costs?

_____

_____

5. Of what significance is the percentage of the gross domestic product represented by health care spending?

_____

_____

providers for holding fees down. Over time, however, when reimbursement for health care costs—either through individual health insurance payments or through employer-provided health insurance payments—became routine, health care costs rose. Government financing mechanisms, such as Medicaid and Medicare, also added to health care costs.

In the 1980s, as health care costs continued to spiral upward, managed care organizations were formed as a means of containing costs. Under the managed care system, clients prepaid for health care services, and managed care organizations restricted reimbursement to health care providers according to certain guidelines. In most cases, for example, patients who belong to managed care organizations are required to see primary, or gatekeeper, physicians who control access to specialists. Furthermore, managed care organizations typically do not pay for medical treatments classified as experimental, and new treatments and procedures often fall within this category.

Managed care clients have often been dissatisfied with reimbursement restrictions, however, and their dissatisfaction has led to continually evolving reimbursement arrangements between health care providers and managed care payers.

ACCESS

Access to health care is determined by availability as well as by the ability to pay for the service. The U.S. Department of Health and Human Services, Health Resources and Services Administration, has determined that 20 percent of the nation's population resides in areas where physicians, dentists, and other health care practitioners are in short supply. Shortages of medical facilities such as community clinics and hospitals are also a factor in determining access to health care. Medically underserved areas can include urban as well as rural areas, entire counties, sections within counties, groups of counties, and other designated areas. Medically underserved populations include groups of persons who face economic, cultural, or linguistic barriers to health care.

Government and employers are the largest purchasers of health care for a majority of working adults—but what happens when individuals are working for small employers who do not provide health care benefits, are too young for Medicare, are earning too much money for Medicaid but not enough to purchase private health insurance, are unemployed, or are otherwise ineligible for dependable health care benefits? Access to health care services, in these cases, is typically available only sporadically—through emergency room visits, free clinics, free immunizations, and so on—or not at all.

Some argue that access to health care services is a basic human right, and should not be denied to anyone, regardless of social or employment status. The fact remains, however, that health care services are not free—so who will pay the bill? This remains the crucial question for Congress and for all health care stakeholders as the twenty-first century progresses.

Government Attempts to Reform Health Care

Presidents Truman, Nixon, and Carter said that health care reform was a priority for their administrations, but no reforms were passed during their years in office. Legislation to substantially reform the American health care industry was introduced during the Clinton presidential administration, in the form of the Health Security Act of 1993. The act included the following provisions:

▪ It guaranteed health insurance benefits to all Americans, with no lifetime limits on coverage.

▪ It provided a comprehensive package of medical services delivered in hospitals, clinics, professional offices, and other sites.

▪ It provided for one uniform, comprehensive benefit package that would replace hundreds of different insurance products on the market.

▪ Health insurance premiums would pay the cost of the new system, but enforceable caps would be placed on the rate of increase in premium prices.

The structure of the proposed new health care system consisted of an independent National Health Board that would act as the board of directors for the health care system, setting national standards and overseeing implementation of reform. It also provided for alliances—state, regional, corporate, and health plan alliances—that would offer a choice of health insurance plans, including traditional fee-for-service arrangements, preferred provider organizations, and health maintenance organizations.

The Health Security Act of 1993 failed to pass, and there were many reasons for its failure. Among them were these:

▪ Medicare was in place to provide help with health care costs for seniors, and Medicaid provided aid for lower-income and unemployed individuals; therefore, the public did not see the need for drastic health care reform.

▪ The act's basis for reform was *managed competition:* a complicated concept that combined market forces and government regulations. The concept had a narrow bloc of backers among members of Congress and the health care provider community.

The act mandated that everyone have health insurance, with employed individuals paying 80 percent of the cost and employers paying 20 percent. (The government would pay for low-income and unemployed individuals' coverage.)

Since health care reform is consistently on the minds of political candidates and voters, the concept will undoubtedly be revisited as new members of Congress and incoming presidents take office.

QUALITY

Agency for Healthcare Research and Quality (AHRQ) The lead federal agency responsible for tracking and improving the quality, safety, efficiency, and effectiveness of health care for Americans.

The **Agency for Healthcare Research and Quality (AHRQ)** is the lead federal agency responsible for tracking and improving the quality, safety, efficiency, and effectiveness of health care for Americans.

Since 2003, the AHRQ has studied the health care industry and tracked quality of health care. The agency's findings are published in an annual report, The National Healthcare Quality Report (NHQR). The first NHQR, issued in 2003, found certain key issues to be problematic, as listed below. Findings from the most recent (2006) NHQR follow each key issue that was originally listed:

1. **High-quality health care is not universal.** The public's access to high-quality health care varies with states, cities, and patients' income levels. For measures that had trend data, however, some areas had improved over time. For example, most diabetics had their blood sugar levels checked, most people had blood pressure and cholesterol levels checked, and 85 percent of people experiencing heart attacks received aspirin on arrival at hospitals. Furthermore, the majority of women were screened for breast cancer with mammography, and over 73 percent of children aged 35 months to 19 years had received all recommended vaccinations. Most of the elderly received influenza immunizations.

   2006: The variation in health care quality remained high. The study's core measures across all 50 states showed hospital quality measures improving faster than those for other facilities. In hospitals, care in the following areas was improving:

   ▮ Heart attack—improving at 15 percent per year
   ▮ Pneumonia—improving at 11.7 percent per year
   ▮ Heart failure—improving at 8.4 percent per year
   ▮ Postoperative safety—improving at 7.3 percent per year

2. **Opportunities for preventive care are frequently missed.** The 2003 NHQR found that too great a proportion of medical services focused on treatment after poor health occurs, rather than preventing it before it began. Progress had been made in the treatment of heart attacks, cancer, diabetes, and end-stage renal disease, but health care practitioners neglected opportunities to stop these same diseases before they start, through either patient education or basic screening tests. Areas where more focus on prevention could save more lives and resources were smoking cessation counseling and screening more people for high cholesterol and for colorectal cancer.

   2006: Prevention continued to lag behind treatment for illness, but improvement in some areas had occurred. New measurements for showing improvement in prevention and treatment were added to the 2006 report:

- How often was advice from health care practitioners on eating, exercise, and vision care given to patients?
- Were occurrences of asthma, administration of hospice care, and treatments emphasizing patient-centeredness recorded in hospitals?
- Were occurrences of postoperative complications, adverse events, and other patient safety concerns recorded?

3. **Management of chronic diseases presents unique quality challenges.** Most of the conditions covered in the report were chronic, and included cancer, chronic kidney disease (CKD), diabetes, HIV and AIDS, depression, asthma, and congestive heart failure. NHQR found considerable variation in the delivery of chronic care tests and treatment.

    2006: NHQR found that especially in hospitals, acute care measures showed higher improvement rates than preventive and chronic care measures. Improvements in hospital care may have been due to public reporting of health care quality, in-house and government quality improvement programs, and policies supporting improvement initiatives.

4. **There is more to learn.** In 2003, there was no one national survey tracking quality of health care in America. The first NHQR relied on a variety of national data sources in compiling the report, and the result was uneven coverage of selected report measures. Rapid advances in knowledge and limitations and advances in information technology also led to uneven tracking of health care quality measures.

    2006: The NHQR has become an annual event, allowing for continuous tracking of certain health care measures. Aspects of health care that had significantly improved by 2006 were the following:

    - Patient-centeredness, or the measure of communication between patients and health care providers. Patients were asked whether or not health care providers sometimes or never listened carefully, explained things clearly, respected what patients had to say, and spent enough time with them. Parents of children who were patients were asked the same questions regarding health care providers' interaction with children.
    - Treatment for respiratory diseases. More tuberculosis patients completed curative courses of treatment within 12 months of initiation, and the percentage of visits at which antibiotics were prescribed for children with common colds decreased.
    - Treatment for diabetes. More adults with diabetes received important screening tests for the management of the disease, and hospital admissions for lower-extremity amputation in diabetic patients decreased.
    - Prevention of heart disease. More smokers receiving routine checkups were advised to quit smoking.

Two measures showed deterioration: the percentage of emergency room visits in which the patient left without being seen had increased in 2006, and the national suicide death rate had also increased.

Both the 2003 and the 2006 reports emphasized that greater improvement in health care quality in the United States is possible and crucial to extending life expectancy and maintaining a healthy quality of life for the nation's population.

Life expectancy, or the number of years an individual can expect to live, calculated from his or her birth, is currently about 78 years in the United States, placing the United States 44th when compared with other countries. Residents of Andorra, a small republic in the eastern Pyrenees between Spain and France, have the world's highest life expectancy, at

life expectancy The number of years an individual can expect to live, calculated from his or her birth.

6. Check the 10 amendments to the United States Constitution called the Bill of Rights at http://usinfo. state.gov/usa/infousa/facts/funddocs/billeng.htm. Is health care listed as a right for all Americans?

_____

_____

7. List three areas where the National Healthcare Quality Report (NHQR) determined improvement had occurred between 2003 and 2006.

_____

_____

8. In your opinion, why is the United States 44th on a list of life expectancies in various countries?

_____

_____

83.5 years, and residents of Swaziland, a monarchy in southeastern Africa, have the lowest, at 32.23 years.

Access to universal health care is not necessarily a contributing factor to longer life expectancies. Factors that determine life expectancy vary greatly even within the United States, according to race, income level, geography, and such preventable risk factors as smoking, drug and alcohol abuse, obesity, high blood pressure, elevated cholesterol levels, poor diet, and physical inactivity.

HEALTH CARE FORECASTS

Experts predict that the key health care issues of cost, access, and quality will continue to be of concern for Americans within the health care system, and will probably be joined by a new group of issues that, according to _Health & Health Care 2010: The Forecast, The Challenge,_ will include the following:

▮ Security of benefits—ensuring that employees do not lose health care benefits when they lose their jobs or go to work for smaller employers.

▮ Monitoring and organizing increasing numbers of managed care organizations, insurers, intermediaries (case managers, provider partners, fee-for-service brokers, and safety-net funders) and providers.

▮ Including consumers in health care decision making.

medical management The management of patient care and populations.

▮ Determining responsibility for **medical management** (the management of patient care and populations in order to lower costs, ensure access, and increase quality of health care). Medical management will involve patients, providers, employers, health plans and governments, and will consist of managing disease states for the acutely sick and chronically ill, as well as managing disease prevention in the generally well.

▮ Improving health behaviors of the American people.[2]

_____

[2]Institute for the Future, _Health & Health Care 2010: The Forecast, The Challenge,_ 2nd ed. (Princeton, NJ: Jossey-Bass, 2003). Reprinted with permission, John Wiley & Sons.

Of course, medical technologies and health information technologies will continue to improve rapidly.

Medical Technologies

New medical technologies are a major driving force within the health care industry. According to *Health & Health Care 2010,* advanced medical technologies that will affect patient care over the next decade include, but are not limited to, the following:

- Rational drug design—use of computers to create drugs designed to attack specific diseased cells or to otherwise pinpoint delivery and enhance efficacy.
- Continuing advancement in imaging equipment and techniques.
- Minimally invasive surgery, such as highly developed arthroscopic and laparoscopic techniques.
- Genetic mapping and testing.
- Gene therapy.
- New and improved vaccines.
- Artificial blood.
- Xenotransplantation.
- Use of stem cells.

Rational Drug Design

Rational drug design refers to the use of increasingly powerful computers to develop new drugs by looking at the molecular structure and chemical composition of target cells and creating substances that will bind to certain molecules, affecting their function inside the body. For example, drugs now in development for antiviral use will prevent viruses from using the body's protease enzymes to chop up amino acids for viruses to use as building blocks for replicating. These new antiviral drugs may be used to combat such diseases as HIV, encephalitis, measles, and influenza.

Drugs are also in development that can bind with receptors for various neurotransmitters in the nervous system, helping to reduce symptoms in patients suffering from neurological and mental diseases.

Similarly, drugs in development to combat cancer will target cancer cells for destruction, but will not destroy normal cells in the body, thus eliminating many of the noxious side effects cancer patients often suffer during chemotherapy.

Advances in Imaging

The improvement of computers is also leading to advances in imaging equipment and techniques.

Energy sources currently used for imaging include X-rays, ultrasound, electron beams, positrons, magnets, and radio frequencies. By precisely pinpointing areas of the body to be imaged and closely focusing the energy source, new imaging devices will be better able to avoid damaging normal tissue. The use of concentrated ultrasound energy to destroy kidney stones is one example of a relatively new technique now in use.

Future imaging equipment will also take advantage of the trend toward smaller, yet more powerful, computerized devices. Smaller magnetic resonance imaging (MRI) machines, for example, will soon be available for use in orthopedics, neurology, and mammography, which developers predict will not only provide clearer, more detailed images, but also lower purchasing and operating costs.

Minimally Invasive Surgery

Minimally invasive surgery involves corrective surgical techniques that do not require large incisions into body cavities. Such techniques include arthroscopic knee surgery, some types of vascular and brain surgeries, coronary angioplasty, and laparoscopic surgeries such as appendectomy (Figure 12-5) and cholecystectomy (removal of the gall bladder).

As a result of minimally invasive surgery, ambulatory surgery centers will continue to increase in number. Since minimally invasive surgeries usually require short hospital stays or no stays at all, and recuperation times are shorter than with traditional surgical procedures, these techniques may also contribute significantly to lowering health care costs.

Genetic Mapping and Testing

The Human Genome Project, discussed in Chapter 10, "The Beginning of Life and Childhood," launched an era of unprecedented interest in mapping the human genome. The project was begun in 1990 and progressed so quickly that it was ended ahead of schedule, in mid-2000. During that time, scientists identified approximately 20,000 to 25,000 genes present in human DNA. They also developed protocols for researching DNA, and passed their acquired knowledge on to other scientists.

The project's results have led to applications in **pharmacogenomics,** the science that defines how individuals are genetically programmed to respond to drugs. The results have also speeded the development of specific tests for genes causing cancers of the breast, colon, and prostate, and have added to scientists' knowledge of how genes cause the expression of certain traits in individuals—a science called **genometrics.**

The Human Genome Project also revealed future ramifications of genetic testing, including social and ethical implications. If a health insurance company obtains a client's genetic testing results, for example, and learns that he or she is at risk to develop a genetic disease, can the company drop coverage for the client? Will reproductive rights of certain individuals be restricted if genetic testing reveals that their offspring are at risk for inherited disabilities or diseases? Will prenatal genetic testing result in "designer" children for many couples? Will self-administered genetic testing kits eventually become available, bypassing valuable genetic counseling for consumers?

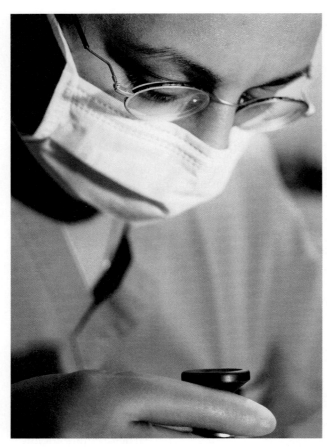

FIGURE 12-5 A surgeon performing laparoscopic surgery.

pharmacogenomics The science that defines how individuals are genetically programmed to respond to drugs.

genometrics The science of determining how genes cause the expression of certain traits in individuals.

Gene Therapy

Gene therapy, which involves correcting defective genes responsible for disease, is also on the horizon for the future. Researchers may use one of several approaches for correcting faulty genes:

▌ A normal gene may be inserted into a nonspecific location within the genome to replace a nonfunctional gene. This approach is most common.

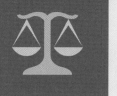

Court Case

Gene Therapy Case Settled

In 1999, physician-researchers at the University of Pennsylvania conducted gene therapy experiments designed to treat a disease called ornithine transcarbamylase (OTC) deficiency, which inhibits the liver's ability to process proteins. Researchers sought out adult subjects for the study who were carriers of the disease (all carriers are women) or who exhibited milder forms of the disease. Jesse Gelsinger, an 18-year-old who allegedly fit the subject search, participated in the study and received treatment. On September 17, 1999, Gelsinger died, allegedly as a direct result of the gene therapy treatment. On September 18, 2000, Gelsinger's father filed a lawsuit against the University of Pennsylvania; researchers James M. Wilson, Steven E. Raper, and Mark L. Batshaw; Arthur Caplan, director of the university's Center for Bioethics; and others.

The lawsuit was settled out of court in February 2005. Under the terms of the settlement, Wilson, Raper, and Batshaw did not admit any wrongdoing. The university and the Children's Hospital of Philadelphia, where Batshaw was affiliated, were to strengthen their research oversight and pay fines of $517,496 and $514, 622, respectively.

The plaintiffs in the case also settled a second lawsuit which the U.S. Justice Department initiated, alleging breach of the False Claims Act. Under terms of this settlement, Wilson was required to wait until 2010 before again leading research on humans. In the meantime, he would also undergo training and education relating to research on human subjects, work under enhanced oversight and monitoring, and lecture and write an article on "lessons learned."

Since the Gelsinger case was settled, other ethical lapses have been alleged in additional lawsuits filed by study participants, including unreported deaths of monkeys given similar gene therapy treatments; failure to inform the FDA, as required, when patients became so ill from the treatment that the study should have been suspended; and researchers' failure to disclose opportunities to profit if the treatment were successful.

John Gelsinger as Administrator and Personal Representative of the Estate of Jesse Gelsinger and Paul Gelsinger, in his own right v. The Trustees of the University of Pennsylvania, James Wilson, M.D., Genovo, Inc., Steven Raper, M.D., Mark Batshaw, M.D., William Kelley, M.D., Children's Hospital of Philadelphia, Children's National Medical Center, and Arthur Caplan, Ph.D.

- A normal gene could be substituted for an abnormal gene through an exchange of sections of chromosomes during meiosis.
- The abnormal gene could be repaired through selective reverse mutation, which returns the gene to its normal function.
- The regulation (the degree to which a gene is turned on or off) of a particular gene could be altered.

Both genetic testing and gene therapy are in evolving stages of development. Widespread utilization of the science will require practicing health care practitioners to acquire the knowledge and techniques necessary to practice genomic medicine—a field in which specialists are currently limited in number.

Improved Vaccines

The most common use of vaccines over time has been to prevent disease. Live or weakened forms of disease organisms are injected, and then stimulate the patient's immune system to produce antibodies against the disease organism. Infectious diseases such as whooping cough, diphtheria, measles, smallpox, polio, and influenza are prevented in this manner.

Another, more current, use of vaccines is to prevent the growth of small metastatic (spreading) tumors in cancer patients. Vaccinations to prevent

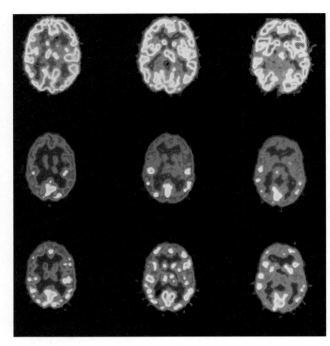

FIGURE 12-6 X-rays of brain activity during cocaine use.

various forms of cancer from developing are also in the works. For example, the vaccine for the human papilloma virus (HPV), which can cause cervical cancer, is now available for use, and is one example of a twenty-first-century vaccine that may significantly reduce cancer in the United States.

Furthermore, recently two medical researchers from Baylor University in Houston, Texas, have reported progress in developing a vaccine to prevent or cure an addiction to cocaine (Figure 12-6). Inactivated drug molecules are bonded with inactivated cholera molecules and injected into the body. The body releases antibodies against the cholera molecule, which also act to prevent the drug from entering the brain, where it can activate an addiction response. The liver metabolizes the drug molecules and they are excreted from the body. When the drug no longer produces a high, addicts may lose interest and stop taking the drug. Scientists theorize that if the FDA approves the vaccine, it may also be developed to cure addiction to other drugs, such as nicotine.

Artificial Blood

When a patient loses a large volume of blood, the loss is significant on two fronts:

1. Loss of plasma, the liquid portion of the blood that consists mostly of water and carries nutrients, hormones, and waste, causes reduced blood volume.

2. Loss of the formed elements in blood—including red and white blood cells, platelets that aid in clotting, and parts of cells that float in the plasma—means that oxygen is not reaching the damaged tissue, and the tissue can die.

For the millions of traumatic brain injury (TBI) and spinal cord injury patients that are rushed to emergency rooms every year, tissue death is especially drastic, because it usually causes paralysis, coma, or even death. Physicians treating such patients have found that administering an artificial blood substitute can restore oxygen circulation to damaged tissue faster than transfusing whole blood, without the necessity for cross-typing or screening for disease organisms.

Pharmaceutical companies developed several varieties of artificial blood in the 1980s and 1990s, but early formulas were abandoned when they caused heart attacks, strokes, and deaths in human trials. Some early formulas also caused capillaries to collapse and blood pressure to rise. Recent research, however, has led to several blood substitutes classified into two types: hemoglobin-based oxygen carriers (HBOCs) and perfluorocarbons (PFCs), which are entirely synthetic and have the highest gas-dissolving capacity of any liquid. Some of these blood substitutes are already in use, and others are nearing the end of their FDA-required testing phases and may soon be available to hospitals.

Xenotransplantation

As discussed in Chapter 10, "The Beginning of Life and Childhood," xenotransplantation involves transplanting animal tissue into human patients.

Two documented cases of xenotransplantation in the 1980s and 1990s involved the use of baboon organs. In 1984, Dr. Leonard Bailey transplanted a baboon's heart into Baby Fae, a newborn with a severe heart defect known as left hypoplastic heart. Bailey had theorized that the baby's underdeveloped immune system would not attack the foreign tissue. Baby Fae did well for a few days; then, her body mounted a massive immune reaction to the baboon heart that subsequently caused her death.

A baboon was the organ source again in 1992, when surgeons at the University of Pittsburgh Medical Center replaced a man's diseased liver with a healthy baboon liver. The patient had Hepatitis B and was not considered a good transplant prospect because the disease was likely to occur in the new, healthy liver, as well. Surgeons hoped the baboon liver would survive, because baboons are not susceptible to the Hepatitis B virus. Again, however, the patient died from a massive immune reaction.

The most successful uses of xenotransplantation to date have involved transplanting into human patients certain pig tissues, such as skin and nervous tissue. Pigs have been chosen as an object of study for possible xenotransplantation of whole organs, various tissues, and cells, since the sizes of their organs and cells closely match those of humans.

A strain of genetically engineered pigs has been raised that lacks the gene responsible for alpha-1, 3-galactosyltransferase (GT), a sugary substance normally present in the pig vascular system. Since humans have natural, preformed antibodies to GT, transplants of pig tissue have, in the past, often resulted in immediate rejection. Scientists are hopeful that tissues and organs in the genetically engineered pigs will more readily be accepted by human transplantation patients.

Use of Stem Cells

The largest barrier to using stem cells to treat disease has been public objection, on religious and ethical grounds, to the destruction of human embryos that are most useful in stem cell research. President George W. Bush felt so strongly about this issue that his administration prohibited federal funding of embryonic stem cell research, which slowed the progress of such research.

In 2007, however, researchers announced that human skin cells had been used to produce the stem cells that might someday be useful to patients with spinal cord injuries, Parkinson's disease, diabetes, damaged hearts, and other diseases or conditions. Skin and bone cells have been among the initial cell-building successes, but the potential for large-scale stem cell use is huge. Political and ethical issues seem the most formidable barriers to use of stem cell technology in the future.

Health Information Technologies

Polls indicate that most Americans believe that their health care providers routinely use computer technology for storing and managing their medical records. Unfortunately, too often this is not the case. The health care industry has lagged behind other industries in adopting technology for performing daily business chores. For instance, many physicians' offices still keep reams of paper patient files, filled with hastily scrawled notes, test results, X-rays, illegible copies of prescriptions written, and other materials that are subject to fire, flood (witness the Katrina disaster), rot, and other natural forces.

Over the next decade, advances in these areas of communications and information technology will significantly affect the health care industry:

Computer hardware. Faster microprocessors and larger memory capabilities will make managing health care information faster and easier for HCI specialists.

Data storage. Nearly unlimited digital storage capabilities will make it possible to store a population's health care data in smaller and smaller spaces.

Wireless technology. Health care practitioners currently use handheld computers as study aids and to access digitalized patient records, and such use will increase in the future.

Networking bandwidths and data compression. Faster networking systems with larger information transmission capabilities will be the rule, increasing the use of these technologies.

Data storage retrieval. Programs that can find and retrieve information—from digitalized libraries, search engines, government collections, and other sources—will become more efficient and easier to use, thus increasing their popularity.

Security and encryption. Privacy of health care information is a major concern as information technology becomes more sophisticated and more widely used. HIPAA's requirements concerning electronic health care records have spurred hospitals and other medical facilities to move toward digital transmission and storage, and the movement will progress as security and encryption methods become more reliable.

Internet. The Internet and the World Wide Web are currently popular sources for medical information, and the trend will continue as the Internet continues to evolve.

3-D computing. Interior designers, architects, car and equipment designers, animated movie makers, and others in various design fields have access to computer programs, called computer-aided design (CAD) programs, that let them work in 3-D. In the future,

CHECK YOUR PROGRESS

Choose three of the medical technologies listed above that are forecast to improve or otherwise change in the future, and give one specific example of how each might be applied in medical situations.

9. _____

_____

10. _____

_____

11. _____

_____

Choose three of the health information technologies listed above that are forecasted to improve in the future, and give one specific example of how each might be applied in medical situations.

12. _____

_____

13. _____

_____

14. _____

_____

CAD programs will become more readily available to health care practitioners, as a means both of visualizing medical procedures and of displaying large amounts of information at one time.

Database software. Already used extensively in business, database software will evolve into new classes that will increase the capacity to store, present, sort, and analyze data.

Sensors. Just as implanted pacemakers and insulin pumps sense when a patient's heart rate or insulin levels must be adjusted, future devices will allow health care practitioners to monitor and adjust a wider range of patient symptoms and events.

As all of the above devices and systems become less expensive, larger numbers of health care practitioners and facilities will adopt them for routine use.

REFORMING THE HEALTH CARE SYSTEM

Some states have taken the initiative in health care reform, but at the national level, because many of the stakeholders in the health care industry do not want change, reform has been an unpopular issue. Suggestions such as these for reform, however, have come from national organizations, policy analysts, and recent presidential and congressional candidates, and cover cost, access, and quality:

- Charge Medicare beneficiaries more.
- Create a dedicated federal health tax to cover all government health spending, such as Medicare and Medicaid. The tax could be an energy tax, a payroll tax, or an income surtax. If health spending rose, the tax would increase.
- Eliminate the income tax exclusion for employer-paid insurance and replace it with a tax credit of lesser value.
- Provide access through public financing for Americans living at or below poverty levels.
- Provide extensive education to consumers concerning living a healthy lifestyle.
- Disclose and reward quality-based medical practice.
- Support and reinvigorate through government financing the nation's deteriorating public health system.
- Require all Americans to have health insurance coverage, available through public and private plan options made available through the existing Federal Employees Health Benefit Program (FEHBP).

State Children's Health Initiative Program (SCHIP)
A program enacted by the Balanced Budget Act of 1997 to help low-income children under 19 who are not covered by Medicaid.

The **State Children's Health Initiative Program (SCHIP)** was enacted by the Balanced Budget Act of 1997 to help ensure health care for low-income children under 19 who are not covered by Medicaid. SCHIP is jointly financed by the federal and state governments and is state-administered. Within broad federal guidelines, each state determines the design of its program, eligibility groups, benefit packages, payment levels for coverage, and administrative and operating procedures. SCHIP provides a capped amount of funds to states on a matching basis for federal funds. Variations of the SCHIP program are in effect in all 50 states, but Congress must periodically pass legislation reauthorizing federal funding, and the president must sign the reauthorization laws to keep the program funded.

As a health care practitioner, not only is it your responsibility to offer patient-centered, thoughtful, professionally competent care; it is also your duty to stay abreast of current trends in the health care industry and to know what is forecast for the future.

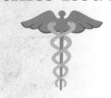

Ethics Issues

Health Care Trends and Forecasts

Jean Connor of Cambridge, Massachusetts, was the 2007–2008 president of the Chicago-based American Dental Hygienists' Association (ADHA). She also works as a practicing dental hygienist. Connor, who says she especially likes the variety of patients she sees, emphasizes that dental hygienists work under the supervision of their dentist-employers. "We may not agree with the dentist's opinions, but they are the opinions that count," she says. "State dental boards may help us with ethical dilemmas, but these types of issues are so subjective, it's often difficult to resolve them.

"It helps if the office where you work has set procedures and standards that you can rely on," Connor continues. Don't take a job just because there was an opening; check the policy and procedures manual before you agree to work for an employer, to be sure you and the potential employer are a good fit.

ETHICS ISSUE 1: You are an LPN employed in a medical office. Medicare payments to the physicians who work in the clinic have been cut, so policy has changed to "no new Medicare patients will be accepted."

DISCUSSION QUESTIONS

1. Do you believe the policy stated above is ethical? Why or why not?

_____

_____

2. You are accompanying an older relative visiting the above clinic for the first time, and your relative has been turned away as a patient. What is your reaction to the clinic's stated policy?

_____

_____

3. Imagine that *you* are the older person visiting the above clinic for the first time, and you are turned away as a patient. Will your reaction be the same as in Question 2 above? Explain your answer.

_____

_____

ETHICS ISSUE 2: Higher health insurance costs limit wage and salary gains, because as insurance costs go up, employers who provide health care benefits raise the amount employees must pay for health insurance.

DISCUSSION QUESTION

1. Do you believe it is ethical for employers to increase employees' share of health insurance premiums when health care costs rise? Explain your answer.

_____

_____

ETHICS ISSUE 3: Health insurance costs rise when health care becomes more costly. Patients who cannot afford to pay more for health insurance may then become underinsured or uninsured.

DISCUSSION QUESTION

1. Do you believe health care practitioners have an ethical obligation to hold down or reduce the fees they charge, considering the millions of people in the United States who are underinsured or uninsured? Why or why not?

_____

_____

ETHICS ISSUE 4: Connor, the dental hygienist quoted above, says that her association is concerned that access to the care dental hygienists provide is decreasing. One reason is lack of insurance coverage, but another is that dental hygienists who retire or leave the profession early are not being replaced.

DISCUSSION QUESTION

1. Do you believe the health care industry has an ethical obligation to actively recruit health care practitioners who are in short supply? Explain your answer.

_____

_____

ETHICS ISSUE 5: Laura Swisher, an associate professor in the physical therapy department at the University of South Florida, says physical therapists are moving toward more autonomy, which creates new ethical issues. For example, in the past it was unethical for physical therapists to diagnose a patient. Now, however, patients have direct access to physical therapists, who often diagnose conditions and refer patients to physicians.

DISCUSSION QUESTION

1. Since a physical therapist may see a patient before he or she visits a physician, does the PT have an ethical obligation to ask this patient about health (e.g., Do you get regular physical exams? Are your immunizations up to date? Have you had health problems in other areas lately?)? Explain your answer.

_____

_____

ETHICS ISSUE 6: The trend in hospital staffing is to hire many temporary workers. This, according to Swisher, raises the continuity of care issue. (James, the physical therapist featured at the beginning of this chapter, is also a temporary worker, filling in where PT shortages exist in many locations.)

DISCUSSION QUESTIONS

1. What is the responsibility for continuity of care for the patients a temporary health care worker sees, when that worker may be gone tomorrow?

_____

_____

2. Do you see an ethical solution to the continuity of care issue regarding temporary health care practitioners? Explain your answer.

_____

_____

Go to www.mhhe.com/judson5e to practice your case review skills. Then read on for more information

CHAPTER 12 REVIEW

Applying Knowledge

Match each definition that follows with the correct term by writing the appropriate letter in the space provided.

_____1. American's total income for all goods and services

_____2. Science that defines how individuals are genetically programmed to respond to drugs

_____3. Science of determining how genes cause the expression of certain traits in individuals

_____4. Federal program designed to provided health insurance for children

_____5. Federal agency that is responsible to study issues in the quality of health care

_____6. Legislation to reform the health care industry

_____7. A report issued annually that discusses improvement in health care in the United States

a. NHQR

b. AHRQ

c. Health Security Act

d. Pharmacogenomics

e. GDP

f. Genometrics

g. SCHIP

Answer the following questions in the spaces provided.

An article by Robert J. Samuelson in the December 10, 2007, issue of *Newsweek* stated, "The politics of health care rests on a mass illusion: Most Americans think that someone else pays for their care."

8. As an employee working in a job with health care benefits, who pays for your care?

_____

9. Who pays for the health care of the uninsured?

_____

10. As the number of people 65 and older increases, who will pay for higher Medicare spending?

_____

11. In your opinion, what are the implications for future health care practitioners in the United States if health care costs continue to rise?

_____

_____

12. How can the major stakeholders in the American health care system work to improve the system?

_____

_____

13. How do increasing numbers of uninsured Americans add to health care costs?

_____

_____

Case Study

Medical tourism is a recent trend in health care. Patients go to a different country for either urgent or elective medical procedures. The procedures are the same procedures being done in United States hospitals and outpatient surgery centers, often by American-trained physicians who have moved back home. Medical tourism is fast becoming a worldwide, multibillion-dollar industry. In fact, some insurance companies are paying for the cost of the procedures, as costs are far less than those charged in the United States. Sometimes the insurance company even pays for the plane fare and hotel costs—so a patient gets a vacation in addition to the needed surgical procedure. The reasons patients travel for treatment vary from the lower costs (for Americans) to shorter waiting times (for those in countries where there is national health insurance). There is no regulation by the United States government of medical tourism. Many patients come back enthusiastic about not only the success of their treatment, and the integrity and skill of all the providers, but also the high-class hotel-like accommodations while in the foreign hospital. India is one of the major countries advertising these services.

14. If other countries are able to do similar procedures as those done in the United States for lower fees, and with the same or better outcomes, why can't the United States offer the same services?

_____

_____

15. If your insurance company wanted you to go to another country for a procedure because it was less expensive, would you do it? Explain your answer.

_____

_____

In 2007, American patients with recurring head and neck cancers were traveling to China to receive gene therapy via a drug designed to activate the p53 gene, which is supposed to turn off cells that multiply abnormally, but often malfunctions, letting cancerous tumors grow. Since the drug was not FDA–approved in the United States, patients traveled to China to receive it, at a cost of $20,000 for the two-month treatment. No studies had yet been conducted to determine the efficacy of the treatment, but many patients believed their tumors were receding. A genetic research company in the United States was threatening to sue the Chinese company manufacturing the drug, alleging patent infringement.

16. In your opinion, should American patients be prohibited from traveling to foreign countries to receive unproven and possibly dangerous medical treatment? Explain your answer.

_____

_____

17. In your opinion, was it ethical for the Chinese company to charge $10,000 per month for the treatment? Explain your answer.

_____

_____

Internet Activities

Complete the activities and answer the questions that follow.

18. Visit the Web sites for the major political parties in this country. The American public repeatedly state in surveys that they want to see the health care system changed. However, it does not appear that we can agree on what that change should be. What are the positions of the major political parties with regard to changing the health care system in America? Are they clearly stated? Do you agree or disagree with the political parties' statements?

_____

_____

_____

_____

19. Visit the Kaiser Family Foundation Web site (www.kff.org) or the Commonwealth Health Foundation Web site (www.commonwealthfund.org). Review the organization's research and position papers, selecting one to summarize and present to your class. Are their reports easy to understand and summarize? Explain your answer.

_____

_____

20. Visit the Centers for Disease Control, National Center for Health Statistics Web site (www.cdc.gov/nchs). List those reports that you think might be helpful to you if you had to prepare a report on the latest trends in health care.

_____

_____

STATE MEDICAL BOARDS

Contact information for each state's medical board is listed online on the Web site of the Federation of State Medical Boards at www.fsmb.org/.

The following list was taken from that site. Check the Web site periodically for updates on contact information.

Alabama State Board of Medical Examiners
P.O. Box 946
Montgomery, AL 36101-0946
(street address: 848 Washington Ave.)
(334) 242-4116 / Fax: (334) 242-4155
(800) 227-2606
www.albme.org

Alaska State Medical Board
550 West Seventh Ave., Suite 1500
Anchorage, AK 99501
(907) 269-8163 / Fax: (907) 269-8196
www.dced.state.ak.us/occ/pmed.htm

Arizona Medical Board
9545 East Doubletree Ranch Road
Scottsdale, AZ 85258-5514
(480) 551-2700 / Fax: (480) 551-2704
www.azmd.gov

**Arizona Board of Osteopathic Examiners
    in Medicine and Surgery**
9535 East Doubletree Ranch Road
Scottsdale, AZ 85258-5539
(480) 657-7703 Fax: (480) 657-7715
www.azdo.gov

Arkansas State Medical Board
2100 Riverfront Dr.
Little Rock, AR 72202-1793
(501) 296-1802 / Fax: (501) 603-3555
www.armedicalboard.org

Medical Board of California
2005 Evergreen Street, Suite 1200
Sacramento, CA 95815
(916) 263-2389 / Fax: (916) 263-2387
(800) 633-2322
www.caldocinfo.ca.gov

Osteopathic Medical Board of California
2720 Gateway Oaks Dr., Suite 350
Sacramento, CA 95833-3500
(916) 263-3100 / Fax: (916) 263-3117
www.dca.ca.gov/osteopathic

Colorado Board of Medical Examiners
1560 Broadway, Suite 1300
Denver, CO 80202-5140
(303) 894-7690 / Fax: (303) 894-7692
www.dora.state.co.us/medical

Connecticut Medical Examining Board
P.O. Box 340308
Hartford, CT 06134-0308
(street address: 410 Capitol Ave., MS #13PHO)
Licensing/Examinations, (860) 509-8374
Administrative (860) 509-7648 / Fax: (860) 509-7553
www.dph.state.ct.us

Delaware Board of Medical Practice
P.O. Box 1401
Dover, DE 19903
(street address: 861 Silver Lake Blvd., Cannon Building,
    Suite 203, 19904)
(302) 739-4522 / Fax: (302) 739-2711
www.dpr.delaware.gov

District of Columbia Board of Medicine
717 14th Street, NW Suite 600
Washington DC 20005
(202) 724-4900/Fax: (202) 727-8471
dchealth.dc.gov

Florida Board of Medicine
Department of Health
4052 Bald Cypress Way, BIN #C03
Tallahassee, FL 32399-3253
(850) 245-4131/ Fax: (850) 488-9325
www.doh.state.fl.us

Florida Board of Osteopathic Medicine
4052 Bald Cypress Way, BIN C06
Tallahassee, FL 32399-1753
(850) 245-4161 / Fax: (850) 487-9874
www.doh.state.fl.us/mqa/osteopath/

Georgia Composite State Board of Medical Examiners
2 Peachtree Street, NW, 36th Floor
Atlanta, GA 30303
(404) 656-3913 / Fax: (404) 656-9723
www.medicalboard.state.ga.us

Guam Board of Medical Examiners
Health Professional Licensing Office
123 Chalan Kareta South Route 10
Margilao, Guam 96913-6304
(011) 671-735-7406-8 / Fax: (011) 671-735-7413

Hawaii Board of Medical Examiners
Department of Commerce and Consumer Affairs
P.O. Box 3469
Honolulu, HI 96813
(street address: 335 Merchant St.,
    Room 301, 96813)
(808) 586-3000 / Fax:(808) 586-2874
www.hawaii.gov/dcca/pvl

Idaho State Board of Medicine
1755 Westgate Drive, Suite 140
Boise, ID 83704
(208) 327-7000 / Fax:(208) 327-7005
www.bom.state.id.us

**Illinois Department of Financial
    and Professional Regulation**
Division of Professional Regulation,
Chicago Office (disciplinary issues)
Doris Barnes, Disciplinary Board Liaison
James R. Thompson Center
100 W. Randolph Street, Suite 9-300
Chicago, IL 60601
(312) 814-4500 / Fax: (312) 814-1837
www.idfpr.com

**Illinois Department of Financial
    and Professional Regulation**
Division of Professional Regulation,
Springfield Office (licensure issues)
Sandra Dunn, Licensure Manager
320 W. Washington St., 3rd Floor
Springfield, IL 62786
(217) 785-0800 / Fax: (217) 524-2169
www.idfpr.com

Indiana Professional Licensing Agency
402 W. Washington St., Room W072
Indianapolis, IN 46204
(317) 232-2960 / Fax: (317) 233-4236
www.in.gov/pla/bandc/mlbi

Iowa Board of Medicine
400 Southwest Eighth Street, Suite C
Des Moines, IA 50309-4686
(515) 281-5171 / Fax: (515) 242-5908
www.docboard.org/ia/ia_home.htm

Kansas Board of Healing Arts
235 South Topeka Blvd.
Topeka, KS 66603-3068
(785) 296-7413 / Fax: (785) 296-0852
www.ksbha.org

Kentucky Board of Medical Licensure
Hurstbourne Office Park
310 Whittington Parkway, Suite 1B
Louisville, KY 40222-4916
(502) 429-7150 / Fax: (502) 429-7158
kbml.ky.gov

Louisiana State Board of Medical Examiners
P.O. Box 30250
New Orleans, LA 70190-0250
(street address: 630 Camp St., 70130)
(504) 568-6820 / Fax: (504) 568-8893
www.lsbme.louisiana.gov

Maine Board of Licensure in Medicine
137 State House Station (U.S. mail)
161 Capitol Street (delivery service)
Augusta, ME 04333
(207) 287-3601 / Fax: (207) 287-6590
www.docboard.org/me/me_home.htm

Maine Board of Osteopathic Licensure
142 State House Station
Augusta, ME 04333-0142
(207) 287-2480 (207) 287-3015
http://www.maine.gov/osteo/

Maryland Board of Physicians
P.O. Box 2571
Baltimore, MD 21215-0095
(street address: 4201 Patterson Ave.,
    fourth floor, 21215)
(410) 764-4777 / Fax: (410) 358-2252
(800) 492-6836
www.mbp.state.md.us/

**Massachusetts Board of Registration
    in Medicine**
560 Harrison Ave., Suite G-4
Boston, MA 02118
(617) 654-9800 / Fax: (617) 451-9568
(800) 377-0550
www.massmedboard.org

Michigan Board of Medicine
P.O. Box 30670
Lansing, MI 48909-8170
(street address: 611 W. Ottawa St,
    1st floor, 48933)
(517) 335-0918 / Fax: (517) 373-2179
www.michigan.gov/healthlicense

**Michigan Board of Osteopathic
    Medicine and Surgery**
P.O. Box 30670
Lansing, MI 48909-8170
(street address: 611 W. Ottawa St, 1st floor, 48933)
(517) 335-0918 / Fax: (517) 373-2179
www.michigan.gov/healthlicense

Minnesota Board of Medical Practice
University Park Plaza
2829 University Ave. SE, Suite 500
Minneapolis, MN 55414-3246
(612) 617-2130 / Fax: (612) 617-2166
Hearing impaired 1-800-627-3529
www.bmp.state.mn.us

Mississippi State Board of Medical Licensure
1867 Crane Ridge Drive, Suite 200B
Jackson, MS 39216
(601) 987-3079 / Fax: (601) 987-4159
www.msbml.state.ms.us

**Missouri State Board of Registration for
the Healing Arts**
3605 Missouri Blvd.
Jefferson City, MO 65109
(573) 751-0098 / Fax: (573) 751-3166
www.pr.mo.gov/healingarts.asp

Montana Board of Medical Examiners
P.O. Box 200513
Helena, MT 59620-0513
(406) 841-2300 / Fax: (406) 841-2363
http://mt.gov/dli/bsd/license/bsd_boards/med_board/
board_page.asp

Nebraska Board of Medicine and Surgery
Health and Human Services
Regulation and Licensure Credentialing Division
P.O. Box 94986
Lincoln, NE 68509-4986
(402) 471-2118 / Fax: (402) 471-3577
www.hhs.state.ne.us/

Nevada State Board of Medical Examiners
1105 Terminal Way, Suite 301
Reno, NV 89502
(775) 688-2559 / Fax: (775) 688-2321
www.medboard.nv.gov

Nevada State Board of Osteopathic Medicine
2860 E. Flamingo Rd., Suite D
Las Vegas, NV 89121
(702) 732-2147 / Fax: (702) 732-2079
www.bom.nv.gov

New Hampshire State Board of Medicine
2 Industrial Park Drive, Suite 8
Concord, NH 03301-8520
(603) 271-1203 / Fax: (603) 271-6702
complaints (800) 780-4757
www.state.nh.us/medicine

New Jersey State Board of Medical Examiners
P.O. Box 183
Trenton, NJ 08625-0183
(609) 826-7100 / Fax: (609) 826-7117
www.state.nj.us/lps/ca/medical.htm#bme5

New Mexico Medical Board
2055 S. Pacheco, Building 400
Santa Fe, NM 87505
(505)476-7220 / Fax: (505) 476-7237
www.nmmb.state.nm.us

New Mexico Board of Osteopathic Medical Examiners
2550 Cerrillos Road
Santa Fe, NM 87501-5101
(505) 476-4654 / Fax: (505) 476-4645
www.rld.state.nm.us/b&c/Osteo

New York State Board for Medicine (Licensure)
89 Washington Avenue, 2nd Floor, West Wing
Albany, NY 12234
(518) 474-3817 Ext. 560 / Fax: (518) 486-4846
www.op.nysed.gov

**New York State Board for Professional
Medical Conduct (Discipline)**
Department of Health
Office of Professional Medical Conduct
433 River St., Suite 303
Troy, NY 12180-2299
(518) 402-0855 / Fax: (518) 402-0866
www.health.state.ny.us/

North Carolina Medical Board
P.O. Box 20007
Raleigh, NC 27619
(919) 326-1100 / Fax: (919) 326-1130
www.ncmedboard.org

North Dakota State Board of Medical Examiners
City Center Plaza
418 E. Broadway, Suite 12
Bismarck, ND 58501
(701) 328-6500 / Fax: (701) 328-6505
www.ndbomex.com

Northern Mariana Islands
Health Care Professions Licensing Board
P.O. Box 501458, CK
Saipan, MP 96950
(670) 664-4811 / Fax: (670) 664-4813
www.cnmiguide.com

State Medical Board of Ohio
30 E. Broad St. 3rd Floor
Columbus, OH 43215-6127
(614) 466-3934 / Fax: (614) 728-5946
(800) 554-7717
www.med.ohio.gov

**Oklahoma State Board of Medical Licensure
and Supervision**
P.O. Box 18256
Oklahoma City, OK 73154-0256
(405) 848-6841 / Fax: (405) 848-8240
(800) 381-4519
www.okmedicalboard.org

Oklahoma State Board of Osteopathic Examiners
4848 N. Lincoln Blvd., Suite 100
Oklahoma City, OK 73105-3335
(405) 528-8625 / Fax: (405) 557-0653
www.docboard.org/ok/ok.htm

Oregon Medical Board
1500 SW 1st Ave., Suite 620
Portland, OR 97201-5847
(971) 673-2700 / Fax: (971) 673-2670
www.oregon.gov/BME

Pennsylvania State Board of Medicine
P.O. Box 2649
Harrisburg, PA 17105-2649
(717) 787-2381 / Fax: (717) 787-7769
www.dos.state.pa.us

Pennsylvania State Board of Osteopathic Medicine
P.O. Box 2649
Harrisburg, PA 17105-2649
(street address: 124 Pine St., 17101)
(717) 783-4858 / Fax: (717) 787-7769
www.dos.state.pa.us

Board of Medical Examiners of Puerto Rico
P.O. Box 13969
San Juan, PR 00908
(787) 782-8937 / Fax: (787) 706-0304

Rhode Island Board of Medical Licensure and Discipline
Department of Health
Cannon Building, Room 205
Three Capitol Hill
Providence, RI 02908-5097
(401) 222-3855 / Fax: (401) 222-2158
http://www.health.ri.gov/hsr/bmld/

South Carolina Board of Medical Examiners
Department of Labor, Licensing and Regulation
110 Centerview Drive, Suite 202
Columbia, SC 29210-1289
(803) 896-4500 / Fax: (803) 896-4515
www.llr.state.sc.us/pol/medical

South Dakota State Board of Medical and Osteopathic Examiners
125 S. Main Ave.
Sioux Falls, SD 57104
(605) 367-7781 / Fax: (605) 367-7786
medicine.sd.gov

Tennessee Board of Medical Examiners
227 French Landing, Suite 300 Heritage Place
MetroCenter
Nashville, TN 37243
(800) 778-4123 / Fax: (615) 253-4484
http://health.state.tn.us

Tennessee Board of Osteopathic Examination
227 French Landing, Suite 300 Heritage Place
MetroCenter
Nashville, TN 37243
(800) 778-4123 / Fax: (615) 253-4484
http://health.state.tn.us

Texas Medical Board
P.O. Box 2018
Austin, TX 78768-2018
(512) 305-7010 / Fax: (512) 305-7008
Disciplinary Hotline (800) 248-4062
Consumer Complaint Hotline (800) 201-9353
www.tmb.state.tx.us

Utah Department of Commerce
Division of Occupational and
   Professional Licensure
Physicians Licensing Board
160 E. 300 South, 84102, Heber M.
   Wells Building, 4th Floor
Salt Lake City, UT 84114
(801) 530-6628 / Fax: (801) 530-6511
www.dopl.utah.gov

Utah Department of Commerce
Division of Occupational and
   Professional Licensure
Board of Osteopathic Medicine
160 E. 300 South, 84102, Heber M.
   Wells Building, 4th Floor
Salt Lake City, UT 84114
(801) 530-6628 / Fax: (801) 530-6511
www.dopl.utah.gov

Vermont Board of Medical Practice
108 Cherry Street
Burlington, VT 05401
(802) 657-4220 / Fax: (802) 657-4227
www.healthvermont.gov

Vermont Board of Osteopathic Physicians and Surgeons
Administrative Assistant
Office of Professional Regulation
National Life Bldg., North Fl 2
Montpelier, VT 05620-3402
802-828-1134
www.vtprofessionals.org

Virgin Islands Board of Medical Examiners
Department of Health
48 Sugar Estate
St. Thomas, VI 00802
(340) 774-0117/ Fax: (340) 777-4001
Medical Licensure Requirements

Virginia Board of Medicine
Perimeter Center
9960 Mayland Drive, Suite 300
Richmond, VA 23233-1463
Phone:(804) 367-4600
Fax Licensing Unit:(804) 527-4426 , Fax Discipline
    Unit:(804) 527-4429
www.dhp.virginia.gov

Washington Medical Quality Assurance Commission
Department of Health
310 Israel Road, SE
MS 47866
Tumwater, WA 98501
(360) 236-4788 / Fax: (360) 236-4768
www.doh.wa.gov

**Washington State Board of Osteopathic Medicine
    and Surgery**
Department of Health
P.O. Box 47866
Olympia, WA 98504-7866
(360) 236-4945 / Fax: (360) 236-2406
www.doh.wa.gov

West Virginia Board of Medicine
101 Dee Drive, Suite 103
Charleston, WV 25311
(304) 558-2921 / Fax: (304) 558-2084
www.wvdhhr.org/wvbom

West Virginia Board of Osteopathy
334 Penco Rd.
Weirton, WV 26062
(304) 723-4638 / Fax: (304) 723-6723
www.wvbdosteo.org

Wisconsin Medical Examining Board
Department of Regulation and Licensing
1400 E. Washington Ave.
Madison, WI 53703
(608) 266-2112 / Fax: (608) 261-7083
www.drl.state.wi.us

Wyoming Board of Medicine
320 West 25th St., Suite 103
Cheyenne, WY 82002
(307) 778-7053 / Fax: (307) 778-2069
wyomedboard.state.wy.us

APPENDIX 2

HEALTH CARE PROFESSIONAL ORGANIZATIONS

Equal Employment Opportunity Field Offices

Visit www.eeoc.gov/offices.html for an up-to-date list of all EEOC field offices.
Web site address for each EEOC field office is www.eeoc.gov/city/index.html.
For example, the Web site address for the Albuquerque district office is www.eeoc.gov/albuquerque/index.html

The general EEOC Web site address listed first above displays a map of the United States with addresses for field offices in each state. Simply click on the map to locate the EEOC field office near your location. If the URL has changed, do an Internet search for "EEOC Offices."

Workers' Compensation Offices

For an updated list of all state workers' compensation offices, see www.dol.gov/esa/regs/compliance/owcp/wc.htm. This federal government Web site provides direct links to each state's workers' compensation office. If the URL has changed, do an Internet search for "State Workers' Compensation Offices."

Professional Organizations for Health Care Practitioners

Anesthesiology
American Society of Anesthesiologists: www.asahq.org/
American Association of Nurse Anesthetists: www.aana.com/
American Society of Critical Care Anesthesiologists: www.gasnet.org/societies/ascca/
American Society of Dentist Anesthesiologists: www.asdahq.org/
Ophthalmic Anesthesia Society: www.eyeanesthesia.org/
The Society for Ambulatory Anesthesia: www.sambahq.org/

Anesthesiozogist assistant
American Academy of Anesthesiologist Assistants: www.anesthetist.org/

Art therapist
American Art Therapy Association: www.arttherapy.org/

Athletic trainer
National Athletic Trainers' Association: www.nata.org/

Audiologist
American Speech-Language-Hearing Association: www.asha.org/

Blindness and visual impairment professions
Association for Education and Rehabilitation of the Blind and Visually Impaired: www.aerbvi.org/modules.php?name=Content&pa=showpage&pid=1

Blood bank technology, specialist in
American Association of Blood Banks: www.aabb.org/content

Cardiovascular technologist
Society for Vascular Ultrasound: www.svunet.org/
American Society of Echocardiography: www.asecho.org/
Alliance of Cardiovascular Professionals: www.acp-online.org/
Society of Invasive Cardiovascular Professionals: www.sicp.com/

Clinical laboratory science/ medical technology
American Medical Technologists: www.sicp.com/
American Society for Clinical Laboratory Science: www.sicp.com/
American Society for Clinical Pathology: www.ascp.org/

Association of Genetic Technologists: www.agt-info.org/

Counseling-related occupations
American Counseling Association: www.counseling.org/

Cytotechnologist
American Society of Cytopathology: www.cytopathology.org/website/article.asp?id=1199

Dance/movement therapist
American Dance Therapy Association: www.adta.org/

Dental assistant
American Dental Assistants Association: www.dentalassistant.org/

Dental hygienist
American Dental Hygienists' Association: www.adha.org/

Dental laboratory technician
National Association of Dental Laboratories: www.nadl.org/

Diagnostic medical sonographer
Society of Diagnostic Medical Sonographers: www.sdms.org/

Dietician and nutritionist, dietetic technician
American Dietetic Association: www.eatright.org
American Society for Nutritional Sciences: www.asns.org/
Dietary Managers Association: www.dmaonline.org/
American Society for Clinical Nutrition: www.ascn.org/

Electroneurodiagnostic technology
American Society of Electroneurodiagnostic Technologists: www.aset.org/i4a/pages/index.cfm?pageid=1

Emergency medical technician-paramedic
National Association of Emergency Medical Technicians: www.naemt.org/

Genetics counselor and other genetics professionals
American Board of Genetic Counseling: www.abgc.net
American Society of Gene Therapy: www.asgt.org/
American Society of Human Genetics: www.ashg.org/
Association of Genetic Technologists: www.agt-info.org/
Genetics Society of America: www.genetics-gsa.org/
National Society of Genetic Counselors: www.nsgc.org/

Health and fitness specialist
International Fitness Professionals Association: www.ifpa-fitness.com/
American Fitness Professionals and Associates: www.afpafitness.com/

Health information manager
American Health Information Management Association: www.ahima.org/

Histologic technician/histotechnologist
National Society for Histotechnology: www.nsh.org/organizations.php3?action=printContentItem&orgid=111&typeID=1234&itemID=19243

Kinesiotherapist
American Kinesiotherapy Association: www.akta.org/

Massage therapist
American Massage Therapy Association: www.amtamassage.org/

Medical assistant
American Association of Medical Assistants: www.aama-ntl.org/
American Medical Technologists: www.amt1.com/

Medical illustrator
Association of Medical Illustrators: www.ami.org/ECOMAMI/timssnet/common/tnt_frontpage.cfm

Medical librarian
Medical Library Association: www.mlanet.org/

Music therapist
American Music Therapy Association: www.musictherapy.org/

Nuclear medicine technologist
Society of Nuclear Medicine—Technologist Section: www.snm.org/

Nurse
American Academy of Nursing: www.aannet.org/
American Nurses Association: www.nursingworld.org/index.htm
National League for Nursing: www.nln.org/
Note: Each nursing specialty also has its own professional organization.

Occupational therapist
American Occupational Therapy Association: www.aota.org/

Ophthalmic dispensing optician
Opticians Association of America: www.oaa.org/index.shtml

Opthalmic laboratory technician
Optical Laboratories Association: www.ola-labs.org/i4a/pages/index.cfm?pageid=1

Opthalmic medical technician/technologist
Joint Commission on Allied Health Personnel in Opthalmology: www.jcahpo.org/newsite/index.htm

Orthoptist
American Orthoptic Council: www.orthoptics.org/

Orthotic and prosthetic professionals
American Orthotic and Prosthetic Association: www.aopanet.org/

Pathologists' assistant
American Association of Pathologists' Assistants: www.pathologistsassistants.org/Home.aspx?n=hm

Perfusionist
American Society of Extra-Corporeal Technologists: www.amsect.org/

Pharmacy technician
American Association of Pharmacy Technicians: www.pharmacytechnician.com/

Physical therapist, physical therapist assistant
American Physical Therapy Association: www.apta.org/AM/Template.cfm?Section=Home

Physician
American College of Physicians: www.acponline.org/
American Medical Association: www.ama-assn.org

Physician assistant
American Academy of Physician Assistants: www.apta.org/AM/Template.cfm?Section=Home

Radiation therapist, radiographer
American Society of Radiologic Technologists: www.asrt.org/

Rehabilitation counselor
National Rehabilitation Counseling Association: http://nrca-net.org/

Respiratory therapist, respiratory therapy technician
American Association for Respiratory Care: www.aarc.org/

Speech-language pathologist
American Speech-Language-Hearing Association: www.asha.org/default.htm

Surgical assistant
National Surgical Assistant Association: www.nsaa.net/

Surgical technologist
Association of Surgical Technologists: www.ast.org/

Therapeutic recreation specialist
American Therapeutic Recreation Association: http://atra-online.com/cms/

ASSOCIATIONS FOR MAJOR DISEASES

AIDS

Foundation for AIDS Research: www.amfar.org/cgi-bin/iowa/index.html

Allergies

Food Allergy & Anaphylaxis Network: www.foodallergy.org/

Cancer

National Cancer Institute: www.cancer.gov/

Cancer Net—for people living with cancer: www.cancer.net/portal/site/patient

National Comprehensive Cancer Network: www.nccn.org/

Digestive and Metabolic Disorders

American Association of Kidney Patients: www.aakp.org/

American Diabetes Association: www.diabetes.org

American Kidney Fund: www.kidneyfund.org/

American Liver Foundation: www.liverfoundation.org/

National Diabetes Information Clearinghouse: http://diabetes.niddk.nih.gov/

National Graves' Disease Foundation: www.ngdf.org/

National Institute of Diabetes and Digestive and Kidney Diseases: www.nhlbi.nih.gov/

National Kidney Foundation: www.kidney.org/

Eating Disorders

Eating Disorder Education Organization: www.edeo.org/

Genetics

Human Genome Project: www.ornl.gov/sci/techresources/Human_Genome/posters/chromosome/index.shtml

Heart Disease

American Heart Association: www.americanheart.org

American Stroke Association: www.strokeassociation.org/

National Heart, Lung and Blood Institute: www.nhlbi.nih.gov/

Lung and Breathing Disorders (including Asthma)

American Academy of Allergy, Asthma & Immunology: www.aaaai.org/

American Lung Association: www.lungusa.org/

Asthma & Allergy Foundation of America: www.aafa.org/

Mental Health

Anxiety Disorders Association of America: www.adaa.org/

Rare Diseases

National Organization for Rare Disorders: www.rarediseases.org/

Skin Conditions

National Psoriasis Foundation: www.psoriasis.org/home/

Note: Voice 4 Patients is a Web site that provides links to the Web sites for a wide variety of disease information sites: www.voice4patients.com/patient%20services.htm.

GLOSSARY

A

Abandonment The suspension of treatment of a patient without justification and proper notification.

Acceptance Agreement to an offer as stated in a contract.

Access The availability of health care and the means to purchase health care services.

Accessory One who contributes to or aids in the commission of a crime, either by a direct or an indirect act.

Accomplice One who directly participates in the commission of a crime.

Accreditation Official authorization or approval for conforming to a specified standard.

Active Euthanasia A conscious medical act that results in death.

Administer To instill a drug into the body of a patient.

Administrative Law Enabling statutes enacted to define powers and procedures when an agency is created.

Advance Directive A document that makes one's wishes known concerning medical life-support measures in the event that one is unable to speak for oneself.

Adverse Event Any patient-involving, unforeseen, damaging event occurring within a medical facility.

Affidavit A sworn, written statement made under oath or an affirmation before an authorized magistrate or officer of the court.

Affirmative Action Programs that use goals and quotas to provide preferential treatment for minority persons determined to have been underutilized in the past.

Affirmative Defenses Defenses used by defendants in medical professional liability suits that allow the accused to present factual evidence that the patient's condition was caused by some factor other than the defendant's negligence.

Age Discrimination in Employment Act A federal act passed in 1967 making it illegal for employers with 20 or more employees working at least 20 weeks a year to discriminate against workers aged 40 years or older.

Age of Majority The age at which full civil rights are accorded.

Agency The relationship between a principal and his or her agent.

Agency for Healthcare Research and Quality (AHRQ) The lead federal agency responsible for tracking and improving the quality, safety, efficiency, and effectiveness of health care for Americans.

Agent One who acts for or represents another. In performing workplace duties, the employee acts as the agent, or authorized representative, of the employer.

Allopathic Literally, "different suffering"; referring to the medical philosophy that dictates training physicians to intervene in the disease process, through the use of drugs and surgery.

Alternative Dispute Resolution (ADR) Settlement of civil disputes between parties using neutral mediators or arbitrators without going to court.

Ambulatory Care Setting Medical care provided in a facility such as a medical office, clinic, or outpatient surgical center for patients who can walk and are not bedridden.

Amendments to the Older Americans Act A 1987 federal act that defines elder abuse, neglect, and exploitation, but does not deal with enforcement.

American Medical Association Principles A code of ethics for members of the American Medical Association written in 1847.

Americans With Disabilities Act Applying to employers with 15 or more employees who work at least 20 weeks a year, Titles I and III of this act took effect in January 1992 and lessened discrimination toward the disabled in the workplace and mandated full access in all public places.

Amniocentesis A test whereby the physician withdraws a sample of amniotic fluid (the fluid surrounding the developing fetus inside the mother's womb) from the uterus of a pregnant woman. The fluid is then tested for genetic or other conditions that may lead to abnormal development of the fetus.

Anesthesiologist Assistant Assists the anesthesiologist in developing and implementing an anesthesia care plan. Duties can include preoperative and postoperative tasks, as well as operating room assistance.

Appeals Phase The phase of a trial, after the verdict, during which appeals may be submitted.

Arbitration The hearing and determination of a case in controversy by a third party, chosen by the parties concerned or appointed under statutory authority.

Arraigned The process by which a person charged with a crime is allowed to answer the indictment in court by pleading guilty, not guilty, or *nolo contendere*.

Artificial Insemination The mechanical injection of viable semen into the vagina.

Assault The open threat of bodily harm to someone.

Associate Practice A medical management system in which two or more physicians share office space and employees but practice individually.

Assumption of Risk A legal defense that holds the defendant is not guilty of a negligent act, since the plaintiff knew of and accepted beforehand any risks involved.

Athletic Trainer Works with attending and/or consulting physicians as an integral part of the health care team associated with physical training and sports.

Audiologist A health care practitioner who is educated in the science of hearing and is qualified to test patients' hearing and to prescribe some types of therapy for hearing problems.

Autopsy A postmortem examination to determine the cause of death or to obtain physiological evidence, as in the case of a suspicious death.

B

Baby Boom Generation Those individuals born between 1946 and 1964.

Battery Any bodily contact without permission.

Bilateral Agreement An agreement between two parties that is mutually acceptable.

Bioethicists Specialists who consult with physicians, researchers, and others to help them make difficult ethical decisions regarding patient care.

Bioethics A discipline dealing with the ethical implications of biological research methods and results, especially in medicine.

Biotechnology Applied biological science.

Bloodborne Pathogen Standard The authority by which OSHA can levy fines, based upon guidelines of the Centers for Disease Control.

Brain Death Final cessation of bodily activity, used to determine when death actually occurs; circulatory and respiratory functions have irreversibly ceased, and the entire brain (including the brain stem) has irreversibly ceased to function.

Breach of Confidentiality Failure to keep private information entrusted to a health care professional by a patient.

Breach of Contract Failure of either party to comply with the terms of a legally valid contract.

Burden of Proof The task of presenting testimony to prove guilt or innocence in a trial.

C

Capital Punishment Government-sanctioned death by execution of those convicted of certain crimes.

Capitation A uniform per capita payment or fee that a managed care plan pays to physicians.

Cardiovascular Technologist Works under the supervision of physicians to perform diagnostic and therapeutic examinations in the cardiology (heart) and vascular (circulation) areas.

Case Law Law established through common law and legal precedent.

Case Manager A health practitioner affiliated with a managed care health plan who is responsible for coordinating the medical care of individuals enrolled in the plan.

Certification A voluntary credentialing process whereby applicants who meet specific requirements may receive a certificate.

Checks and Balances The system established by the U.S. Constitution that keeps any one branch of government from assuming too much power over the other branches.

Chemical Hygiene Plan The Standard for Occupational Exposures to Hazardous Chemicals in Laboratories, which clarifies the handling of hazardous chemicals in medical laboratories.

Child Abuse Prevention and Treatment Act A federal law passed in 1974 requiring physicians to report cases of child abuse and to try to prevent future cases.

Chiropractor One who is trained to provide a system of manipulative treatments for diseases caused by impingement on spinal nerves.

Chromosome A microscopic structure found within the nucleus of a plant or animal cell that carries genes responsible for the organism's characteristics.

Civil Law Law that involves wrongful acts against persons.

Civil Rights Act of 1964 Title VII of the act makes discrimination in the workplace illegal, for reasons of race, color, religion, sex, or national origin; applies to businesses with 15 or more employees who work at least 20 weeks a year.

Claims-Made Insurance A type of liability insurance that covers the insured only for those claims made (not for any injury occurring) while the policy is in force.

Clinical Exercise Specialist One who specializes in exercise testing, prescription, leadership, emergency procedures, and health education.

Clinical Investigation The process by which research is conducted to produce data that are scientifically valid and significant.

Clinical Laboratory Improvement Act (CLIA) Also called Clinical Laboratory Improvement Amendments. Federal statutes passed in 1988 that established minimum quality standards for all laboratory testing.

Clone An organism begun asexually, usually from a single cell of the parent.

Code of Ethics A system of principles intended to govern behavior—here, the behavior of those entrusted with providing care to the sick.

Code Set Under HIPAA, terms that provide for uniformity and simplification of health care billing and record keeping.

Coma A condition of deep stupor from which the patient cannot be roused by external stimuli.

Commission on Accreditation of Allied Health Education Programs (CAAHEP) Accredits programs in 18 allied health professions and provides information concerning duties, education requirements, and sources for further information about the profession and the location of schools offering the accredited programs.

Common Law The body of unwritten law developed in England, primarily from judicial decisions based on custom and tradition.

Common Sense Sound practical judgment.

Comparative Negligence An affirmative defense claimed by the defendant, alleging that the plaintiff contributed to the injury by a certain degree.

Compassion The identification with and understanding of another's situation, feelings, and motives.

Compensatory Damages Monetary damages awarded to the plaintiff in a civil suit. May be general—to compensate for injuries or losses due to a violation of the plaintiff's rights—or special—to compensate for losses not directly caused by the wrong.

Competency The state of having requisite or adequate ability, skills, or qualities.

Confidentiality The act of holding information in confidence, not to be released to unauthorized individuals.

Confidentiality of Alcohol and Drug Abuse, Patient Records A federal statute that protects patients with histories of substance abuse regarding the release of information about treatment.

Conflict of Interest A situation in which a person is faced with choosing between financial gain and his or her duty to provide the best possible medical care to patients.

Consent Permission from a patient, either expressed or implied, for something to be done by another. For example, consent is required for a physician to examine a patient, to perform tests that aid in diagnosis, and/or to treat for a medical condition.

Consequential Damages Monetary award to a plaintiff based on losses caused indirectly by a product defect.

Consideration Something of value bargained for as part of a contractual agreement.

Constitutional Law Law that derives from federal and state constitutions.

Contingent Dependent on or conditioned by something else.

Contract A voluntary agreement between two parties in which specific promises are made for a consideration.

Contributory Negligence An affirmative defense that alleges that the plaintiff, through a lack of care, caused or contributed to his or her own injury.

Controlled Substances Act The federal law giving authority to the Drug Enforcement Administration to regulate the sale and use of drugs.

Coroner A public official who investigates and holds inquests over those who die from unknown or violent causes; he or she may or may not be a physician, depending upon state law.

Corporation A body formed and authorized by law to act as a single person.

Cost In this context, the amount individuals, employers, state and federal governments, HMOs, and insurers spend on health care in the United States.

Counteroffer An alternative offer made by one who has rejected an earlier, unsatisfactory offer.

Courtesy The practice of good manners.

Covered Entity Health care providers and clearinghouses that transmit HIPAA transactions electronically, and must comply with HIPAA standards and rules.

Covered Transactions Electronic exchanges of information between two covered-entity business partners using HIPAA-mandated transaction standards.

Crime An offense against the state or sovereignty, committed or omitted, in violation of a public law forbidding or commanding it.

Criminal Law Law that involves crimes against the state.

Critical Thinking The ability to think analytically, using fewer emotions and more rationality.

Curative Care Treatment directed toward curing a patient's disease.

Cybermedicine A form of telemedicine that involves direct contact between patients and physicians over the Internet, usually for a fee.

Cytology The study of the structure and function of cells.

Cytotechnologist Works with pathologists to microscopically examine body cells, in order to detect changes that may help to diagnose cancer and other diseases.

D

Damages Monetary awards sought by plaintiffs in lawsuits.

Defamation of Character Damaging a person's reputation by making public statements that are both false and malicious.

Defendant The person or party against whom criminal or civil charges are brought in a lawsuit.

Defensive Medicine The practice of ordering and/or performing medical tests and procedures simply to protect against future liability and to construct for patients a medical record that documents the health care provider's judgment.

De-identify To remove all information that identifies patients from health care transactions.

Denial A defense that claims innocence of the charges or that one or more of the four Ds of negligence are lacking.

Dental Assistant One who serves as a chair-side assistant to a dentist/employer within a dental office.

Dental Hygienist A health care practitioner who performs clinical and educational duties related to hygiene of the mouth and teeth, usually for dentist/employers within a dental office. A dental hygienist may work for one dentist or for several dentists at varying locations.

Deposition Sworn testimony given and recorded outside the courtroom during the pretrial phase of a case.

Designated Record Set Records maintained by or for a HIPAA-covered entity.

Diagnostic Medical Sonographer Administers ultrasound examinations under the supervision of a physician responsible for the use and interpretation of ultrasound procedures.

Dietician One who works closely with physicians and other medical practitioners to educate and assist patients with special dietary and nutritional needs.

Discrimination Prejudiced or prejudicial outlook, action, or treatment.

Dispense To deliver controlled substances in some type of bottle, box, or other container to a patient.

DNA (Deoxyribonucleic Acid) The combination of proteins, called nucleotides, that is arranged to make up an organism's chromosomes.

Doctrine of Common Knowledge Literally, "the thing speaks for itself"; also known as the doctrine of *res ipsa loquitur*. Under this principle, an act of negligence was obviously under the control of the defendant, the patient did not contribute to the accident, and it is apparent the patient would not have been injured if reasonable care had been used.

Doctrine of Informed Consent The legal basis for informed consent, usually outlined in a state's medical practice acts.

Doctrine of Mature Minors A principle that allows minors to make their own decisions regarding medical treatment if they are mature enough to comprehend a physician's recommendations and give informed consent.

Doctrine of Professional Discretion A principle under which a physician can exercise judgment as to whether to show patients who are being treated for mental or emotional conditions their records. Disclosure depends on whether, in the physician's judgment, such patients would be harmed by viewing the records.

Do-Not-Resuscitate Orders (DNR) Orders written at the request of patients or their authorized representatives that cardiopulmonary resuscitation not be used to sustain life in a medical crisis.

Drug Enforcement Administration A branch of the U.S. Department of Justice that regulates the sale and use of drugs.

Durable Power of Attorney An advance directive that confers upon a designee the authority to make a variety of legal decisions on behalf of the grantor, usually including health care decisions.

Duty of Care The obligation of health care professionals to patients and, in some cases, nonpatients.

E

E-Health Term used for the use of the Internet as a source of consumer information about health and medicine.

Electrocardiogram (ECG) The recording made by an instrument that measures the electrical activity of the heart.

Electrocardiogram (ECG) Technician A health care practitioner who, under the direct supervision of physicians, operates electrocardiogram equipment to measure and record the electrical activity of the heart.

Electroencephalogram (EEG) The recording made by an instrument that measures the electrical activity of the brain.

Electroencephalogram Technician and Technologist A health care practitioner who works under the supervision of physicians to operate EEG equipment used to perform patient diagnostic tests.

Electroneurodiagnostic Technologist Involves the study and recording of the electrical activity of the brain and nervous system. Electroneurodiagnostic technologists work in collaboration with EEG technicians and technologists.

Electronic Data Interchange (EDI) The use of uniform electronic protocols to transfer business information between organizations via computer networks.

Electronic Transmission The sending of information from one network-connected computer to another.

Emancipated Minors Individuals in their mid- to late teens who legally live outside of their parents' or guardians' control.

Emergency A type of affirmative defense in which the person who comes to the aid of a victim in an emergency is not held liable under certain circumstances.

Emergency Medical Technician (EMT) A paramedic who most often works from an ambulance or in a hospital emergency room to provide life-support care to critically ill and injured patients.

Employment-at-Will A concept of employment whereby either the employer or the employee can end the employment at any time, for any reason.

Encryption The scrambling or encoding of information before sending it electronically.

Endorsement The process by which a license may be awarded based on individual credentials judged to meet licensing requirements in a new state.

Equal Employment Opportunity Commission (EEOC) A federal agency that enforces provisions of the Civil Rights Act, the Age Discrimination in Employment Act, the Equal Pay Act, and the Rehabilitation Act.

Ethics Standards of behavior, developed as a result of one's concept of right and wrong.

Ethics Committee Committee made up of individuals who are involved in a patient's care, including health care practitioners, family members, clergy, and others, with the purpose of reviewing ethical issues in difficult cases.

Ethics Guidelines Publications that detail a wide variety of ethical situations that professionals (in this case, health care practitioners) might face in their work and offer principles for dealing with the situations in an ethical manner.

Etiquette Standards of behavior considered to be good manners among members of a profession as they function as individuals in society.

Euthanasia The practice of willfully ending life in an individual with an incurable disease or condition.

Executive Branch That branch of government responsible for administering the law. The president is the chief executive of the executive branch at the federal level; governors preside at the state level.

Executive Order A rule or regulation issued by the president of the United States that becomes law without the prior approval of Congress.

Expert Testimony Trial testimony provided by recognized authorities in a particular field.

Expressed Contract A written or oral agreement in which all terms are explicitly stated.

F

Fair Debt Collection Practices Act (FDCPA) A federal statute prohibiting certain unfair and illegal practices by debt collectors and creditors. It prohibits certain methods of debt collection, including harassment, misrepresentation, threats, disseminating false information about the debtor, and engaging in unfair or illegal practices in attempting to collect a debt.

False Imprisonment The unlawful violation of the personal liberty of another.

Federal False Claims Act A law that allows for individuals to bring civil actions on behalf of the United States government for false claims made to the federal government, under a provision of the law called *qui tam* (from Latin meaning "to bring an action for the king and for oneself").

Federal Register A U.S. government publication that contains all administrative laws.

Federal Trade Commission Act A federal statute that established the Federal Trade Commission (FTC), which prohibits unfair or deceptive acts in advertising and other trade areas.

Federal Unemployment Tax Act (FUTA) The act that requires employers to contribute to a fund that is paid out to eligible unemployed workers.

Fee Splitting Payment by one physician to another solely for the referral of a patient, or payment from a source for using its services or supplies.

Felony An offense punishable by death or by imprisonment in a state or federal prison for more than one year.

Fiduciary Duty A physician's obligation to his or her patient, based upon trust and confidence.

Firewall Hardware, software, or both designed to prevent unauthorized persons from accessing electronic information.

Food and Drug Administration (FDA) A federal agency within the Department of Health and Human Services that oversees drug quality and standardization and must approve drugs before they are released for public use.

Forensics A division of medicine that incorporates law and medicine and involves medical issues or medical proof at trials having to do with malpractice, crimes, and accidents.

Four Cs of Medical Malpractice Prevention Caring, Communication, Competence, and Charting.

Four Ds of Negligence Elements necessary to prove negligence: duty, derelict, direct cause, and damages.

Fraud Dishonest or deceitful practices in depriving, or attempting to deprive, another of his or her rights.

G

Gatekeeper Physician The primary care physician who directs the medical care of HMO members.

Gene A tiny segment of DNA found on a chromosome in a cell. Each gene holds the formula for making a specific molecule.

Gene Therapy The insertion of a normally functioning gene into cells in which an abnormal or absent element of the gene has caused disease.

General Duty Clause A section of the Hazard Communication Standard which states that any equipment that may pose a health risk must be specified as a hazard.

General Liability The legal responsibility for personal acts borne by all competent adults, both on the job and in their private lives.

Genetic Counseling The process by which prospective parents at risk for passing on genetic disorders to their offspring are screened.

Genetic Counselor An expert in human genetics who is qualified to counsel individuals who may have inherited genes for certain diseases or conditions.

Genetic Discrimination Differential treatment of individuals based on their actual or presumed genetic differences.

Genetic Engineering Manipulation of DNA within the cells of plants and animals, through synthesis, alteration, or repair, to ensure that certain harmful traits will be eliminated in offspring and that desirable traits will appear and be passed on.

Genetics The science that accounts for natural differences and resemblances among organisms related by descent.

Genome   All the DNA in an organism, including its genes.

Genometrics   The science of determining how genes cause the expression of certain traits in individuals.

Germ Line Therapy   A procedure in which a replacement gene is put into human gametes, resulting in expression of the new gene in the patient's offspring.

Good Samaritan Acts   State laws protecting physicians and sometimes other health care practitioners and laypersons from charges of negligence or abandonment if they stop to help the victim of an accident or other emergency.

Gross Domestic Product (GDP)   America's total income for all goods and services.

Group Model HMO   A type of HMO that contracts with independent groups of physicians to provide coordinated care for large numbers of HMO patients for a fixed, per-member fee.

Group Practice   A medical management system in which a group of three or more licensed physicians share their collective income, expenses, facilities, equipment, records, and personnel.

H

Hazard Communication Standard (HCS)   An OSHA standard intended to increase health care practitioners' awareness of risks, to improve work practices and appropriate use of personal protective equipment, and to reduce injuries and illnesses in the workplace.

Health and Fitness Specialist   Professionals qualified to assess, design, and implement exercise and fitness programs.

Healthcare Integrity and Protection Data Bank (HCIPDB)   A national health care fraud and abuse data collection program established by HIPAA for the reporting and disclosure of certain adverse actions taken against health care providers, suppliers, or practitioners.

Health Care Practitioners   Those who are trained to administer medical or health care to patients.

Health Care Proxy   A durable power of attorney issued for purposes of health care decisions only.

Health Care Quality Improvement Act of 1986 (HCQIA)   A federal statute passed to improve the quality of medical care nationwide. One provision established the National Practitioner Data Bank.

Health Information Administrator   Manages health information and systems used to collect, store, process, retrieve, analyze, disseminate, and communicate health information.

Health Information Technician   A health care practitioner who may have full responsibility for the records department of a medical office, clinic, hospital, or other health care institution. Duties include organizing, analyzing, and preparing health information about patients, usually for use by patients, patients' physicians, and the health care facility.

Health Information Technology (HIT)   The application of information processing, involving both computer hardware and software, that deals with the storage, retrieval, sharing, and use of health care information, data, and knowledge for communication and decision making.

Health Insurance Portability and Accountability Act of 1996 (HIPAA)   A federal law passed in 1996 to protect privacy and other health care rights for patients. The act helps workers keep continuous health insurance coverage for themselves and their dependents when they change jobs, and protects confidential medical information from unauthorized disclosure and/or use. It was also intended to help curb the rising cost of health care fraud and abuse.

Health Maintenance Organization (HMO)   A health plan that combines coverage of health care costs and delivery of health care for a prepaid premium.

Heredity   The process by which organisms pass genetic traits on to their offspring.

Heterologous Artificial Insemination   The process in which donor sperm is mechanically injected into a woman's vagina to fertilize her eggs.

Hippocratic Oath   A pledge for physicians, developed by the Greek physician Hippocrates circa 400 B.C.

Homologous Artificial Insemination   The process in which a husband's sperm is mechanically injected into his wife's vagina to fertilize her eggs.

Hospice   A facility or program (often carried out in a patient's home) in which teams of health care practitioners and volunteers provide a continuing environment that focuses on the emotional and psychological needs of the dying patient.

Hostile Environment   An antagonistic work environment that has been created by, among other things, sexual harassment.

Human Genome Project   A scientific project funded by the U.S. government, begun in 1990 and successfully completed in 2000, for the purpose of mapping all of a human's genes. This Web site is an excellent resource: www.ornl.gov/sci/techresources/Human_Genome/home.shtml.

I

Implied Contract   An unwritten and unspoken agreement whose terms result from the actions of the parties involved.

Implied Limited Contract   A contract created when a physician or other health care worker treats a patient in an emergency situation. The agreement does not extend to the relationship after the emergency ends.

Incapacity   A lack of physical or intellectual power, or of natural or legal qualifications.

Incompetent   Lacking the qualities or skills necessary for effective action.

Indemnity   A traditional form of health insurance that covers the insured against a potential loss of money from medical expenses resulting from an illness or accident.

Indicted   Charged with a crime.

Individual (or Independent) Practice Association (IPA)   A type of HMO that contracts with groups of physicians who practice in their own offices and receive a per-member payment (capitation) from participating HMOs to provide a full range of health services for HMO members.

Infertility   The failure to conceive for a period of 12 months or longer due to a deviation from or interruption of the normal structure or function of any reproductive part, organ, or system.

Informed Consent   The patient's right to receive all information relative to his or her condition and then to make a decision regarding treatment based upon that knowledge.

Intentional Tort   *See* "Tort."

Interrogatory   A written set of questions requiring written answers from a plaintiff or defendant under oath.

Invasion of Privacy   Intrusion into a person's seclusion or into his or her private affairs.

In Vitro Fertilization (IVF)   Fertilization that takes place outside a woman's body, literally, "in glass," as in a test tube.

Involuntary Euthanasia   The act of ending a terminal patient's life by medical means without his or her permission.

J

Judicial Branch   That branch of government responsible for interpreting laws; the court system and judges.

Judicial Council Opinions   A publication of the American Medical Association, issued for the purpose of defining ethics for physicians in all situations common to the practice of medicine.

Jurisdiction   The power and authority given to a court to hear a case and to make a judgment.

Just Cause   An employer's legal reason for firing an employee.

K

Kinesiology   The study of muscles and muscle movement.

Kinesiotherapist   Works under a physician's supervision, using therapeutic exercise and education to treat the effects of disease, injury, and congenital disorders on body movement.

L

Law   Rule of conduct or action prescribed or formally recognized as binding or enforced by a controlling authority.

Law of Agency   The law that governs the relationship between a principal and his or her agent.

Legal Precedents   Decisions made by judges in the various courts that become rule of law and apply to future cases, even though they were not enacted by legislation.

Legislative Branch   The Senate and the House of Representatives, responsible for creating laws.

Liability Insurance   Contract coverage for potential damages incurred as a result of a negligent act.

Liable   Accountable under the law.

Libel   Expressing through publication in print, writing, pictures, or signed statements that injure the reputation of another.

Licensed Practical Nurse (LPN)   A health care practitioner who performs many of the same duties as a registered nurse.

Licensure   A mandatory credentialing process established by law, usually at the state level, that grants the right to practice certain skills and endeavors.

Lien   A charge upon real or personal property for the satisfaction of a debt or duty owed by law.

Life Expectancy   The number of years an individual can expect to live, calculated from his or her birth.

Limited Data Set   Protected health information from which certain specified, direct identifiers of individuals have been removed.

Limited Practitioner   A provider licensed to provide specific treatment or treatments specific to certain body parts.

Litigious   Prone to engage in lawsuits.

Living Will   An advance directive that specifies an individual's end-of-life wishes.

M

Malfeasance   The performance of a totally wrongful and unlawful act.

Managed Care   A system in which financing, administration, and delivery of health care are combined to provide medical services to subscribers for a prepaid fee.

Material Safety Data Sheet (MSDS)   A sheet that identifies each hazardous chemical used in the workplace and lists safety precautions necessary for its use, storage, and disposal; manufacturers must supply an MSDS upon request for each hazardous chemical used.

Mature Minors   Individual in their mid- to late teens, who, for health care purposes, are considered mature enough to comprehend a physician's recommendations and give informed consent.

Medical Assistant   One who performs administrative and clinical duties for a physician/employer within a medical office.

Medical Boards   Bodies established by the authority of each state's medical practice acts for the purpose of protecting the health, safety, and welfare of health care consumers through proper licensing and regulation of physicians and other health care practitioners.

Medical Ethicists   Specialists who consult with physicians, researchers, and others to help them make difficult ethical decisions regarding patient care.

Medical Examiner   A physician who investigates suspicious or unexplained deaths.

Medical Illustrator   Creates illustrations for science and medical texts and other publications, and may also function in administrative, consultative, and advisory capacities.

Medical Laboratory Technician (MLT)   A health care practitioner who performs simple tests in hematology, serology, blood banking, urinalysis, microbiology, and clinical chemistry.

Medical Management   The management of patient care and populations.

Medical Massage Therapist   One who uses massage to relieve pain and help patients with recovery and rehabilitation.

Medical Practice Acts   State laws written for the express purpose of governing the practice of medicine.

Medical Record   A collection of data recorded when a patient seeks medical treatment.

Medical Technologist (MT)   A health care provider who supervises technicians and assistants and performs more complicated, analytical laboratory tests than a medical laboratory technician.

Medical Transcriptionist   One who keys material dictated by physicians, to be placed with patients' medical records.

Medical Waste Tracking Act   The federal law that authorizes OSHA to inspect hazardous medical wastes and to cite offices for unsafe or unhealthy practices regarding these wastes.

Mentally Incompetent   Unable to fully understand all the terms and conditions of a transaction, and therefore unable to enter into a legal contract.

Minimum Necessary   Term referring to the limited amount of patient information that may be disclosed, depending on circumstances.

Minor   Anyone under the age of majority: 18 years in most states, 21 years in some jurisdictions.

Misdemeanor   A crime punishable by fine or by imprisonment in a facility other than a prison for less than one year.

Misfeasance   The performance of a lawful act in an illegal or improper manner.

Moral Values   One's personal concept of right and wrong, formed through the influence of the family, culture, and society.

Mutual Assent   An understanding and consent to the terms of an agreement by both parties in order for the contract to be legally valid.

N

National Childhood Vaccine Injury Act   A federal law passed in 1986 that created a no-fault compensation program for citizens injured or killed by vaccines, as an alternative to suing vaccine manufacturers and providers.

National Vaccine Injury Compensation Program (VICP)   A no-fault federal system of compensation for individuals or families of individuals injured by childhood vaccination.

National Organ Transplant Act Passed in 1984, a statute that provides grants to qualified organ procurement organizations and established an Organ Procurement and Transplantation Network.

National Practitioner Data Bank A repository of information about health care practitioners, established by the Health Care Quality Improvement Act of 1986.

Negligence An unintentional tort alleged when one may have performed or failed to perform an act that a reasonable person would not or would have done in similar circumstances.

Nominal Damages A token court-awarded payment, usually one dollar, which recognizes that the legal rights of the plaintiff were violated but that no actual loss was proved.

Nonfeasance The failure to act when one should.

Notice of Privacy Practices A written document detailing a health care provider's privacy practices.

Nurse Practitioner A registered nurse who has completed a graduate degree program and is skilled in physical diagnosis, psychosocial assessment, and primary health care management. He or she may work independently.

Nursing Assistant A health care practitioner who provides routine patient care under the direct supervision of registered nurses.

O

Occupational Exposure to Bloodborne Pathogen Standard An OSHA regulation designed to protect health care workers from the risk of exposure to bloodborne pathogens.

Occupational Safety and Health Act (OSHA) Established by the Occupational Safety and Health Act of 1970, it enforces compulsory standards for health and safety in the workplace.

Occupational Safety and Health Administration Established by the Occupational Safety and Health Act, the organization that is charged with writing and enforcing compulsory standards for health and safety in the workplace.

Occupational Therapist One who works with clients who are mentally, physically, developmentally, and/or emotionally disabled to help these individuals become more independent and productive.

Occupational Therapy Assistant Works under the supervision of licensed occupational therapists.

Occurrence Insurance A type of liability insurance that covers the insured for any claims arising from an incident that occurred, or is alleged to have occurred, during the time the policy is in force, regardless of when the claim is made.

Officers of the Court Those individuals charged with specific responsibilities in the conduct of court cases.

Open Access A managed care feature whereby subscribers may see any in-network health care provider without a referral.

Ophthalmic Medical Technician/ Technologist Assists ophthalmologists by performing such tasks as collecting data, administering diagnostic tests, and administering some treatments ordered by the supervising ophthalmologist.

Ophthalmologist A physician who specializes in the treatment of disorders and diseases of the eye.

Optician One who is licensed to sell or make optical materials.

Optometrist One who is trained and licensed to examine the eyes in order to determine the presence of vision problems and to prescribe and adapt lenses to preserve or restore maximum efficiency of vision. The optometrist's professional degree is doctor of optometry (O.D.).

Organ Transplantation The process by which a patient (recipient) surgically receives a body organ from a living or dead donor.

Orthotist and Prosthetist Works directly with physicians and others to rehabilitate people with disabilities. The orthotist designs and fits devices (orthoses) for patients with disabling conditions of the limbs and spine. The prosthetist designs and fits devices (prostheses) for patients who have partial or total absence of a limb.

P

Palliative Care Treatment of a terminally ill patient's symptoms in order to make dying more comfortable; also called comfort care.

Parens Patriae A legal doctrine that gives the state the authority to act in a child's best interest.

Partnership A form of medical practice management system whereby two or more parties practice together under a written agreement specifying the rights, obligations, and responsibilities of each partner.

Passive Euthanasia The act of allowing a patient to die naturally, without medical interference.

Pathogen   Disease-causing organism.

Patient Self-Determination Act   A federal law passed in 1990 that requires hospitals and other health care providers to provide written information to patients regarding their rights under state law to make medical decisions and execute advance directives.

Patient's Bill of Rights   A statement approved by the American Hospital Association in 1973, guaranteeing an individual's rights to certain courtesies and considerations while a hospital patient.

Peer Review   The process by which professional colleagues may review and judge one another's actions.

Perfusionist   Operates transfusion equipment when necessary and consults with physicians in selecting the appropriate equipment, techniques, and transfusion media to be used, depending upon the patient's condition.

Permissions   Reasons under HIPAA for disclosing patient information.

Persistent Vegetative State (PVS)   Severe mental impairment characterized by irreversible cessation of the higher functions of the brain, most often caused by damage to the cerebral cortex.

Pharmacogenomics   The science that defines how individuals are genetically programmed to respond to drugs.

Phlebotomist   One who draws blood from patients or donors for diagnostic testing or other medical purposes.

Physical Therapist (PT)   A health care practitioner who helps patients restore function to muscles, nerves, joints, and bones after impairment due to illness or injury.

Physical Therapy Assistant   Works under the supervision of licensed physical therapists.

Physician-Hospital Organization (PHO)   A health care plan in which physicians join with hospitals to provide a medical care delivery system and then contract for insurance with a commercial carrier or an HMO.

Physician Assistant (PA)   One who performs routine diagnostic and treatment procedures for the physician/employer.

Plaintiff   The person bringing charges in a lawsuit.

Pleadings Phase   That time before a trial when a complaint is filed, a summons is issued, an answer filed, and a counter-complaint made.

Point-of-Service (POS) Plan   A health care plan that allows members to seek health care from non-network physicians but pays the highest benefits for care when it is given by the primary care physician (PCP) or via a referral from the PCP.

Polysomnographic Technologist   Performs sleep diagnostics and clinical evaluation for patients with sleep disorders.

Precedent   Decisions made by judges in the various courts that become rule of law and apply to future cases, even though they were not enacted by a legislature; also known as case law.

Preferred Provider Organization (PPO)   A network of independent physicians, hospitals, and other health care providers who contract with an insurance carrier to provide medical care at a discount rate to patients who are part of the insurer's plan. Also called **preferred provider association (PPA).**

Prepaid Group Practice (PGP)   A group model HMO in which physicians are salaried employees, usually practice in facilities provided by the HMO, and share in profits at the end of the year.

Prescribe   To issue a medical prescription for a patient.

Pretrial Discovery Phase   That period before a trial begins when a trial date is set by the court and pretrial motions are made and decided. Discovery procedures may be used to uncover evidence that will support the charges when the case comes to court, subpoenas are issued, depositions are taken, and pretrial conferences are called by the judge to discuss the issues in the case.

Primary Care Physician (PCP)   The physician responsible for directing all of a patient's medical care and determining whether the patient should be referred for specialty care.

Privacy   Freedom from unauthorized intrusion.

Prior Acts Insurance Coverage   A supplement to a claims-made policy that can be purchased when health care practitioners change insurance carriers.

Privileged Communication   Information held confidential within a protected relationship.

Procedural Law   Law that defines the rules used to enforce substantive law.

Professional Courtesy   The practice of treating other physicians and their families free of charge or at a reduced fee.

Professional Liability   One's legal accountability regarding all actions performed as a member of a certain profession.

Proposed Guidelines for Universal Precautions   A list of general precautions issued by the Centers for Disease Control to promote safety and prevent contamination in the workplace.

Prosecution   The government as plaintiff in a criminal case.

Protected Health Information (PHI)   Information that contains one or more patient identifiers.

Protocol   A code prescribing correct behavior in a specific situation, such as a situation arising in a medical office.

Public Policy   The common law concept of wrongful discharge when an employee has acted for the "common good."

Punitive Damages   Monetary award to the plaintiff in a lawsuit by the court, intended to serve as punishment for the defendant's act.

Q

Quality   The degree of excellence of health care services offered.

Quality Assurance   *See* **quality improvement.**

Quality Improvement (QI)   A program of measures taken by health care providers and practitioners to uphold the quality of patient care. Also called **quality assurance.**

Quid Pro Quo   Literally, "something for something"; a concept in the commission for sexual harassment in which an employee is expected to exchange sexual favors for workplace advantages.

R

Radiologic, or Medical Imaging, Technologist   A health care practitioner who positions patients for X-rays, operates the X-ray equipment, develops exposed X-ray film, and maintains records and films.

Reasonable Person Standard   That standard of behavior that judges a person's actions in a situation according to what a reasonable person would or would not do under similar circumstances.

Reciprocity   The process by which a professional license obtained in one state may be accepted as valid in other states by prior agreement without reexamination.

Referral   The act of recommending to a patient the diagnostic or therapeutic services of another physician.

Registered Nurse (RN)   A nurse who has completed a university or associate degree program.

Registration   A credentialing procedure whereby one's name is listed on a register as having paid a fee and/or met certain criteria within a profession.

Rehabilitation Act of 1973   An act that requires federal contractors to take affirmative action to hire the disabled, requires federal contractors to implement affirmative action plans in hiring and promoting disabled employees, and prohibits discrimination against the disabled in programs that receive federal funds.

Release of Tortfeasor   A technical defense to a lawsuit that prohibits a lawsuit against the person who caused an injury (the tortfeasor) if he or she was expressly released from further liability in the settlement of a suit.

Res Ipsa Loquitur   Literally, "the thing speaks for itself"; a situation that is so obviously negligent that no expert witnesses need be called. Also known as the doctrine of common knowledge.

Res Judicata   Literally, "the thing has been decided"; legal principle that a claim cannot be retried between the same parties if it has already been legally resolved.

Respiratory Technician or Therapist   A health care practitioner who works under a physician's supervision to assist patients with breathing disorders.

Respondeat Superior   Literally, "let the master answer." A doctrine under which an employer is legally liable for the acts of his or her employees, if such acts were performed within the scope of the employees' duties.

Revocation   The cancellation of a professional license.

Right-to-Know Laws   State laws that allow employees access to information about toxic or hazardous substances, employer duties, employee rights, and other workplace health and safety issues.

Risk Contract   An arrangement in which a health provider agrees to provide medical services to a set population of patients for a prepaid fee. The physician is responsible for managing the care of these patients and risks losing money if total expenses exceed prepaid fees.

Risk Management   The taking of steps to minimize danger, hazard, and liability.

Rule   A document that includes the HIPAA standards or requirements.

S

Safe Haven Laws   State laws that allow mothers to abandon newborns to designated safe facilities without penalty.

Security   The use of policies and procedures to protect electronic information from unauthorized access.

Self-Insurance Coverage   An insurance coverage option whereby insured subscribers contribute to a trust fund to be used in paying potential damage awards.

Sexual Harassment   A form of sexual discrimination in the workplace, in which an employee is expected to exchange sexual favors for employment advantages or must work in a hostile environment.

Sexual Misconduct   An unethical sexual relationship between medical supervisors and trainees or between health care providers and patients.

Slander   The speaking of defamatory words intended to prejudice others against an individual in a manner that jeopardizes his or her reputation or means of livelihood.

Sole Proprietorship   A form of medical practice management in which a physician practices alone, assuming all benefits and liabilities for the business.

Somatic Cell Therapy   A procedure in which human cells other than germ cells (eggs and sperm) are genetically altered.

Specialist in Blood Bank Technology   Performs both routine and specialized tests in blood bank immunohematology and performs transfusion services. Must have a bachelor's degree and certification in medical technology and must have completed the required course of study in blood bank technology.

Staff Model HMO   A type of HMO that employs salaried physicians and other health practitioners who provide care solely for members of one HMO.

Staff Privileges   The right to practice at a particular hospital.

Stakeholders   Those who have a vested interest in the health care industry in the United States, and in any efforts to reform the industry.

Standard   A general requirement under HIPAA.

Standard of Care   The level of performance expected of a health care worker in carrying out his or her professional duties.

State Children's Health Initiative Program (SCHIP)   A program enacted by the Balanced Budget Act of 1997 to help low-income children under 19 who are not covered by Medicaid.

State Preemption   If a state's privacy laws are stricter than HIPAA privacy standards, state laws take precedence.

Statute of Frauds   State legislation governing written contracts.

Statute of Limitations   That period of time established by state law during which a lawsuit may be filed.

Statutes   Laws enacted by state or federal legislatures.

Statutory Law   Law passed by the U.S. Congress or state legislatures.

Stem Cells   Cells that have the potential to become any type of body cell.

Subpoena   A legal document requiring the recipient to appear as a witness in court or to give a deposition.

Subpoena *Duces Tecum*   A legal document requiring the recipient to bring certain written records to court to be used as evidence in a lawsuit.

Substantive Law   The statutory or written law that defines and regulates legal rights and obligations.

Summary Judgment   A decision made by a court in a lawsuit in response to a motion that pleads there is no basis for a trial.

Summons   A written notification issued by the clerk of the court and delivered with a copy of the complaint to the defendant in a lawsuit, directing him or her to respond to the charges brought in a court of law.

Surety Bond   A type of insurance that allows employers, if covered, to collect up to the specified amount of the bond if an employee embezzles or otherwise absconds with business funds.

Surgical Technologist   Works closely with surgeons, anesthesiologists, nurses, and other surgical personnel before, during, and after surgery.

Surrogate Mother   A woman who becomes pregnant, usually by artificial insemination or surgical implantation of a fertilized egg, and bears a child for another woman.

Suspension   The temporary withdrawal of a professional license.

T

Tail Coverage An insurance coverage option available for health care practitioners: when a claims-made policy is discontinued, it extends coverage for malpractice claims alleged to have occurred during those dates that claims-made coverage was in effect.

Technical Defenses Defenses used in a lawsuit that are based upon legal technicalities.

Telemedicine Remote consultation by patients with physicians or other health professionals via telephone, closed-circuit television, or the Internet.

Terminally Ill Referring to patients who are expected to die within six months.

Termination The ending of a contract between a physician and a patient, usually because all treatment has been completed and the bill has been paid.

Tertiary Care Settings Those care settings providing highly specialized services.

Testimony Statements sworn to under oath by witnesses testifying in court and giving depositions.

Thanatology The study of death and of the psychological methods of coping with it.

Therapeutic Abortion A medical termination of pregnancy performed to save the life of the mother.

Third Party Payor Contract A written agreement signed by a party other than the patient who promises to pay the patient's bill.

Title VII of the Civil Rights Act of 1964 A law that makes discrimination in the workplace illegal.

Tort A civil wrong committed against a person or property, excluding breach of contract.

Tortfeasor The person guilty of committing a tort.

Transaction Transmission of information between two parties for financial or administrative activities.

Transmission Sending information electronically.

Treatment, Payment, and Healthcare Operations (TPO) A HIPAA term for qualified providers, disclosure of PHI to obtain reimbursement, and activities and transactions among entities. *Treatment* means that a health care provider can provide care; *payment* means that a provider can disclose PHI to be reimbursed; *health care operations* refers to HIPAA-approved activities and transactions.

Trial Phase That point in a lawsuit when the actual court trial begins, wherein evidence is heard and a verdict reached.

Truth-in-Lending Act A law that specifies those collection agreements that must be in writing and lists items that must be included in such contracts; also known as Regulation Z of the Consumer Protection Act of 1968.

U

Unborn Victims of Violence Act Also called Laci and Conner's Act, a federal law passed in 2004 that provides for the prosecution of anyone who causes injury to or the death of a fetus in utero.

Unemployment (or Reemployment) Insurance Under the Federal Unemployment Tax Act (FUTA), employers contribute to a fund that is paid out to eligible unemployed workers. Each state also provides for unemployment insurance.

Uniform Anatomical Gift Act A national statute allowing individuals to donate their bodies or body parts, after death, for use in transplant surgery, tissue banks, or medical research or education.

Uniform Determination of Death Act A proposal that established uniform guidelines for determining when death has occurred.

Uniform Rights of the Terminally Ill Act A federal statute passed in 1989 to guide state legislatures in constructing laws to address advance directives.

Unintentional Tort *See* "Tort."

Universal Precautions Guidelines of the Centers for Disease Control and Prevention (CDC) that deal with handling body fluids.

V

Verification The requirement under HIPAA that a patient's identity be verified before protected health information is released.

Vital Statistics Numbers collected for the population of live births, deaths, fetal deaths, marriages, divorces, induced terminations of pregnancy, and any change in civil status that occurs during an individual's lifetime.

Void Without legal force or effect.

Voidable Able to be set aside or to be revalidated at a later date.

Voluntary Euthanasia The act of ending a patient's life by medical means with his or her permission.

W

Waiver   The act of intentionally relinquishing a known right, claim, or privilege.

Withholding   Deductions made from an employee's paycheck.

Workers' Compensation   A form of insurance established by federal and state statutes that provides reimbursement for workers who are injured on the job.

Wrongful Death Statutes   State statutes that allow a person's beneficiaries to collect for loss to the estate of the deceased for future earnings when a death is judged to have been due to negligence.

Wrongful Discharge   A concept established by precedent that says an employer risks litigation if he or she does not have just cause for firing an employee.

X

Xenotransplantation   Transplantation of animal tissues and organs into humans.

PHOTO CREDITS

Chapter 1
Opener: © BrandX122/Getty RF; 1.4: © BrandX 128/Getty RF; 1.5: © ImageSource/Jupiter RF.

Chapter 2
Opener: © Vol. 59 PhotoDisc/Getty RF; 2.1: © Vol. 40 PhotoDisc/Getty RF; 2.2: © Stockbyte/Punchstock RF.

Chapter 3
Opener: © Royalty-Free/Corbis RF; 3.2: © Comstock/Punchstock RF; 3.6: © Vol. 86 PhotoDisc/Getty RF.

Chapter 4
Opener: © BrandX128/Getty RF; 4.1: © Image Source/Jupiter RF; 4.3: © Royalty-Free/Corbis.

Chapter 5
Opener: © BrandX/Punchstock RF; 5.1: © VL08/Getty RF; 5.2: © OS47 PhotoDisc/Getty RF.

Chapter 6
Opener: © Royalty-Free/Corbis; 6.1: © Dynamic Graphics/Jupiter RF; 6.3: © The McGraw-Hill Companies, Inc./Rick Brady, photographer.

Chapter 7
Opener: © Comstock/PictureQuest RF; 7.1: © Dynamic Graphics/Jupiter RF.

Chapter 8
Opener: © Royalty-Free/Corbis; 8.3, 8.5: Centers for Disease Control and Prevention.

Chapter 9
Opener: © Stockbyte/Punchstock RF; 9.1: © Royalty-Free/Corbis; 9.2: © Digital Vision/Punchstock RF.

Chapter 10
Opener: © Royalty-Free/Corbis; 10.1: © Vol. 72 PhotoDisc/Getty RF; 10.2: © The McGraw-Hill Companies, Inc./Joe DeGrandis, photographer.

Chapter 11
Opener: © Creatas/Punchstock RF; 11.1: © Royalty-Free/Corbis; 11.2: © The McGraw-Hill Companies, Inc./Rick Brady, photographer; 11.6: © Royalty-Free/Corbis.

Chapter 12
Opener: © BrandX/Punchstock RF; 12.5: © Royalty-Free/Corbis; 12.6: © Vol. 54 PhotoDisc/Getty RF.

COURT CASES IN
ALPHABETICAL ORDER INDEX

Right to Die Precedent, 283
Right to Privacy Decided, The, 174

S

State Board of Nursing Finds Nurse Incompetent, 42
State Law Mandates Notification of Sexual Partners
    by HIV Carrier, 216
Supreme Court Shields Medical Devices from Lawsuits, 7

U

U.S. Attorney General Denied Medical
    Records, 186

W

Wrongful Death and Physician-Patient Relationship
    Both at Issue in Lawsuit, 107–108

COURT CASES BY SUBJECT INDEX

Tortfeasor

Wrongful Death

INDEX

("b" indicates boxed material; "f" indicates a figure; "t" indicates a table)